Brain Aging and Therapeutic Interventions

Mahendra K. Thakur · Suresh I. S. Rattan
Editors

Brain Aging and Therapeutic Interventions

Springer

Editors
Mahendra K. Thakur
Banaras Hindu University
Varanasi
India

Suresh I.S. Rattan
Aarhus University
Denmark

ISBN 978-94-007-5236-8   ISBN 978-94-007-5237-5 (eBook)
DOI 10.1007/978-94-007-5237-5
Springer Dordrecht Heidelberg London New York

Library of Congress Control Number: 2012953201

Printed on acid-free paper

Springer is part of Springer Science+Business Media (www.springer.com)

Editorial: Maintaining Brain Health Throughout Life

The idea of compiling this book was conceived during a satellite symposium on "Brain Aging and Dementia: Basic and Clinical Aspects", following the 5th Congress of the Federation of Asian and Oceanian Neuroscience Societies(FAONS) on Nov 26–28, 2010 at Hotel Clarks Avadh, Lucknow, India. The satellite symposium was held at Banaras Hindu University, Varanasi and sponsored by the Department of Biotechnology, Government of India. One of the main inspiring forces behind this idea was Padmashri Professor M.S. Kanungo, respected as the "Father of Biogerontology in India", who, unfortunately, could not see the result of his inspiration, as he passed away in July 2011. Therefore, we dedicate this book to the memory of Professor Kanungo, who was the mentor of numerous biogerontologists, several of whom are the contributors of articles in this book.

Maintaining physical and mental health throughout life is the ideal goal of all biomedical research. This becomes even more challenging and imminent in a rapidly changing demographic scenario throughout the world, which has significantly increased the proportion of the elderly in a population. However, this great success in the extension of lifespan has been accompanied by a parallel increase in the incidence of neurological and psychiatric disorders in old age. Therefore, understanding brain aging and testing, developing and applying novel methods of prevention and treatment of brain disorders is a high priority area.

Recently, there have been enormous advances in the understanding of brain aging and related disorders facilitated by the advancement in neuroimaging and other techniques. The brain undergoes a number of structural and functional changes with increasing age and these changes vary greatly from one person to the next. In particular, studies have focused on basic mechanisms of brain aging, pathogenesis of brain disorders and development of therapeutic strategies. A common concern in old age is the decline in cognitive functions, particularly the decrease in efficiency to learn new skills and difficulty in retrieving the memory stored throughout the life. Hence, researchers have been analysing the mechanisms of memory formation and its impairment and devise the strategies to improve the cognitive functions.

This book is our attempt to bring together information on different aspects of brain aging and on the strategies for intervention and therapy of age-related brain disorders. It includes 18 chapters written by leading researchers in the field on different aspects of brain aging and on therapeutic interventions. Each chapter is a comprehensive and critical review of the topic in question, discusses the current scenario and focuses on future perspectives. The target readership for this collection of articles is the undergraduate and graduate students in the universities, in medical and nursing colleges, along with the post-graduate researchers taking up research projects on different aspects of brain aging, and practicing clinicians who would like to know about the latest developments in the field of neurodegenerative disorders and their therapeutic interventions. This book will also be important for the college and university libraries maintaining a good database in biology, medical and biomedical sciences. This book will be of much interest to pharmaceutical, nutrition and healthcare industry for an easy access to accurate and reliable information in the field of aging research and intervention.

As editors, we are grateful to all the authors for their valuable contributions, timely submission of chapters and making revisions as suggested by the reviewers. We are also grateful to Padma Vibhusan Professor P.N. Tandon for his constant support and encouragement during the preparation of this book.

M. K. Thakur and Suresh I. S. Rattan
Editors

Contents

Contributors

Lorena Arranz Departamento de Fisiología (Fisiología Animal II), Facultad de Ciencias Biológicas, Universidad Complutense, 28040 Madrid, España
e-mail: mondelaf@bio.ucm.es

Maheep Bhatnagar Faculty of Science, University College of Science, MLS University, Udaipur 313001, India
e-mail: mbhatnagar@yahoo.com

Sasanka Chakrabarti Department of Biochemistry, Institute of Post-Graduate Medical Education and Research, Kolkata, India
e-mail: profschakrabarti95@gmail.com

Abha Chauhan NYS Institute for Basic Research in Developmental Disabilities, 1050 Forest Hill Road, Staten Island, NY 10314, USA
e-mail: abha.chauhan@opwdd.ny.gov

Ved Chauhan NYS Institute for Basic Research in Developmental Disabilities, 1050 Forest Hill Road, Staten Island, NY 10314, USA
e-mail: abha.chauhan@opwdd.ny.gov

S. Asha Devi Laboratory of Gerontology, Department of Zoology, Bangalore University, Bangalore 560056, Karnataka, India
e-mail: asuba@blr.vsnl.net.in; sambe.ashadevi@gmail.com

Shogo Endo Aging Regulation Research Team, Tokyo Metropolitan Institute of Gerontology, Itabashi, Tokyo 173-0015, Japan
e-mail: sendo@tmig.or.jp

Mónica De la Fuente Departamento de Fisiología (Fisiología Animal II), Facultad de Ciencias Biológicas, Universidad Complutense, 28040 Madrid, España
e-mail: mondelaf@bio.ucm.es

Akash Gautam Brain Research Centre, Biochemistry and Molecular Biology Laboratory, Department of Zoology, Banaras Hindu University, Varanasi 221005, India
e-mail: mktian2007@gmail.com; mkt_bhu@yahoo.com

Mahdi Hasan Department of Anatomy, CSM Medical University, Lucknow 226003, India
e-mail: drmahdihasan36@gmail.com

Kalpana Barhwal Hota Department of Cognitive Sciences, High Altitude Physiology Division, Defence Institute of High Altitude Research, C/o-56 APO, Leh, Ladakh, India
e-mail: drsunilhota@hotmail.com

Sunil Kumar Hota Department of Cognitive Sciences, High Altitude Physiology Division, Defence Institute of High Altitude Research, C/o-56 APO, Leh, Ladakh, India
e-mail: drsunilhota@hotmail.com

Yasuyuki Ishikawa Core Research for Evolutional Science and Technology (CREST), Japan Science and Technology Agency (JST), Kawaguchi, 332-0012, Japan

Laboratory of Functional Neuroscience, Nara Institute of Science and Technology, 8916-5, Takayama, Ikoma, Nara 630-0192, Japan

Anita Jagota Neurobiology and Molecular Chronobiology laboratory, Department of Animal Sciences, School of Life Sciences, University of Hyderabad, Hyderabad 500046, India
e-mail: ajsl@uohyd.ernet.in; anita_jagota@yahoo.com

Ayushi Jain Faculty of Science, University College of Science, MLS University, Udaipur 313001, India
e-mail: mbhatnagar@yahoo.com

Neha Jaiswal Faculty of Science, University College of Science, MLS University, Udaipur 313001, India
e-mail: mbhatnagar@yahoo.com

Marian Joels Department of Neuroscience and Pharmacology, Division of Neuroscience, UMC Utrecht, Rudolf Magnus Institute, Utrecht, The Netherlands

Sunil C. Kaul National Institute of Advanced Industrial Science & Technology (AIST), Central 4, 1-1-1 Higashi, Tsukuba, Ibaraki 305-8562, Japan
e-mail: renu-wadhwa@aist.go.jp

Gurcharan Kaur Department of Biotechnology, Guru Nanak Dev University, Amritsar, Punjab, India
e-mail: kgurcharan.neuro@yahoo.com

Masami Kojima Bio-interface Research Group, Health Research Inst., National Institute of Advanced Industrial Science and Technology (AIST), 1-8-31, Midorioka, Ikeda, Osaka, 563-8577, Japan
e-mail: m-kojima@aist.go.jp

Core Research for Evolutional Science and Technology (CREST), Japan Science and Technology Agency (JST), Kawaguchi, 332-0012, Japan

Arpita Konar Brain Research Centre, Biochemistry and Molecular Biology Laboratory, Department of Zoology, Banaras Hindu University, Varanasi 221005, India
e-mail: mktian2007@gmail.com; mkt_bhu@yahoo.com

Harmen J. Krugers Swammerdam Institute of Life Sciences, Center for Neuroscience, University of Amsterdam, Science Park 904, 1098 XH, Amsterdam, The Netherlands
e-mail: h.krugers@uva.nl

Pavan Kumar Department of Anatomy, All India Institute of Medical Sciences, New Delhi 110029, India
e-mail: rdmehra98@hotmail.com

Debomoy K. Lahiri Department of Psychiatry, Institute of Psychiatric Research, Indiana University School of Medicine, 791 Union Drive, Indianapolis, IN 46202, USA
e-mail: dlahiri@iupui.edu

Sukhwinder S. Lakhman Department of Pharmaceutical, Social and Administrative Sciences, DYC School of Pharmacy, Buffalo, USA

Abbas A. Mahdi Department of Biochemistry, CSM Medical University, Lucknow 226003, India

Raj D. Mehra Department of Anatomy, All India Institute of Medical Sciences, New Delhi 110029, India
e-mail: rdmehra98@hotmail.com

Kalluri Subba Rao Centers for Biotechnology and Innovative Research, Institute of Science and Technology, Jawaharlal Nehru Technological University Hyderabad 500085, India

Chavi Sharma Faculty of Science, University College of Science, MLS University, Udaipur 313001, India
e-mail: mbhatnagar@yahoo.com

Shashi Bala Singh Defence Institute of Physiology & Allied Sciences (DIPAS), Defence R & D Organisation, Lucknow Road, Timarpur, Delhi 110054, India
e-mail: drsunilhota@hotmail.com

Maitrayee Sinha Department of Biochemistry, Institute of Post-Graduate Medical Education and Research, Kolkata, India
e-mail: sasanka_c54@rediffmail.com

Pooja Suvalka Faculty of Science, University College of Science, MLS University, Udaipur 313001, India
e-mail: mbhatnagar@yahoo.com

Umakanta Swain School of Medical Sciences, University of Hyderabad Hyderabad 500046, India
e-mail: ksrbrain@gmail.com; ksrsl@yahoo.com

Mahendra K. Thakur Brain Research Centre, Biochemistry and Molecular Biology Laboratory, Department of Zoology, Banaras Hindu University, Varanasi 221005, India
e-mail: mktian2007@gmail.com; mkt_bhu@yahoo.com

Sandeep Tripathi Department of Biotechnology (IAST), NIMS University, Jaipur 303121, India

Department of Biochemistry, CSM Medical University, Lucknow 226003, India

Mukesh K. Varshney Department of Anatomy, All India Institute of Medical Sciences, New Delhi 110029, India
e-mail: rdmehra98@hotmail.com

Renu Wadhwa National Institute of Advanced Industrial Science & Technology (AIST), Central 4, 1-1-1 Higashi, Tsukuba, Ibaraki 305-8562, Japan
e-mail: renu-wadhwa@aist.go.jp

Keith A. Wesnes Bracket, Goring-on-Thames, RG80EN, UK

Centre for Human Psychopharmacology, Swinburne University, Melbourne, Australia

Andrea Zangara SOHO-Flordis International, Level 4, 156 Pacific Highway St Leonards, NSW 2065 Australia
e-mail: andre.zangara@sfihealth.com

Centre for Human Psychopharmacology, Swinburne University, Melbourne, Australia

Chapter 1
Brain Aging: A Critical Reappraisal

Mahendra K. Thakur, Arpita Konar and Akash Gautam

Abstract Despite remarkable scientific advancements in recent years, much about the human brain still remains a mystery, particularly in the context of brain aging and associated disorders. Understanding of the factors that influence brain integrity late in life will help to maintain healthy brain functions. This is indeed a difficult task because in several cases, normal brain aging switches to pathological aging associated with drastic deterioration in cognitive abilities, motor skills and mood resulting in neurological diseases, ranging from late onset neurodegenerative diseases such as Alzheimer's and Parkinson's to early onset neuropsychiatric disorders such as schizophrenia and bipolar disorder. Brain aging is accompanied by several anatomical, cellular and molecular alterations including reduction in brain volume, protein turnover, increase in protein aggregation, impairment in neural plasticity, perturbed calcium homeostasis, neuronal survival and neuroinflammation, eventually affecting brain functions with increased incidence of neurological disorders. Factors like stress, depression, hypertension as well as obesity accelerate the aging of brain contributing to neurodegeneration and associated cognitive deficits. During the past decades, technical advances including microarray, neuroimaging and behavioral paradigms have helped to get a holistic picture of age-associated alterations in the brain. Here we review the current understanding of age-related structural and functional changes in the brain and how these changes might contribute to vulnerability for developing age-related neurological diseases and designing potential therapeutic avenues. Taken together, the findings suggest that adoption of certain neuroprotective strategies like dietary restriction, antioxidant supplementation, low alcohol intake, less exposure to stressors, environmental enrichment and lifestyle modulations involving exercise and intellectual brain training programs can be beneficial to delay the loss of brain integrity during aging.

M. K. Thakur (✉) · A. Konar · A. Gautam
Brain Research Centre, Biochemistry and Molecular Biology Laboratory,
Department of Zoology, Banaras Hindu University, Varanasi 221005, India
e-mail: mktian2007@gmail.com; mkt_bhu@yahoo.com

M. K. Thakur, S. I. S. Rattan (eds.), *Brain Aging and Therapeutic Interventions*,
DOI 10.1007/978-94-007-5237-5_1,

Keywords Aging • Cognition • Diet • Environment • Epigenetics • Genes • Hormones • Neurodegeneration • Neuroimaging • Therapeutics

1.1 Introduction

Brain aging is characterized by several anatomical, molecular and functional changes leading to enhanced vulnerability to a number of insults and diseases. Structural changes include shrinkage in total brain volume and morphological changes in specific regions. Besides loss of structural integrity and neural plasticity, progressive deterioration of cellular homeostatic reserves and alterations in calcium dependent signaling mechanisms have been proposed as the key events associated with brain aging (Yankner et al. 2008). Other chemical and molecular changes associated with brain aging include changes in neurotransmitter and hormone levels, increased reactive oxygen species production, mitochondrial dysfunction (see Chap. 4), accumulation of nuclear and mitochondrial DNA damage accompanied by age-related decline in DNA repair (see Chap. 2), and intracellular and extracellular protein aggregates. Such drastic changes at cellular and molecular levels are reflected in the impairment of various functions like sleep, attention, speech, language, decision making and cognitive abilities like working memory and long term memory. If the brain cells fail to adapt to these age-related changes, the normal aging process will gradually transit to pathological conditions resulting in brain tumours (Weller et al. 2011), stroke, white matter lesions and neurodegenerative disorders like Alzheimer's disease (AD) and Parkinson's disease (PD). Besides pharmacological and molecular interventions (see Chap. 15), protective factors like regular exercise (Kohman et al. 2011), a healthy diet (see Chaps. 16 and 17), low to moderate alcohol consumption, intake of herbal products (see Chaps. 9 and 18) and a blissful environment (see Chap. 6) aid to retard brain aging. Increased cognitive effort in the form of education or occupational attainment also helps in healthy brain aging. A healthy life both physically and mentally may be the best defence against the changes in aging brain.

1.2 Changes During Brain Aging

With advancing age, brain shows various anatomical, molecular and functional changes and severity of such alterations leads to increased incidence of neurological disorders (Shetty et al. 2011) and traumatic brain injuries (Sivanandam and Thakur 2012). Constantly emerging neuroimaging (Ketonen 1998), neurogenomic (Lee et al. 2000) and neuroproteomic (Vanguilder and Freeman 2011) techniques demonstrate that brain aging involves loss of structural integrity, alteration in levels of enzymes, hormones, genetic and epigenetic modulation, dysregulated metabolism, increased oxidative stress, altered protein processing and synaptic function, and these changes together lead to decline in physiological and cognitive functions.

1.2.1 Anatomical Changes

Age-related decline in brain volume is predominant in frontal cortex, temporal cortex, putamen, thalamus and nucleus accumbens. Recent MRI analysis revealed that grey matter volume reduces (Taki et al. 2011) while white matter volume increases in frontal, parietal and temporal cortices (Berti et al. 2011), insula and superior parietal gyri (Taki et al. 2011) in both genders. However, there is a debate about the age- related effects on white matter. Schmidt et al. (2011) show differential changes in white matter in different regions of the brain during aging. Also the regional variation in brain volume is not uniform as there are reports of shrinkage of some brain regions at a rate of up to 1 % per year, whereas others remain relatively stable until the end of life-span (Beason-Held et al. 2008). These volumetric reductions occur due to neuronal shrinkage, reduction of synaptic spines, lower number of synapses and reduced length of myelinated axons (Dickstein 2007). Dendritic arbors and spines of cortical pyramidal neurons decrease in size and/or number in humans and primates as a result of age. Electron microscopic studies reveal 50 % loss in spines on the apical dendritic tufts of pyramidal cells in prefrontal cortex of old monkeys (27–32 years) as compared to young ones (6–9 years old) (Barnes 2011). Similarly, 46 % decrease in spine number and density has been reported in humans older than 50 years as compared with younger individuals. Cortical lining is also diminished during aging with annual reduction between 0.5 % and 1.0 % in most brain areas. Studies from computed tomography show that the cerebral ventricles enlarge with progression of age, and this process is called as ventriculomegaly and has been studied biomechanically in detail with its applications to hydrocephalus (Wilkie et al. 2012). The permeability of blood-brain barrier also increases with advancing age (Farall and Wardlaw 2007). Functional MRI studies have demonstrated relative increase or decrease in brain activity when comparing old with young individuals (Beason-Held et al. 2008), and alteration in hemispheric lateralization in prefrontal cortex in aged brain (Woodard and Sugarman 2012).

1.2.2 Molecular Changes

Integrating age-related neuroanatomical changes with underlying molecular alterations including changes in neurochemicals, genetic and epigenetic factors and identification of biomarkers might have profound consequences for retarding brain aging and associated disorders.

1.2.2.1 Chemical Changes

Brain aging involves marked alteration in levels of neurotransmitters, enzymes, hormones and metabolites (Smith et al. 2005). Dopamine levels decline by around 10 % per decade from early adulthood due to loss of dopaminergic neurons between frontal cortex and striatum or reduction in number and binding affinity of dopamine receptors (Ota et al. 2006). Decrease in dopamine level is associated with age-related decline in cognitive and motor performance. Serotonin (Yamamoto et al. 2001) and glutamate (Chang et al. 2009) levels also fall with increasing age and are implicated in the loss of synaptic plasticity in old brain. Activities of enzymes regulating neurotransmitters like monoamine oxidase increase with age and may liberate free radicals from reactions that exceed the inherent antioxidant reserves (Esiri 2007).

Another important factor influencing aging brain and its cognitive performance is hormone. While majority of hormones like growth hormone, thyroxine, melatonin and sex hormones including testosterone, DHEA, estrogen and progesterone (Veiga et al. 2004; Schumacher et al. 2003) decline during aging, stress hormone cortisol shows significant increase (Lupien et al. 2009) and is considered to be a serious risk factor for cardiovascular disorders, obesity and rapid brain aging. Age-related structural and functional changes are attributed largely to modulation in the level of estrogen which acts mainly through its intracellular receptors, estrogen receptor (ER)α and ERβ. The expression of these receptors is regulated by several factors including their own ligand estrogen, and others such as growth hormone and thyroid hormone. The levels of these factors decrease during aging which in turn influence estrogen signaling leading to alterations in brain functions (Thakur and Sharma 2006). Recent report that ER β interacts with casein kinase2, phosphokinase C and N-myristoylation sites present in mitochondrial and nuclear proteins might be useful to regulate estrogen dependent gene regulation in brain for therapeutics (Paramanik and Thakur 2012).

Insulin and Insulin-like growth factors (IGFs) have been increasingly documented as significant molecules in modulating the speed of aging in humans (Sonntag et al. 2000). Increase in insulin level and resistance with advancing age affects synaptic integrity, brain vascular function and energy metabolism and imposes the risk of developing dementia in late life. The aging brain may also suffer from impaired glucose metabolism or a reduced input of glucose due to fall of cerebrovascular efficiency (Cohen and Dillin 2008). Recent studies reveal that high lactate level in the brain caused by a shift in the lactate dehydrogenase A/B ratio is a hallmark of aging (Ross et al. 2010). They show that elevation of lactate levels occurs before other indicators in the prematurely aged mitochondrial DNA mutator mouse and most probably a similar pattern may characterize normal aging.

1.2.2.2 Genetic Changes

Advancement in gene expression studies such as genomic microarray analysis has helped to understand the molecular mechanisms underlying changes that occur during brain aging. Majority of gene expression studies in brain across the lifespan reveal alterations in molecules related to stress (see Chap. 7), inflammation, immune response, mitochondrial functions, growth factors, neuronal survival, synaptic plasticity (see Chap. 3) and calcium homeostasis (Lu et al. 2004). Comparative analysis of phylogenetically distant organisms has revealed a few broadly conserved functional categories of genes with age-dependent expression changes (Loerch et al. 2008). While genes related to stress response, inflammation and DNA repair are upregulated, mitochondrial genes are repressed during aging in almost all the organisms studied (Yankner et al. 2008). In a transcriptional profiling study of the aging cortex in mice, rhesus macaques and humans, the greatest conserved change was age-dependent upregulation of the apolipoprotein D gene13 that functions as a lipid antioxidant conferring resistance and is induced in the brain of individuals with AD (Bishop et al. 2010). Recent studies reveal that gene expression changes during aging are region specific and exhibit sexual dimorphism (Berchtold et al. 2008). Different regions of the forebrain exhibit substantially different gene profile changes with age. For instance, superior frontal gyrus shows remarkable alteration in gene expression while changes in entorhinal cortex are moderate. Prominent changes occurring in 60–70 years old individuals across the entire cortical region suggest it to be a critical transition point in brain aging. In hippocampus, CA1 region is more susceptible to aging and exhibits a greater number of altered genes relative to CA3 and the dentate gyrus (DG), and an enrichment of genes related to the immune response and apoptosis (Zeier et al. 2011).

As the sexual dimorphism is concerned, males show more gene changes than females across all brain regions. Male brain is characterized by global decrease in catabolic and anabolic capacity with aging, and down-regulation of genes involved in energy production and protein synthesis/transport. Increased immune activity is a prominent feature of aging in both sexes, with proportionally greater activation in the female brain. Besides regional and gender differences, gene expression has also been shown to be specific for neurons and glia. It is suggested that glial-enriched genes largely associated with immune system and complement activation are up-regulated, whereas neuronal-enriched genes related to synaptic structure and function, calcium regulation, signal transduction and transmembrane receptors, are largely down-regulated with age. Even among glial genes, astrocytic markers are up-regulated while oligodendrocytic genes are repressed during aging (Loerch et al. 2008). Few examples of genes that undergo age dependent alteration in humans have been enlisted in Table 1.1.

1.2.2.3 Epigenetic Changes

Besides genetic alterations, the emerging field of epigenetics indicates that accumulation of aberrant epigenetic marks including histone and DNA modifications may be a driver of aging-related cellular and physiological changes. Studies of Zeng et al. (2011) reveal that age-dependent deficits in long-term synaptic plasticity and loss of hippocampal dendritic spines in the aged Fischer 344 rats are closely asso-

Table 1.1 Gene expression changes during brain aging

SN	Category	Example
Genes upregulated		
1	Stress response	Heat shock 70kD protein 2, mortalin, crystallin alpha B, hypoxia inducible factor1α (HIF1α), HIF-1 responsive RTP801, transglutaminase 2, p53 binding protein 2, retinoblastoma-associated protein 140
2	DNA repair	8-oxoguanine DNA glycosylase, uracil-DNA glycosylase, topoisomerase I binding protein
3	Mitochondrial function	Mitochondrial 3-oxoacyl-CoenzymeA thiolase
4	Inflammatory response	TNF-α, C type lectin, H factor (complement)-1, interferon gamma-inducible protein 16, interferon regulatory factor 7, integrin α5, integrinβ1
5	Growth factors	Vascular endothelial growth factor, FGF receptor 2, FGF receptor 3
6	Synaptic transmission	SNAP23, synaptophysin-like protein
7	Myelin related proteins/ lipid metabolism	Amyloid precursor protein[a], oligodendrocyte lineage transcription factor 2, peripheral myelin protein 22, proteolipid protein 1, fatty acid desaturase 1, apolipoprotein D, low density lipoprotein receptor related protein 4, sterol carrier protein 2
8	Metal ion homeostasis	Metallothionein 1G, metallothionein 1B, metallothionein 2A, haem binding protein 2, haemoglobin β, hephaestin
Genes downregulated		
1	Synaptic plasticity	BDNF, neurexin 1, synaptobrevin1,synapsin II b, growth associated protein 43 (GAP-43), activity regulated cytoskeletal protein (Arc)
2	Synaptic transmission	NMDA receptor, serotonin receptor 2A; GABA A receptor subunits α1, α5, β3; GABA biosynthetic enzymes glutamate decarboxylase 1 and 2 (GAD1&GAD2), glutamate receptor subunits
3	Vesicular transport	GABA vesicular transporter (SLC32A1), kinesin 1B, sortilin, dynein (DNCH1), dynamin, trans Golgi network protein 2, Golgi reassembly stacking protein 2, phosphatidylinositol transfer protein β, clathrin
4	Neuronal survival	Presenilin (PS)1[b] MADS box transcription enhancer factor 2C (MEF2C), inositol polyphosphate-4-phosphataseI, inositol 1,4,5 trisphosphate 3 kinase A
5	Calcium homeostasis	Calmodulin 1 and 3, CAMkinase IIα′ and IV, calcineurin Bα, ATPase Ca^{2+}-transporting, plasma membrane 2 (ATP2B2)
6	Mitochondrial function	ATP synthase H+-transporting mitochondrial F1α1, mitochondrial ribosomal protein L28, S12, cytochrome c synthase, translocase of inner mitochondrial membrane 17A
7	Microtubule structure and function	Microtubule associated protein (MAP)1B, MAP2, tau J, RAN binding protein 9
8	G-protein coupled receptors	Rap2A, regulator of G protein signalling 4, G protein q polypeptide (GNAQ)
9	Protein turnover	ATPase H^+-transporting lysosomal V1 subunit H and A, ubiquitin conjugating enzyme Ubch5, ubiquitin conjugating enzyme E2M, ubiquitin carrier protein

Table 1.1 (continued)

SN	Category	Example
10	Amino acid modification	Protein-L-isoaspartate O-methyltransferase, methionine adenosyltransferase IIα, β-1,3-galactosyltransferase, glutamate decarboxylase 1
11	Kinases and phosphatases	Protein kinase C isoforms (PKCβ1), PKCγ and PKCζ)
12	Stress response	Stress 70 protein chaperone
13	Hormones	Proenkephalin, somatostatin, cholecystokinin B receptor, chromogranin B (secretogranin1)
14	Voltage gated channels	Voltage-gated Na channel II b (SCN2B), voltage-dependent calcium channel b2
Genes unaltered		
1	Lipid transport	ApoE
2	Cytoskeletal elements	βtubulin III, neurofilament L chain, βActin
3	Glycolytic enzyme	GAPDH

[a] Sivanandam and Thakur 2011
[b] Thakur and Ghosh 2007

ciated with reduced histone acetylation, upregulated histone deacetylase (HDAC) 2 and decreased expression of histone acetyltransferase. Further analysis reveals brain-derived neurotrophic factor (BDNF) as one of the key genes affected by such changes. Age-dependent reductions in H3 and H4 acetylation are detected in multiple promoter regions of the BDNF gene, leading to a significant decrease in BDNF expression and impairment of downstream signaling in the aged hippocampus. These deficits could be rescued by enhancing BDNF and trkB expression via HDAC inhibition or by directly activating trkB receptors with 7,8-dihydroxyflavone, a newly identified, selective agonist for trkB. Epigenetic changes in genes like Arc, zif268 and BDNF in vulnerable brain regions of hippocampus and prefrontal cortex are also associated with age-related cognitive deficits (Penner et al. 2010). Dynamic changes in chromatin structure across the lifespan could potentially either counter aging and age-associated diseases in some cases, or contribute to accelerated aging and age-related dysfunctions in other cases. Despite the identification of several genes influencing brain aging and overall lifespan, an important question still remains unanswered whether age-related cognitive changes are mediated by any of the master regulators of aging and lifespan identified in model organisms.

1.2.3 Functional Changes

Aging impacts a variety of brain functions including attention, speech, sleep, decision making, working and long term memory (Hedden and Gabrieli 2004). Experiments with rodent models show that old age exhibits decline in cognition and motivation, decreased interest in novel tasks, motor disabilities and increased anxiety. These changes show corresponding pattern in primates and humans.

Sleep: Sleep dysregulation is a common complaint among the elderly. Age-related sleep changes include circadian advance, sleep fragmentation, insomnia and loss of deep, slow wave sleep while daytime symptoms include sleepiness, increased napping and breakthrough sleep (Buechel et al. 2011). Further, healthy younger adults exposed to experimentally induced selective deprivation of night time (inactive period) deep sleep show some aging-like phenotypes, including daytime sleepiness, biochemical and metabolic dysfunctions and cognitive deficits. Recent studies suggest that deep, slow wave sleep during the inactive period promotes memory, possibly through localized synaptic protein synthesis effects. Thus, the dysregulated slow wave sleep seen with age might contribute to cognitive deficits. Despite the seemingly similar effects of age and sleep dysregulation on cognition, and high prevalence of sleep changes with age, relatively few studies have investigated possible mechanistic links between sleep architecture changes and age related cognitive decline.

Working Memory: Older adults exhibit significant deficits in working memory (Schulze et al. 2011). Although the mechanisms underlying these age-related deficits are still obscure, decline in the activity of prefrontal cortex has been attributed to age dependent deficits in working memory.

Episodic Memory: Aging principally affects episodic memory, namely memory for specific events or experiences that occurred in the past (Fjell and Walhovd 2010). A great problem for older adults is remembering context or source information; where or when something was heard or read, or even whether something actually happened or was just thought about, what has been called "reality monitoring". Although semantic memory is largely preserved during aging, older people provide general information rather than specific details.

Attention: Older adults show significant impairment in attention, which is a cognitive function associated with the frontal lobe that requires dividing or switching of concentration among multiple inputs or tasks (Fjell and Walhovd 2010). Importantly, these types of tasks appear to be amenable to training and show benefits of cardiovascular fitness. Attention deficits can have a significant impact on old person's ability to function adequately and independently in everyday life. One important aspect of daily functioning affected by attention problem is driving, an activity that is essential to independence for many old people. Driving requires a constant switching of attention in response to environmental contingencies. Attention must be divided between driving, monitoring the environment, and sorting out relevant from irrelevant stimuli in a cluttered visual array. Research has shown that divided attention impairments are significantly associated with increased automobile accidents in older adults.

Decision Making: Relatively little research has been done on the effect of aging on decision-making. It has been noticed that while making decision, old people tend to rely more on prior knowledge about the problem domain and less on new information whereas young people are likely to have less knowledge about these issues and tend to sample and evaluate more current information and consider more alternatives before making their decisions.

1.3 Factors Accelerating Brain Aging

Multiple factors affect the rate of brain aging; while some of them accelerate, others slow down age-related deterioration and delay the attainment of pathological levels. Identifying such factors is crucial to design therapeutic strategies. Some of the factors that modify brain aging are discussed below:

Hypertension: Hypertension is a chronic age-related condition associated with multiple changes in the vascular system. Chronic elevation of blood pressure affects structure of brain and persons with medically controlled hypertension are at lower risk for cognitive decline than those who are undiagnosed or untreated. Hypertension accelerates age-related shrinkage of the hippocampus. Persons with hypertension and other vascular disease factors show longitudinal decline in the regions that are usually stable in normal aging, such as the primary visual cortex. Indeed, in contrast to healthy adults, persons with vascular risk factors and vascular disease show rapid expansion in parietal areas and increase in the pace of expansion is associated with higher systolic blood pressure. Unfortunately, little is known about neuroanatomical correlates of hypertension in standard animal models. However, selective vulnerability of the prefrontal regions to hypertension is observed in spontaneously hypertensive rats, and treatment with antihypertensive agents shows notable neuroprotective effect in the prefrontal cortex (Raz and Rodrigue 2006).

In addition to hypertension, metabolic markers of cardiovascular risk may be associated with structural differences in the brain usually attributed to aging. One such marker is homocysteine (Hcy), an amino acid that is synthesized with participation of vitamins of the B-group as co-factors. In healthy adults, Hcy increase is associated with atrophy of the hippocampus, reduced total Grey matter volume and ventriculomegaly. Increased plasma Hcy levels predict cognitive decline in non demented elderly, and is linked to poor performance on a wide range of neuropsychological tests, especially those measuring delayed recall and executive control (Raz and Rodrigue 2006).

Stress and Depression: Another factor that may contribute to variable age-related changes in brain function is individual differences in the stress system which could arise through natural genetic variation or through exposure to a variety of stressors over the lifespan of the individual. Stress has an important influence on the brain throughout the lifespan. Early life stressful experiences initially impair learning and memory processes but enhances emotional memory formation later in life (see Chap. 13). Recent research has reported that people with recurrent depression or those exposed to chronic stress exhibit accelerated brain aging. With increasing age, telomeres shorten, and studies have shown that oxidative stress and inflammation accelerate this shortening. On this basis, it has been suggested that telomere length

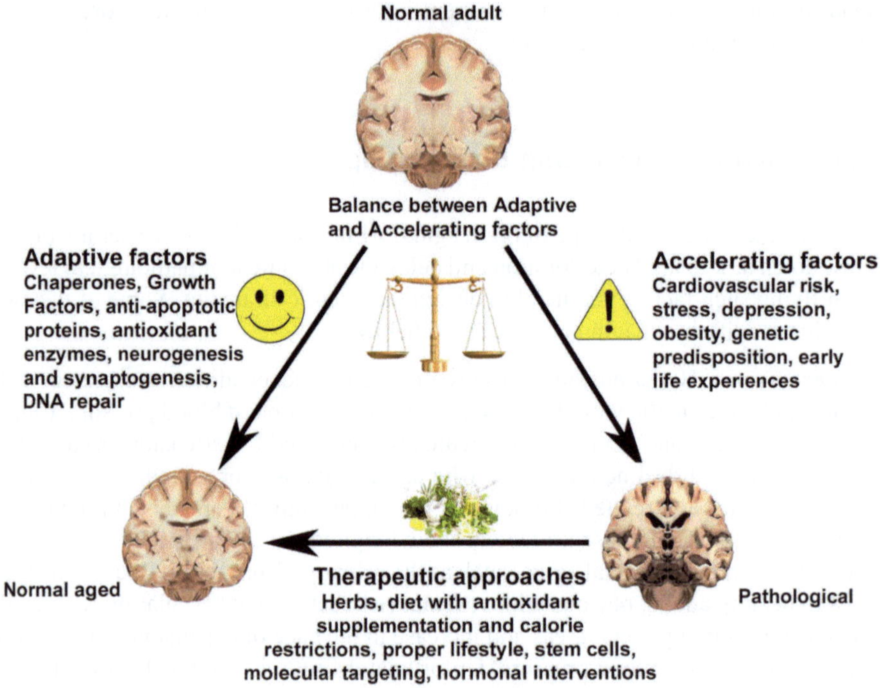

Fig. 1.1 Schematic representation of transition from normal aging brain to pathological brain

is a measure of biological aging, and telomere length has subsequently been linked to age-related diseases, unhealthy lifestyle and longevity. Recent research shows that shorter telomere length is associated with both recurrent depression and cortisol levels indicative of exposure to chronic stress (Wikgren et al. 2012).

1.4 Transition of Normal Brain Aging to Pathological Aging

Neural cells may respond to multiple changes during brain aging adaptively, or they may give rise to neurodegenerative cascades that result in disorders such as AD and PD, commonly termed as pathological aging. Multiple mechanisms are employed to maintain the integrity of nerve cell circuits and to facilitate responses to environmental demands and promote recovery of function after injury. The mechanisms include production of neurotrophic factors and cytokines, expression of various cell survival-promoting proteins (e.g., protein chaperones, antioxidant enzymes, Bcl-2 and inhibitor of apoptotic proteins), preservation of genomic integrity by telomerase and DNA repair proteins, and mobilization of neural stem cells to replace damaged neurons and glia (Fig. 1.1). The aging process challenges neuroprotective and neurorestorative mechanisms. Genetic and environmental factors such as hypoxia (see Chap. 12) and early life experiences (see Chap. 5) superimposed upon the aging process can determine whether brain aging is normal or pathological. Mutations in genes that cause inherited forms of AD (amyloid precursor protein and presenilins), PD (α-synuclein and parkin), and trinucleotide repeat disorders (huntingtin, androgen receptor, ataxin, and others) overwhelm endogenous neuroprotective mechanisms; other genes such as those encoding apolipoprotein E have more subtle effects on brain aging (Singh and Thakur 2011). On the other hand, neuroprotective mechanisms can be bolstered by dietary restriction (see Chap. 10), antioxidant supplementation, herbal interventions (see Chap. 11) and behavioral (intellectual and physical activities) modifications. At the cellular and molecular levels, successful brain aging can be facilitated by activating a hormesis response in which neurons increase production of neurotrophic factors and stress proteins (Stranahan and Mattson 2012). Hormonal interventions, particularly steroids promote successful aging regulating neurotransmitter system, neuronal viability, myelination and cognitive processes. Comparative analysis of neurosteroids in AD patients and age-matched non-demented controls reveals negative correlation between neurosteroid level and biochemical markers like phophorylated tau and beta amyloid peptides in AD (Schumacher et al. 2003). Modulation in estrogen level has also been suggested to play an important role in neuroprotection (see Chap. 14). Hormones like melatonin help to recover age induced disturbance in biological clock (see Chap. 8). Neural stem cells that reside in the adult brain are also responsive to environmental demands and appear capable of replacing lost or dysfunctional neurons and glial cells, perhaps even in the aging brain.

1.5 Therapeutic Interventions

Earlier it was believed that brain aging associated decline in physiological and higher cognitive functions are difficult to combat, but recent advancement in neuroscience research has endeavoured to retard age associated deficits as well as maintain healthy and successful aging. These approaches include a wide variety of herbs as dietary constituents, life style modulations and molecular interventions as mentioned in Table 1.2. From *in vitro* molecular studies to clinical trials, contributions of molecular and cell biology are crucial for all these therapeutic approaches and offer the hope of curative advances that deal with elementary biological processes as well as the clinically significant challenges of brain aging.

1.6 Conclusion

During aging, there is a progressive decline in brain integrity affecting physiological and cognitive functions. Brain may cope up with the adversities of aging by recruiting adaptive cellular responses to strengthen neuronal networks, compensate

Table 1.2 Different therapeutic approaches to retard brain aging associated dysfunctions

Therapy	References	Mode of action	Effect on aging brain
Herbs			
Curcumin	Singh and Aggarwal 1995	Efficient inhibitor of NF-κB and the mTOR signaling pathway, acts as antioxidant, induces heme oxygenase 1 and Phase II detoxification enzymes, protects neurons against different modes of oxidative challenge	Lower old age related disorders like AD incidences, cognitive impairments, etc.
Ginger	Nakatani 2000	Increase in the levels of monoamines [norepinephrine (NE), dopamine (DA) and serotonin 5-HT] and amino acids neurotransmitters—glutamic, aspartic, GABA, glycine and alanine	Counteract age induced deficiency in the brain cortex and hippocampus
Green tea	Mandel et al. 2006	Catechin polyphenols are potent bioactive molecules which act either as antioxidants or modulators of intracellular cell signaling and metabolism	Green tea consumption is inversely correlated with the incidence of dementia, AD and PD
Indian ginseng	Mishra et al. 2000	Withanolides possess anti-oxidant, immunomodulatory and anti stress properties	Retard brain aging and help in regeneration of neural tissues
Chinese ginseng	Peng et al. 2011	Ginsenoside Rg1 improves antioxidation ability, downregulates expressions of aging-associated P16INK4a and P21Cip1/Waf1 mRNA and protein	Produce antistress, adaptogenic and memory enhancing effect
Brahmi	Rastogi et al. 2012	Antioxidant, anti-inflammatory, neuroprotective, pro-cholinergic and anti-acetylcholinesterase properties	Retard age related cognitive deficits
Lifestyle			
Sleep	Buechel et al. 2011	Suprachiasmatic nucleus (SCN) in hypothalamus contains a light entrained circadian clock that regulates melatonin synthesis in the pineal gland in mammals which in turn may regulate SCN through a feedback loop. Serotonin (precursor of melatonin) is a regulator of circadian rhythms	Proper sleep of 6–8 hours produce beneficial effects on cognitive abilities in aged individuals, attenuate brain damage and increase repair abilities of brain

Table 1.2 (continued)

Therapy	References	Mode of action	Effect on aging brain
Exercise	Ahlskog et al. 2011; Lautenschlager et al. 2011	Increase levels of BDNF and other growth factors, stimulate neurogenesis, increase resistance to brain insult, improve learning and mental performance	Maintain brain function and promote brain plasticity, increase oxygen content in blood flow
Caloric restriction	Zeier et al. 2011	Differentially influences genes for synaptic plasticity in CA1 and CA3 of hippocampus, decreases insulin resistance	Slow down the aging process and delay or prevent different age-related diseases
Education and enriched environment	Mattson et al. 2001; Cohen 2000	Balances the effect of subclinical disease in late midlife	Counteracts the deleterious effects of cerebrovascular disease and AD
Diet with low energy and high anti-oxidants	Floyd and Hensley 2002	Has neuroprotective role via actions that enhance neurogenesis, neuronal morphology and/or neurotrophin release	Reduce cerebrovascular risk and support intermediary metabolism
Fish and sea food	Gomez-Pinilla 2008	Decrease stroke	Upregulate cortical synapses and buffer against age related synapse downregulation
Low to moderate alcohol	Herbert et al. 1993	Reduce cardiovascular risk and may stimulate the hippocampus	Moderate drinkers show reduced white matter lesions, infarcts and even dementia
Low stress		Amelioration of stress and depression induced cognitive deficits	
Cellular and molecular targeting			
Short telomeres	Rolyan et al. 2011	Reduces adult neurogenesis, possibly via telomere-dependent effects on microglia activation	Telomere dysfunction delays the progression of AD-associated amyloid pathology in aging mice

Table 1.2 (continued)

Therapy	References	Mode of action	Effect on aging brain
Neurotransmitter signaling interventions	Neill 2012	Alteration in signaling of neurotransmitter agonists or antagonists, positive allosteric modulation and reduction in protein aggregation	Maintain the optimum level of excitatory and inhibitory neurotransmission
Lipoic acid	Hegazy and Ali 2011	Increase the levels of hippocampal monoamines [norepinephrine (NE) and serotonin 5-HT], glutamic, aspartic, GABA and cortical dopamine (DA) and 5-HT, cortical glutamic, aspartic, glycine and alanine	Counteract age induced deficiency via modulating the monoamines and amino acids in the brain cortex and hippocampus
PI3K/AKT/mTOR pathway	Heras-Sandoval et al. 2011	PI3K/AKT pathway has been found to be dysregulated in several models of neurodegenerative diseases associated with aging, suggesting that two or more initiating events may trigger disease formation in an age-related manner	Chemical compounds able to modulate the activity of the PI3K/AKT/mTOR pathway, are key transducer of brain metabolic and mitogenic signals involved in neuronal proliferation, differentiation and survival
Stem cells	Anthony et al. 2005	Surgical replacement of damaged cells in the aging brain by neurogenesis	Replacement of lost cells and recovery of lost function

lost or damaged cells, combat stress and enhance plasticity. If this adaptation does not succeed, age related alterations are accelerated eventually leading to neurodegeneration and death. Successful aging is determined in part by genetic background as well as experiential factors associated with lifestyle and culture. Dietary, behavioral and pharmacological interventions have also been identified as potential means to slow brain aging and treat neurodegenerative diseases. Thus the research in brain aging holds a great promise for the once remote dream of living a healthy and long life free of disease and disability.

Acknowledgements The work cited in this article from authors' laboratory has been supported by grants from the Department of Biotechnology, Department of Science and Technology, Indian Council of Medical Research, Council of Scientific and Industrial Research and University Grants Commission, Government of India.

References

Ahlskog JE, Geda YE, Graff-Radford NR, Petersen RC (2011) Dementia and brain aging. Mayo Clin Proc 86:876–884

Anthony DH, Wagner W, Mahlknecht U (2005) Stem cells and aging. EMBO Rep 6:S35–38

Barnes CA (2011) Secrets of aging: what does a normally aging brain look like? F1000 Biol Rep 3:22

Bishop NA, Lu T, Yankner BA (2010) Neural mechanisms of aging and cognitive decline. Nature 464:529–535

Beason-Held LL, Kraut MA, Resnick SM (2008) Temporal patterns of longitudinal change in aging brain function. Neurobiol Aging 29:497–513

Berchtold NC, Cribbs DH, Coleman PD, Rogers J, Head E, Kim R, Beach T, Miller C, Troncoso J, Trojanowski JQ, Zielke HR, Cotman CW (2008) Gene expression changes in the course of normal brain aging are sexually dimorphic. Proc Natl Acad Sci USA 105:15605–15610

Berti V, Mosconi L, Glodzik L, Li Y, Murray J, De Santi S, Pupi A, Tsui W, De Leon MJ (2011) Structural brain changes in normal individuals with a maternal history of Alzheimer's. Neurobiol Aging 32:2325.e17–2325.e26

Buechel HM, Popovic J, Searcy JL, Porter NM, Thibault O, Blalock EM (2011) Deep sleep and parietal cortex gene expression changes are related to cognitive deficits with age. PLoS One 6:e18387

Chang L, Jiang CS, Ernst T (2009) Effects of age and sex on brain glutamate and other metabolites. Mag Res Ima 27:142–145

Cohen CI (2000) Relation of education to brain size in normal aging. Neurology 54:1207–1208

Cohen E, Dillin A (2008) The insulin paradox: aging, proteotoxicity and neurodegeneration. Nat Rev Neurosci 9:759–767

Dickstein DL, Kabaso D, Rocher AB, Luebke JI, Wearne SL, Hof PR (2007) Changes in the structural complexity of the aged brain. Aging Cell 6:275–284

Esiri MM (2007) Aging and the brain. J Pathol 211:181–187

Farrall AJ, Wardlaw JM (2007) Blood brain barrier: aging and microvascular disease-systemic review and meta-analysis. Neurobiol Aging 30:337–352

Fjell AM, Walhovd KB (2010) Structural brain changes in aging: courses, causes and cognitive consequences. Rev Neurosci 21:187–221

Floyd RA, Hensley K (2002) Oxidative stress in brain aging: Implications for therapeutics of neurodegenerative diseases. Neurobiol Aging 23:795–807

Gomez-Pinilla F (2008) Brain foods: the effects of nutrients on brain function. Nat Rev Neurosci 9:568–578

Hedden T, Gabrieli JDE (2004) Insights into the aging mind: a view from cognitive neuroscience. Nat Rev Neurosci 5:87–97

Hegazy HG, Ali EHA (2011) Modulation of monoamines and amino-acids neurotransmitters in cerebral cortex and hippocampus of female senile rats by ginger and lipoic acid. Afr J Pharm Pharmaco 5:1080–1085

Heras-Sandoval D, Avila-Munoz E, Arias C (2011) The phosphatidylinositol 3-kinase/mTor pathway as a therapeutic target for brain aging and neurodegeneration. Mex Pharma 4:1070–1087

Herbert LE, Scherr PA, Beckett LA, Albert MS, Rosner B, Taylor JO, Evans DA (1993) Relation of smoking and low-to-moderate alcohol consumption to change in cognitive function: a longitudinal study in a defined community of older persons. Am J Epidemiol 137:881–891

Ketonen LM (1998) Neuroimaging of the aging brain. Neurologic Clin 16:581–598

Kohman RA, Sandra LR, Southey BR, Kelley KW, Dantzer R, Rhodes JS (2011) Voluntary wheel running reverses age-induced changes in hippocampal gene expression. PLoS One 6:e22654

Lautenschlager NT, Cox K, Cyarto EV (2011) The influence of exercise on brain aging and dementia. Biochim Biophys Acta 1822:474–481

Lee C, Weindruch R, Prolla TA (2000) Gene-expression profile of the aging brain in mice. Nat Gen 25:294–297

Loerch PM, Lu T, Dakin KA, Vann JM, Isaacs A, Geula C, Jianbin W, Pan Y, Gabuzda DH, Li C, Prolla TA, Yankner BA (2008) Evolution of the aging brain transcriptome and synaptic regulation. PLoS One 3:e3329

Lu T, Pan Y, Kao S, Li C, Kohane I, Chan J, Yankner BA (2004) Gene regulation and DNA damage in the aging human brain. Nat 429:883–891

Lupien SJ, McEwen BS, Gunnar MR, Heim C (2009) Effects of stress throughout the lifespan on the brain, behaviour and cognition. Nat Rev Neurosci 10:434–445

Mandel S, Amit T, Reznichenko, Weinreb O, Youdim MBH (2006) Green tea catechins as brain-permeable, natural iron chelators-antioxidants for the treatment of neurodegenerative disorders. Mol Nutr Food Res 50:229–234

Mattson MP, Duan W, Lee J, Guo Z (2001). Suppression of brain aging and neurodegenerative disorders by dietary restriction and environmental enrichment: molecular mechanisms. Mech Ageing Dev 122:757–778

Mishra LC, Singh BB, Dagenais S (2000) Scientific basis for the therapeutic use of Withania somnifera (Ashwagandha): a review. Alt Med Rev 5:334–346

Nakatani N (2000) Phenolic antioxidants from herbs and spices. Biofactors 13:141–146

Neill D (2012) Should Alzheimer's disease be equated with human brain aging? A maladaptive interaction between brain evolution and senescence. Aging Res Rev 11:104–122

Ota M, Yasuno F, Ito H, Seki C, Kozaki S, Asada T, Suhara T (2006) Age-related decline of dopamine synthesis in the living human brain measured by positron emission tomography with L-[β-11C]DOPA. Life Sci 79:730–736

Paramanik V, Thakur MK (2012) Estrogen receptor β and its domains interact with casein kinase 2, phosphokinase C and N-myristoylation sites of mitochondrial and nuclear proteins in mouse brain. J Biol Chem 287:22305–22316

Peng B, Chen M, Pu Y, Wang Y (2011) Anti-aging effects of ginsenoside Rg1 and its mechanisms on brain aging rats induced by D-galactose. J Chongqing Med Univ 36:419–422

Penner MR, Roth TL, Barnes CA, Sweatt JD (2010) An epigenetic hypothesis of aging-related cognitive dysfunction. Front Aging Neurosci 2:9

Rastogi M, Ojha RP, Prabu PC, Devi BP, Agrawal A, Dubey GP (2012) Prevention of age-associated neurodegeneration and promotion of healthy brain aging in female Wistar rats by long term use of bacosides. Biogerontology 13:183–195

Raz N, Rodrigue KM (2006) Differential aging of the brain: patterns, cognitive correlates and modifiers. Neurosci and Biobehav Rev 30:730–748

Rolyan H, Scheffold A, Heinrich A, Begus-Nahrmann Y, Langkopf BH, Holter SM, Vogt-Weisenhorn DM, Liss B, Wurst W, Lie DC, Thal DR, Biber K, Rudolph KL (2011) Telomere shortening reduces Alzheimer's disease amyloid pathology in mice. Brain 134:2044–2056
Ross JM, Öberg J, Brené S, Coppotelli G, Terzioglu M, Pernold K, Goiny M, Sitnikov R, Kehr J, Trifunovic A, Larsson NG, Hoffer BJ, Olson L (2010) High brain lactate is a hallmark of aging and caused by a shift in the lactate dehydrogenase A/B ratio. Proc Natl Acad Sci USA 107:20087–20092
Schmidt R, Schmidt H, Haybaeck J, Loitfelder M, Weis S, Cavalieri M, Seiler S, Enzinger C, Ropele S, Erkinjuntti T, Pantoni L, Scheltens P, Fazekas F, Jellinger K (2011) Heterogeneity in age-related white matter changes. Acta Neuropathol 122:171–185
Schumacher M, Weill-Engerer S, Liere P, Robert F, Franklin RJM, Garcia-Segura LM, Lambert JJ, Mayoe W, Melcangi RC, Parducz A, Suter U, Carelli C, Baulieu EE, Akwa Y (2003) Steroid hormones and neurosteroids in normal and pathological aging of the nervous system. Prog Neurobiol 71:3–29
Schulze ET, Geary EK, Susmaras MT, Paliga JT, Maki PM, Little DM (2011) Anatomical correlates of age-related working memory declines. J Aging Res 2011:606871
Shetty PK, Galeffi F, Turner Dennis A (2011) Age-induced alterations in hippocampal function and metabolism. Aging Dis 2:196–218
Singh S, Aggarwal BB (1995) Activation of transcription factor NF-κB is suppressed by curcumin (diferuloylmethane). J Biol Chem 270:24995–25000
Singh S, Thakur MK (2011) Age-dependent expression of apolipoprotein E in mouse cerebral cortex. J Mol Neurosci 43:251–256
Sivanandam TM, Thakur MK (2011) Amyloid precursor protein (APP) mRNA level is higher in the old mouse cerebral cortex and is regulated by sex steroids. J Mol Neurosci 43:235–240
Sivanandam TM, Thakur MK (2012) Traumatic brain injury: a risk factor for Alzheimer's disease. Neurosci Biobehav Rev 36:1376–1381
Smith RG, Betancourt L, Sun Y (2005) Molecular endocrinology and physiology of the aging central nervous system. Endocr Rev 26:203–250
Sonntag WE, Lynch C, Thornton P, Khan A, Bennett S, Ingram R (2000) The effects of growth hormone and IGF-1 deficiency on cerebrovascular and brain aging. J Anat 197:575–585
Stranahan AM, Mattson PM (2012) Recruiting adaptive cellular stress responses for successful brain aging. Nat Rev Neurosci 13:209–216
Taki Y, Thyreau B, Kinomura S, Sato K, Goto R, Kawashima R, Fukuda H (2011) Correlations among brain gray matter volumes, age, gender and hemisphere in healthy individuals. PLoS One 6:e22734
Thakur MK, Ghosh S (2007) Age and sex dependent alteration in presenilin expression in mouse cerebral cortex. Cell Mol Neurobiol 27:1059–1067
Thakur MK, Sharma PK (2006) Aging of brain: role of estrogen. Neurochem Res 31:1389–1398
VanGuilder HD, Freeman WM (2011) The hippocampal neuroproteome with aging and cognitive decline: past progress and future directions. Front Aging Neurosci 3:8
Veiga S, Melcangib RC, DonCarlosc LL, Garcia-Seguraa LM, Azcoitiad I (2004) Sex hormones and brain aging. Exp Gerontol 39:1623–1631
Weller M, Platten M, Roth P, Wick W (2011) Geriatric neuro-oncology: from mythology to biology. Curr Opin Neurol 24:599–604
Wikgren M, Maripuu M, Karlsson T, Nordfjäll K, Bergdahl J, Hultdin J, Del-Favero J, Roos G, Nilsson LG, Adolfsson R, Norrback KF (2012) Short telomeres in depression and the general population are associated with a hypocortisolemic state. Biol Psychiatry 71:294–300
Wilkie KP, Drapaca CS, Sivaloganathan S (2012) Aging impact on brain biomechanics with applications to hydrocephalus. Math Med Biol 29:145–161
Woodard JL, Sugarman MA (2012) Functional magnetic resonance imaging in aging and dementia: detection of age-related cognitive changes and prediction of cognitive decline. Curr Top Behav Neurosci 10:113–136
Yamamoto M (2001) Depression in Parkinson's disease: its prevalence, diagnosis, and neurochemical background. J Neurol 248:III5–III11

Yankner A, Lu T, Bruce LP (2008) The aging brain. Annu Rev Pathol Mech Dis 3:41–66
Zeier Z, Madorsky I, Xu Y, Ogle WO, Notterpek L, Foster TC (2011) Gene expression in the hippocampus: regionally specific effects of aging and caloric restriction. Mech Age Dev 132:8–19
Zeng Y, Tan M, Kohyama J, Sneddon M, Watson JB, Sun YE, Xie CW (2011) Epigenetic enhancement of BDNF signaling rescues synaptic plasticity in aging. J Neurosci 31:17800–17810

Chapter 2
Base Excision DNA Repair: The House Keeping Guardian for Genomic Stability in the Brain

Umakanta Swain and Kalluri Subba Rao

Abstract During evolution, organisms have developed a number of strategies to keep the structure of their genetic material intact. However, evolutionary forces keep driving metabolic changes that would lead to more viable progenies for survival and propagation. Thus natural evolution uses two opposing forces to improve the genetic makeup of the species. With the advent of organisms turning aerobic, the advantage of gains in energy production also paved the way to cope up with increasing oxidative damage from within. In response, the system has developed ways and means to offset the possibilities of oxidative damage to macromolecules and in particular, the genetic material, DNA. Of the many pathways of DNA repair, the base excision repair (BER) stands out as the watch dog to alert even a minor modification to a base in DNA and also to initiate the process of repair. Thus, BER plays a seminal role in maintaining the structural integrity of DNA that is quite often threatened from events taking place within the cell itself. Implicit in this crucial role is also the fact that any perturbation in this repair pathway could lead to deleterious consequences—particularly in a post-mitotic tissue like brain. It is becoming increasingly apparent that BER has close correlation with the age-dependent debilities/disorders.

Keywords Base excision repair • Brain • DNA damage • Aging • DNA polymerase β

K. Subba Rao (✉)
Centers for Biotechnology and Innovative Research, Institute of Science and Technology, Jawaharlal Nehru Technological University
Hyderabad 500085, India

U. Swain
School of Medical Sciences, University of Hyderabad
Hyderabad 500046, India
e-mail: ksrbrain@gmail.com; ksrsl@yahoo.com

M. K. Thakur, S. I. S. Rattan (eds.), *Brain Aging and Therapeutic Interventions*,
DOI 10.1007/978-94-007-5237-5_2,

2.1 Introduction

The basic prerequisites for the survival and proper functioning of the living organisms are the accurate maintenance and transmission of the genetic instructions coded in DNA, with the highest possible fidelity. The faithful course of these processes is guaranteed by the genomic stability, which ensures both cellular homeostasis and genetic continuity in multicellular organisms. The integrity of the genetic material is under constant attack by numerous exogenous and endogenous sources. Consequently, formation of DNA damages is a common event in living cells. Accordingly, it is not surprising that during the evolution, an intricate network of sophisticated, interwoven DNA repair systems has developed. The various features of DNA damages require different ways to counteract their deleterious effects. However, mutagenesis is a prerequisite for evolution and some adaptive genomic alterations escape the watchful security of DNA repair system. Sometimes these mutations can lead to increasing vulnerability for diseases like cancer and phenomenon like aging. It thus appears that DNA repair potential in organisms plays a very crucial and fundamental role in conserving the genomic integrity in any given species as well as allowing the evolution as and when necessary.

With the original findings of Alexander (1967) that DNA repair is at a low key once the cells are differentiated into the post-mitotic state, the manner in which the genomic maintenance is achieved in a post-mitotic but metabolically very active organ like brain has become a curious issue. Subsequent studies have indicated, however, that even in adult brain a certain level of DNA repair exists, and it was realized that the terminally differentiated nature of brain cells offers a good model for studying the repair pathways and the accumulation of genomic damage during the lifespan of a given animal.

The purpose of this article is to review an outline of the various types of structural alterations that are known to occur in genomic DNA of mammalian cells and discuss how the base excision repair (BER) pathway operates to counteract such DNA damage, with a special emphasis on the brain tissue.

2.2 The Vulnerable Nervous System

The nervous system consists of two classes of cells, the neurons and glial cells, which include astrocytes, oligodendrocytes and microglial cells. Further, in almost all the species, central nervous system is one of the earliest systems to develop and differentiate. It would therefore follow that a neuronal cell in brain of any species, at any given point of time, is almost as old as the animal itself. An important feature of neuronal cells is their post-mitotic state, i.e., unlike other cell populations (e.g. skin, blood, connective tissue, and even glial cells); neurons are terminally differentiated (i.e. non-dividing), and therefore, devoid of chromosome replication. However, it is also known that neurons are one of the most metabolically active cells in the body.

Hence, they need elaborate, stringent defense mechanisms to ensure their longevity. Neurons display high rates of transcription and translation, which are associated with high rates of metabolism and mitochondrial activity. The amount of oxygen consumed by the brain, relative to its size, exceeds by 20 % that of other organs (Clark and Sokoloff 1999). This high activity, coupled with high oxygen consumption, creates a stressful environment for neurons that includes noxious metabolic by-products, primarily reactive oxygen species (ROS), constantly attacking neuronal genomic and mitochondrial DNA (Barzilai 2007, 2010; Fishel et al. 2007).

2.3 DNA Damage in Brain

DNA is vulnerable to attack by other chemicals, which can result in alterations in its coding properties or normal function in transcription or replication (Subba Rao and Loeb 1992; Lindahl 1993). The native structure of DNA is subject to damage by both endogenous and exogenous events. DNA damage can result in loss or modification of bases, single-strand breaks (SSBs) and double strand breaks (DSBs), the production of mismatched base pairs, DNA-DNA crosslinks and crosslinks between DNA and other cellular constituents (Rao 1993; Barnes and Lindahl 2004). Many of these DNA modifications have been shown to be mutagenic in vitro and in vivo (Loeb 1989). In view of the generally protected situation of brain (including the blood-brain barrier), the main enemy for causing DNA damage in brain cells is from within only. The number of ways the nuclear DNA in brain cells could possibly be damaged is in detail described by Rao (1993).

Endogenous sources of DNA damage and mutations can be classified into three groups. First, DNA is subjected to spontaneous hydrolytic processes, including depurination, depyrimidination, deamination and cleavage of phosphodiester bonds. Of these, depurination is the most frequent process. From the rate of depurination of DNA in aqueous solution under physiological conditions in vitro, it has been estimated that the DNA in each cell undergoes 10,000 depurinations per day (Lindahl and Nyberg 1972). The hydrolytic damage to DNA is the deamination of DNA bases, in particular at cytosine yields uracil, which is recognized by a specific repair enzyme uracil DNA-glycosylase (UDG) and uracil in DNA is known to be removed with very high efficiency. In contrast, deamination of 5-methyl cytosine yields thymine, a normal base in DNA. Possibly, because of this reason, G-T mispairs are repaired rather less efficiently than G-U mispairs and as a consequence, 5-methyl cytosine residues are hot spots for mutation in cells (Duncan and Miller 1980; Ehrlich et al. 1990).

A second major source of damage to cellular DNA is the formation of reactive derivatives of oxygen from normal metabolic process and by exposure of cells to exogenous agents (Demple and Harrison 1994; Barnes and Lindahl 2004). Such ROS includes reactive methyl and ethyl groups, lipid peroxides and oxygen free radicals. It is becoming increasingly apparent that oxidative reactions may be a major source of DNA damage. Oxygen is metabolized by a series of single electron

Table 2.1 Approximate frequencies of occurrence of DNA damages in mammalian cells

Type of damage	Events per day/cell	Reference
Depurination	10,000	Lindahl and Nyberg (1972)
Depyrimidination	500	Lindahl and Karlstorm (1973)
Deamination	100–300	Lindahl and Nyberg (1974)
Base damages (including all types of base damage viz. oxidative damage, adduct formation with reducing sugars, methylation, crosslinks, and so forth)	10,000	Richter et al. (1988)
Single-strand breaks	20,000–40,000	
Double strand breaks	9	Bernstein and Bernstein (1991)
Interstrands crosslinks	8	Bernstein and Bernstein (1991)
DNA protein crosslinks	Unknown	Bernstein and Bernstein (1991)

reductions, yielding highly reactive species including hydroxyl radicals, hydrogen peroxide, superoxide and singlet oxygen. Ionizing radiation can also generate reactive radicals both by direct attack on DNA and by the radiolysis of H_2O (Halliwell 1992; Riley 1994; Bandyopadhyay et al. 1999). The range of DNA lesions generated by ROS is extensive and more than 20 products of base oxidation have been identified (Cooke et al. 2003). Modified purine and pyrimidine bases constitute one of the major classes of hydroxyl radical mediated DNA damage together with oligonucleotide strand breaks, DNA-protein crosslinks and abasic (AP) sites (Cadet et al. 1999). The products of such reactions, e.g., 8-oxoguanine (8-oxoG), formamidopyrimidines and ring-saturated pyrimidines such as thymine glycol, are often mutagenic or cytotoxic (Wilson et al. 2003; Evans et al. 2004). Considering that ROS produces multiple modifications in DNA, it can be estimated that as many as 10^4–10^5 bases in DNA in each human cell are replaced as a result of oxygen free radical damage every day. Third, though neurons are non-replicative cells, DNA synthesis occurs during the repair of DNA damage. This repair synthesis is believed to be catalyzed in part by DNA polymerase β (pol β), the most error prone of the mammalian DNA polymerases (Loeb and Kunkel 1982). Considering that brain is an organ with unusually high oxygen consumption, these aspects of genetic damage can be expected to play a greater role in brain than in other tissues.

The frequency with which the DNA damaging events occur in a mammalian cell has been examined by a number of workers, and this information is summarized in Table 2.1, and some of the DNA base alterations are as shown in Fig. 2.1. Work from our laboratory, using two biochemical approaches, has demonstrated that neurons from different regions of rat brain harbor both SSBs and DSBs in their nuclear DNA, and this strand breaks increase with age of the animal (Mandavilli and Rao 1996a, b). However, we have recently accessed genomic DNA damage of brain cells on a single-cell basis, popularly called "comet assay". By adjusting the pH as well as experimental conditions, the types of DNA lesions that are detectable by comet assay include AP sites (alkali-labile sites), SSBs, DSBs and DNA-protein

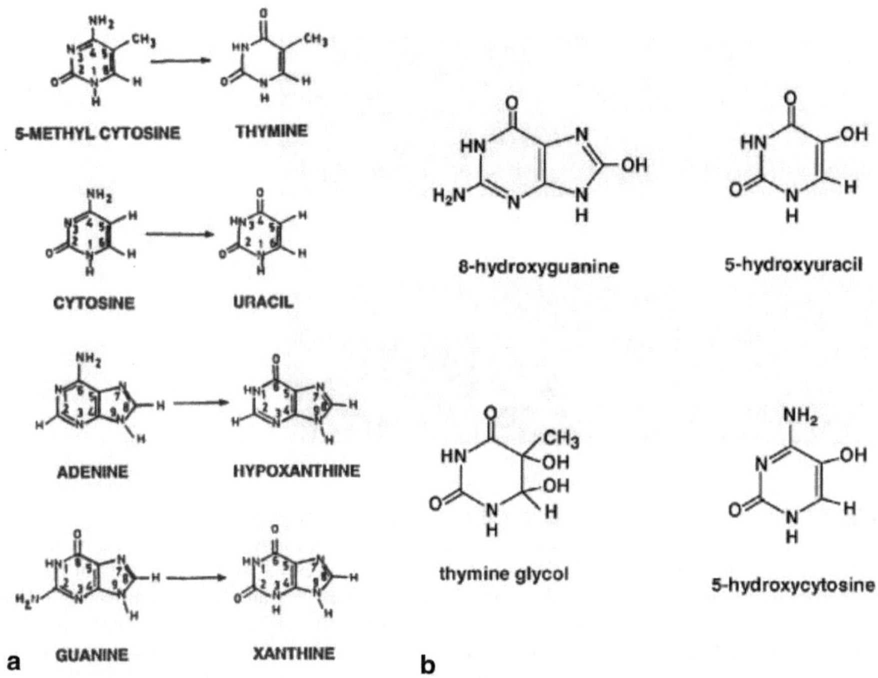

Fig. 2.1 Different forms of DNA damage that could occur due to various endogenous or/and exogenous factors. **a** Some of the deamination product of the DNA bases. **b** Some of the oxidized products of DNA bases

crosslinks (Tice et al. 2000). The alkaline denaturation of DNA and electrophoresis at pH > 13 is generally considered capable of detecting DNA SSBs, AP sites, DNA-DNA/DNA-protein crosslinking, and SSBs associated with incomplete excision repair sites (Singh et al. 1988; Tice et al. 2000). Neutral conditions (pH ~ 8.3) are used to detect mostly DSBs because DNA remains double stranded under this condition, and regions containing DSBs migrate more readily in an electrophoretic field (Ostling and Johanson 1984; Singh et al. 1988; Lemay and Wood 1999).

As it can be seen in Fig. 2.2a, the alkaline version of the comet assay is used to determine the level of DNA strand breaks in isolated neurons prepared from animals of different age groups. After SYBR Green I staining, young neuronal nuclei appeared very bright and round (Fig. 2.2a). Furthermore, very little migration of DNA is evident; suggesting that DNA damage is at its minimum in young neurons. However, with advancement of age (adult and old), there is significant relaxation and migration of DNA from the nucleus, forming a "comet" tail (Fig. 2.2a). It is also clear that the tail moment values increased with age. The tail moment value, in comparison with that in young neurons increased 4.1-fold in adult, and 5.1-fold in old neurons (Fig. 2.2b). Closer evaluation of the data reveals that a considerable

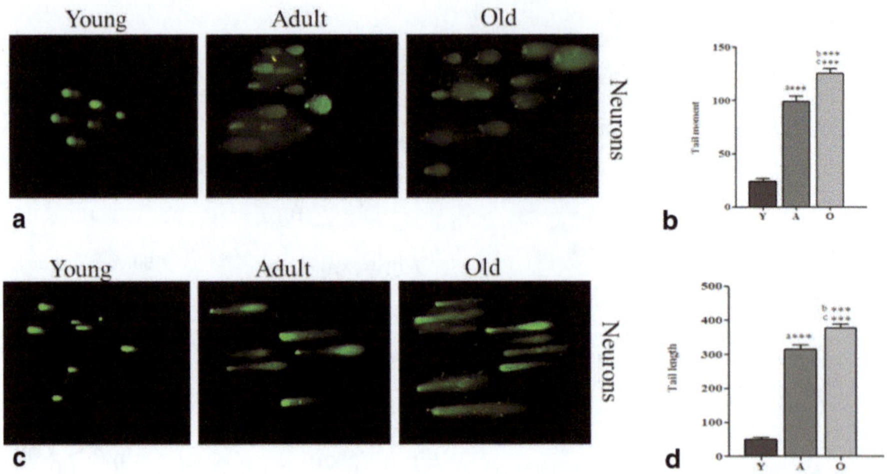

Fig. 2.2 Comet assay of neurons prepared from 'young' (7 days postnatal), 'adult' (6 months) and 'old' (≥24 months) rat brain. **a** Fluorescence photomicrographs showing comets of neurons (alkaline condition). **b** Bar graph showing tail moment expressed in arbitrary units in neurons prepared from young, adult and old rat brain cortex. Values at **a** and **b** are significantly different from the corresponding values at young. **c** is significantly different from the corresponding values at adult. **c** Fluorescence photomicrographs showing comets of neurons (neutral condition). **d** Bar graph showing tail length expressed in arbitrary units in neurons. Values at **a** and **b** are significantly different from the corresponding values at young; **c** is significantly different from the corresponding values at adult. ***$p < 0.001$ (Adapted from Swain and Subba Rao 2011)

number of strands break accumulated by adulthood itself (6 months) with the further increase in the strand breaks in old age in both types of cells.

We have also examined neutral version of the comet assay without treatment with alkaline buffer for electrophoresis. Under these conditions, the comet is considered to detect largely, if not exclusively DSBs. The extent of DNA damage measured as tail length under these conditions also increased in neurons with age (Fig. 2.2c). The tail length value of adult neurons increased 6.2-fold in comparison to that in young while in the case of old neurons, there was a 7.4-fold increase in comparison to young neurons (Fig. 2.2c and d).

The above comet assay method measures different DNA strand breaks by changing the pH condition. Strand breaks cause relaxation of the supercoiling in the DNA, and free DNA loops are pulled towards the anode during electrophoresis giving the appearance of a comet tail. Fluorescence staining enables DNA damage to be visualized and quantified. However, in this method damage or alteration of DNA base could not be quantified. To make the assay more sensitive for determination of damaged base in nuclear DNA specifically, we have modified the alkaline version of the comet assay by incorporating a lesion-specific enzyme which increases its activity through the recognition of the damaged base substrate and thus introducing additional breaks causing enhanced DNA relaxation and migration (Swain and

Table 2.2 Measurement of OGG1 sensitive sites in young (7 days postnatal), adult (6 months) and old (≥2 years) rat brain neurons by FLARE™ comet assay. (Adapted from Swain and Subba Rao 2011)

Sample	Tail moment		
	Mean ± SEM		Net amount of OGG1 sensitive series
	Buffer	hOGG1	
Young neurons	14.46 ± 1.42	22.75 ± 2.96	8.29
Adult neurons	94.76 ± 4.68	138.18 ± 11.04[a***]	43.42
Old neurons	114.01 ± 3.00	175.64 ± 7.77[b, c***]	61.63

a and b are significantly different from the corresponding values at young. c is significantly different from the corresponding values at adult
***$p < 0.001$

Subba Rao 2011). When using lesion-specific enzymes to measure DNA damage, the usual practice is to incubate a slide (two gels) with buffer alone in parallel along with the +enzyme slide, and to subtract the mean comet score of the control (buffer) slide from the mean score of the +enzyme slide (Collins 2009).

We have recently measured the presence of 8-oxoguanine DNA-glycosylase 1 (OGG1) sensitive sites in DNA of neurons by introducing human OGG1 in the assay on naked DNA after lysis was performed.

Human OGG1 initiates the repair of 8-oxoG bases by excising them and cutting the sugar-phosphate backbone of the DNA molecule. Thus additional strand breaks are induced at the location of oxidized base substrate, causing additional DNA relaxation and migration. The outcomes from these studies are shown in Table 2.2. When neurons were incubated with only buffer, an increase of DNA migration in the tail was observed with increasing age of the animal (Table 2.2). This increase in tail movement is taken to indicate increasing DNA damage that occurs due to aging. When the cells were incubated with buffer containing human OGG1, there was a further increase in the tail movement, which must be due to the removal of 8-oxoG residues accumulating in DNA with age. Incubation of the brain cells with human OGG1 represents the increase in the number of OGG1 sensitive sites with age. In neuronal DNA, the content of OGG1 sensitive sites between the young and adult ages has increased by 5.2-fold and between young and old ages by 7.4-fold. Closer observation of the data revealed that accumulations of OGG1 sensitive sites occurred continuously through adulthood and old age unlike the general damage due to overall strand breaks, which occurred mostly by adulthood itself (Table 2.2).

Similarly, the UDG sensitive sites in neurons at these three ages were assessed by the introduction of UDG, which removes uracil and creates AP sites that are cleaved to result in strand breaks during the alkali processing. When neurons were incubated with only buffer, increase of DNA migration in the tail was observed with age of the animal (Table 2.3). This increase in tail movement is taken as increased damage occurring due to aging. When the cells were incubated with buffer containing the UDG, there was a further increase in tail movement, which must be due to the presence of uracil residues accumulating in DNA with age. Essentially the

Table 2.3 Measurement of UDG sensitive sites in young, adult and old rat brain neurons by FLARE™ comet assay. (Adapted from Swain and Subba Rao 2011)

Sample	Tail moment		
	Mean ± SEM		Net amount of UDG sensitive sites
	Buffer	UDG	
Young neurons	14.96 ± 1.70	22.77 ± 2.15	7.81
Adult neurons	115.71 ± 4.35	141.78 ± 9.24[a]***	26.07
Old neurons	134.70 ± 5.91	185.34 ± 10.55[b, c]***	50.64

a and b are significantly different from the corresponding values at young; c is significantly different from the corresponding values at adult|
***$p<0.001$

enhanced tail movement due to the incubation of the neurons with UDG denotes the increase in the number of uracil or other UDG sensitive sites with age. Table 2.3 shows the actual fold increase of such sensitive sites with age in neurons. For example, in neuronal DNA, the content of UDG sensitive sites between the young and adult ages has increased 3.3-fold, and between young and old ages by 6.5-fold. Keen observation of the data suggests that accumulation of UDG sensitive sites in neurons is a gradual process with age (Table 2.3).

A striking feature appears to be that the damage accumulation occurs very rapidly during the first 6 months of life. A somewhat comparable result was noticed in a very early study carried out by Price et al. (1971). It is possible that this phenomenon of significant accumulation of DNA damage coupled with decreased DNA repair, particularly in a post-mitotic tissue, may have something to do with the timing of the attainment of reproductive maturity of the animal (Bernstein and Bernstein 1991). This, however, remains a speculation at this time. It is also possible that during this rapid growth and reproductive phase of the animal, the repair efficiency is not able to match with the accumulation of damage.

2.4 BER Pathway

BER is perhaps the most fundamental and ubiquitous DNA repair mechanism in all-higher organisms that depend on oxygen for the sustenance of life. This pathway has evolved to handle the numerous minor alterations—including spontaneous modification, oxidation, alkylation, deamination and loss of bases—that can occur in the structure of DNA as a result of cellular metabolic activity. This mode of repair is of particular importance in post-mitotic tissues such as those of the brain, where simple base modifications are more likely to occur than is major damage to DNA.

The core BER pathway requires the function of only four enzymes in the basic reaction steps to remove a damaged DNA base and replace it with the correct base. These proteins include a DNA glycosylase, an AP endonuclease or AP lyase, a DNA polymerase, and a DNA ligase. BER is initiated by a lesion-specific DNA glycosylase (mono- or bi- functional) and completed by either of two sub-pathways: short-patch BER (SP-BER); a mechanism whereby only one nucleotide is replaced or long-patch BER (LP-BER); a mechanism whereby 2–13 nucleotides are replaced (Wilson 1998; Fortini et al. 1999; Fortini 2003; Almeida and Sobol 2007; Wilson and Bohr 2007; Hegde et al. 2008; Jeppesen et al. 2011). A currently accepted model for the core BER pathway reveals five distinct enzymatic steps for the repair of damaged bases.

1. Recognition and excision of the damage base,
2. Incision of the DNA adjacent to the resulting abasic site,
3. End cleaning of the DNA termini to produce a 3′-hydroxyl group (3′-OH) and a 5′-phosphate group (5′-P),
4. Repair synthesis, and
5. DNA ligation to seal the nick.

(i) The initiation of BER is performed by a specific DNA glycosylase that recognizes and excises a specific base by catalyzing hydrolysis of the N-glycosylic bond resulting in an AP site. Depending on the types of damaged base, DNA glycosylase can be either monofunctional (such as UDG, has only the glycosylase activity) or bifunctional (such as OGG1 and NEILS, have an intrinsic 3′AP lyase activity in addition to the glycosylase activity).

(ii) The second step consists of incision of DNA strand at 5′ to the AP site by major apurinic endonuclease 1 (APE1), leaving a 5′-deoxyribose phosphate (5′-dRP) and 3′-OH group (Demple et al. 1991; Robson et al. 1992; Seki et al. 1992; Demple and Sung 2005). The bifunctional DNA glycosylase incises the DNA strand at 3′ to the AP site via β- or βδ-elimination, leaving a DNA SSB with a 3′-phospho-α,β-unsaturated aldehyde (3′-PUA) or a 3′-phosphate (3′-P), respectively (Hazra et al. 2002, 2007; Pascucci et al. 2002; Dou et al. 2003).

(iii) The third step in BER is end cleaning of obstructive 3′- and 5′-termini to generate the 3′-OH and 5′-P groups in the gap at the strand break, which is the favorable substrate for DNA pol β. Pol β is a 39 kDa single polypeptide comprising 335 amino acid residues. Both the rat and human enzymes were cloned 15 yrs ago and extensively studied over the years by Wilson and his group (SenGupta et al. 1986) and by Matsukage's group (Date et al. 1988). The structural, catalytic and physiological aspects of pol β have been the subjects of two elegant reviews by Wilson and his associates (Wilson 1998; Idriss et al. 2002). The 5′-dRP group is removed by pol β, by its dRP lyase activity (Matsumoto and Kim 1995; Prasad et al. 1998; Allinson et al. 2001). On the other hand, APE1 removes the 3′-PUA group generated by β-elimination via its 3′-phosphodiesterase activity (Suh et al. 1997; Izumi et al. 2000). The 3′-P group generated by βδ-elimination is a poor substrate for APE1 (Wilson 2003), so such blocking groups are excised primarily by phosphatase activity of polynucleotide kinase 3′-phosphatase (PNKP) (Jilani et al. 1999; Dobson and Allinson 2006).

(iv) In this step, the repair synthesis to replace nucleotide(s), can proceed by one of two sub- pathways, SP-BER or LP-BER., when the 5′-dRP can be efficiently removed by pol β in the previous step (iii), SP-BER is favored. In SP-BER, pol β fills up one nucleotide gap (Sobol et al. 1996), and also interacts with X-ray cross-complementing 1 (XRCC1), a scaffold protein involved in prompting SP-BER by interacting with other proteins (Kubota et al. 1996; Dianova et al. 2004). The majority of BER events are currently thought to occur via SP-BER. LP-BER is initiated in cases where the 5′-dRP group is refractory to the pol β AP lyase activity (for example, reduced AP site) (Podlutsky et al. 2001), the repair synthesis would nevertheless continue but in a strand displacement manner. In LP-BER, the repair synthesis of 2–13 nucleotides is performed by pol β, and/or pol δ/ε coupled with proliferating cell nuclear antigen (PCNA) incorporation with loading factor RFC. The resulting 5′-flap structure formed during repair synthesis is removed by the flap endonuclease 1(FEN1), the activity of which is stimulated by PCNA (Klungland and Lindahl 1997; Fortini et al. 1998; Stucki et al. 1998; Gary et al. 1999). In addition, a number of accessory proteins have been reported to participate in and/or stimulate BER, for example, Poly (ADP-ribose) polymerase-1 (PARP-1) stimulates the strand displacement synthesis of pol β in the presence of FEN1 in LP-BER (Prasad et al. 2001). The Werner syndrome protein helicase (WRN) is also observed to stimulate strand displacement activities of pol β (Harrigan et al. 2003).

(v) The final step in BER is ligation to seal the nick containing a 3′-OH group and a 5′-P group. In SP-BER, the ligation of the final nick is performed by DNA ligase IIIα (LIGIII α) in association with scaffold protein XRCC1 (Caldecott et al. 1994; Cappelli et al. 1997; Tomkinson et al. 2001). In LP-BER, ligation is performed by DNA ligase I (LIGI) with the physical association with PCNA, which helps to stimulate the effective ligation (Levin et al. 2000; Tom et al. 2001; Tomkinson et al. 2001).

SSBs resulting from a variety of causes like ionizing radiation, ROS etc., can also be repaired through BER. Sometimes if the break has a 3′-P or 3′-PUA and 5′-OH then the phosphorylation of 5′-OH and removal of phosphate from 3′-end or removal of 3′-PUA becomes necessary before the break is filled up through BER pathway. This operation is achieved by the enzymes PNKP or APE1. Both enzymes thus carry out important functions of converting the ends of a break in DNA into a repairable mode. If these preparative changes are not taken fast enough, then there is the possibility of undesirable recombination events taking place. In order to avoid this eventuality, PARP-1 provides protection to the DNA SSBs by binding to them (Le Rhun et al. 1998; Ziegler and Oei 2001; Chalmers 2004). There is also a report that PARP-1 interacts with XRCC1 and this interaction accelerates the recruitment of repair proteins involved in BER pathway (Mackey et al. 1999). XRCC1 also stimulates the DNA kinase and DNA phosphatase activities of PNK at damaged DNA termini and thereby accelerates the overall repair process (Whitehouse et al. 2001).

Finally, a newly discovered polymerase is claiming its entry as a possible participant in the BER pathway- DNA polymerase λ (pol λ). Pol λ is a recently described eukaryotic DNA polymerase belonging to Pol X family. It is the closest homologue to pol β, sharing 32 % identity at the protein level. Based on three-dimensional structure modeling, Pol λ is predicted to have a pol β like core formed by two domains: a 31 kDa polymerase domain and 8 kDa domain (Garcia-Diaz et al. 2000;

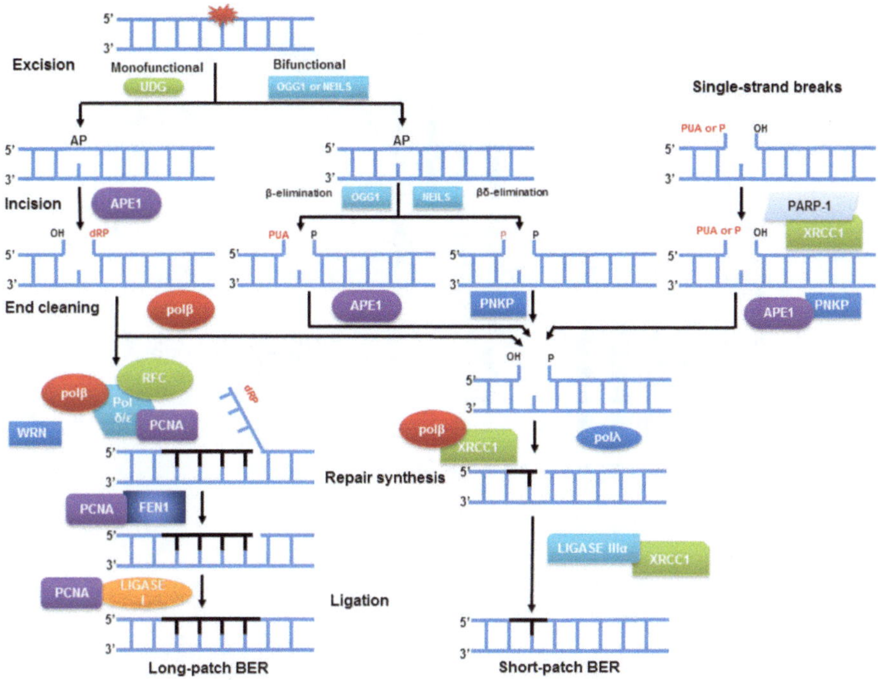

Fig. 2.3 Schematic representation of the mammalian base excision repair and single-strand break repair pathway

DeRose et al. 2003). Recently, Gap-filling DNA synthesis and dRP lyase activities of pol λ have been demonstrated in vitro, suggesting its participation in BER (Garcia-Diaz et al. 2001; Braithwaite et al. 2005). Figure 2.3 shows the BER pathway depicted on the basis of latest information available.

2.5 BER and Brain

In the BER pathway, the actual substrate for pol β is a DNA duplex with one of the strands with a baseless site, which is eventually converted into a gap. Thus, a gap DNA is the most natural substrate for pol β to insert the correct nucleotide using the other strand as the template. In view of this, synthetic oligo duplexes (32-mers) with one or four nucleotide gap in one of the strands were used as substrates and the gap filling activity in young, adult and old neuronal extracts was measured (Krishna et al. 2005). Gap repair involves two steps: the filling of the gap by the addition of the required number of nucleotides followed by the ligation with the 5′ phosphorylated downstream primer. This repair process, if completed properly should give a radioactive spot on the sequencing gel corresponding to the 32-mer.

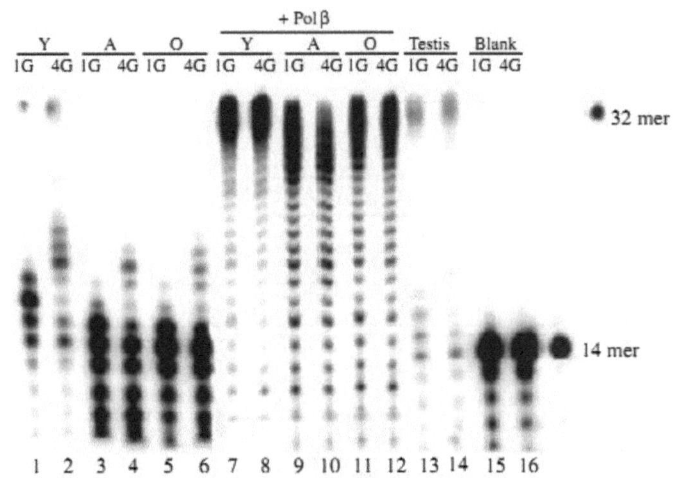

1 Gap Oligo: (14 mer) 32P 5'- cgagccatggccgc -aga tttttgcgg tgcc-3' (17 mer)
3'- gct cggtaccggcgg tc t aaaaaacgccacgg - 5' (32 mer)

4 Gap Oligo: (14 mer) 32P 5'- cgagccatggccgc ---- tttttt gcggtgcc-3' (14 mer)
3'- gct cggtaccggcggtct aaaaa acgccacgg- 5' (32 mer)

Fig. 2.4 Gap repair activity in 'young,' 'adult' and 'old' neuronal extracts and supplemented with recombinant pure rat liver pol β with 5′-PO_4 on the downstream primer. Lanes 1–6 neuronal extracts from young brain (Y, 5 days postnatal), adult brain (A, 6 months) old brain (O, ≥2 years). Lanes 7–12 neuronal extracts supplemented with one unit of pol β. Lanes 13 and 14 are with testis extracts alone as positive control. Lanes 15 and 16 are without any neuronal extracts (enzyme blanks). The mobility of labeled standard, 14-mer and 32-mer is also shown. Lanes 1, 3, 5, 7, 9, 11, 13, 15 are with the one-gap substrate (1G) while lanes 2, 4, 6, 8, 10, 12, 14, 16 are with the four-gap substrate (4G). The oligo duplexes with one and four nucleotide gaps used in the study are also shown. As can be seen one of the strands has a gap of either 1 or 4 nucleotides. These strands are ^{32}P labeled on 5′ end for the subsequent identification on the sequencing gel followed by autoradiography. Furthermore, in either case, the downstream primer after the gap is phosphorylated on 5′ end with non-radioactive phosphate before annealing. (Adapted from Rao 2007)

However, it is seen that only addition of nucleotide has occurred with adult and old neuronal extracts. In the young, addition of nucleotides was seen and ligation to downstream primer also occurred although quite feebly. On the other hand, when the extracts were supplemented with pol β, addition of nucleotides occurred all the way to extend the upstream primer to a 32-mer apparently in a distributive strand displacement manner (Fig. 2.4). On the other hand, when low amounts of pol β were added, addition of just the required number of nucleotides occurred. Even then ligation was achieved only in young extracts, and no ligation could be visualized in adult and old. Finally efficient gap filling followed by ligation, that is complete gap repair, was achieved and for this to happen, conditions required are the presence of

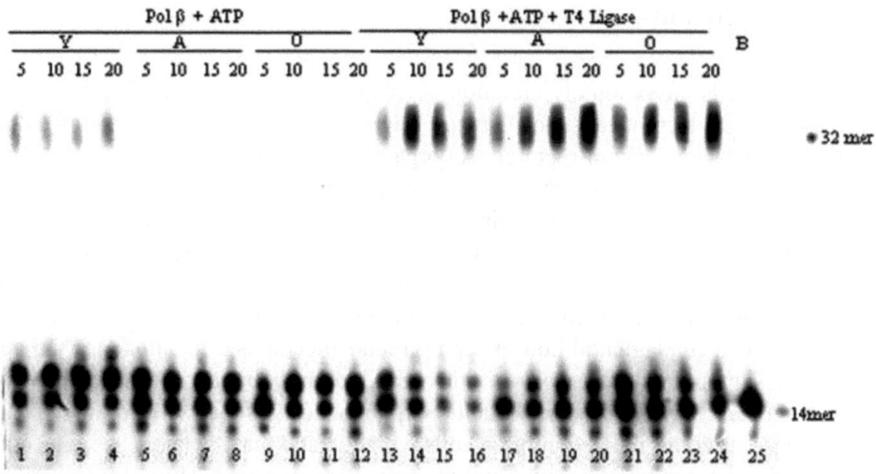

Fig. 2.5 Restoration of the gap repair activity in adult and old rat neuronal extracts when supplemented with limited amounts of pol β (0.2 units) and 20 units of T_4 DNA ligase. All the experimental details and notations are as in Fig. 2.4. Only one gap duplex was used as substrate

5′-PO_4 on the downstream primer, and supplementation of aging neuronal extracts with both pol β and DNA ligase (Fig. 2.5). These studies thus demonstrated that aging neurons are unable to affect BER, due to deficiency of pol β and DNA ligase and fortifying the neuronal extracts from aged animals with these two factors can restore the lost BER activity.

While pol β together with DNA ligase in the case of DNA gap repair could restore the repair activities when supplemented to neuronal extracts from old animals, it is possible that some other polymerases present in neurons may also be functioning in the BER pathway. In recent times many new DNA polymerases, generally error prone and capable of carrying out a variety of other tasks have been discovered (Hubscher et al. 2002; Bebenek and Kunkel 2004). One of them is pol λ belonging to the same family as pol β does, the X-family. The structure and sequence homology of pol λ are similar to pol β and in particular, pol λ contains all the critical residues involved in the DNA binding, nucleotide binding and selection, and catalysis of DNA polymerization, that are conserved in pol β and other DNA polymerases belonging to X-family (Garcia-Diaz et al. 2000), and therefore, emerging as a candidate that could help/substitute pol β in its role in BER (Garcia-Diaz et al. 2005). However, there is no concrete information available about the levels of these novel DNA polymerases in brain. In a preliminary Western blot analysis of pol λ in rodent brain regions, we have noticed the presence of pol λ in brain extracts. Similarly, immunoprecipitated pol λ from brain extract is able to fill one nucleotide gap in one of the strands of DNA oligoduplexes (Swain et al. unpublished observations). A comprehensive study to examine the status of many of these newly discovered DNA polymerases in brain is warranted.

2.6 Conclusions

DNA damage is an extremely common event in all living cells. Both intrinsic as well as extrinsic factors cause the damage. ROS cause a major form of damage that could be deleterious, if not repaired. As organisms age, their DNA repair capacity decreases and this coupled with accumulating damage to DNA may eventually lead to breakdown of the cellular machinery culminating in disease and finally death. Among the various pathways of DNA repair, BER vested with the responsibility of correcting the simple alterations in DNA structure like base modifications and AP sites, essentially resulting from the active metabolism within the cell, can perhaps be viewed as a fundamental housekeeping repair mechanism to safeguard the genomic integrity not only in a post-mitotic organ like brain but in the rest of the body as well. The activity of some important components of this pathway, like pol β and DNA ligase, is compromised in brain cells with age and may be taken as molecular markers for the genomic stability and process of senescence. Thus, any inherited mutational vulnerability in this pathway could display telling effects on the process of aging and associated disorders.

Acknowledgements Umakanta Swain is grateful to University Grants Commission (UGC) for Dr. D.S. Kothari postdoctoral fellowship (Award No. F.4-2/2006(BSR)13-213/2008 (BSR).

References

Alexander P (1967) The role of DNA lesions in the processes leading to aging in mice. Symp Soc Exp Biol 21:29–50

Allinson SL, Dianova II, Dianov GL (2001) DNA polymerase β is the major dRP lyase involved in repair of oxidative base lesions in DNA by mammalian cell extracts. EMBO J 20:6919–6926

Almeida KH, Sobol RW (2007) A unified view of base excision repair: lesion-dependent protein complexes regulated by post-translational modification. DNA Repair (Amst) 6:695–711

Bandyopadhyay U, Das D, Banerjee RK (1999) Reactive oxygen species: Oxidative damage and pathogenesis. Curr Sci 77:658–666

Barnes DE, Lindahl T (2004) Repair and genetic consequences of endogenous DNA base damage in mammalian cells. Annu Rev Genet 38:445–476

Barzilai A (2007) The contribution of the DNA damage response to neuronal viability. Antioxid Redox Signal 9:211–218

Barzilai A (2010) DNA damage, neuronal and glial cell death and neurodegeneration. Apoptosis 15:1371–1381

Bebenek K, Kunkel TA (2004) Functions of DNA polymerases. Adv Protein Chem 69:137–165

Bernstein C, Bernstein H (1991) Aging, sex, and DNA repair. Academic, San Diego

Braithwaite EK, Prasad R, Shock DD, Hou EW, Beard WA, Wilson SH (2005) DNA polymerase lambda mediates a back-up base excision repair activity in extracts of mouse embryonic fibroblasts. J Biol Chem 280:18469–18475

Cadet J, Delatour T, Douki T, Gasparutto D, Pouget JP, Ravanat JL, Sauvaigo S (1999) Hydroxyl radicals and DNA base damage. Mutat Res 424:9–21

Caldecott KW, Mckeown CK, Tucker JD, Ljungquist S, Thompson LH (1994) An interaction between the mammalian DNA-mepair protein Xrcc1 and DNA Ligase-III. Mol Cell Biol 14:68–76

Cappelli E, Taylor R, Cevasco M, Abbondandolo A, Caldecott K, Frosina G (1997) Involvement of XRCC1 and DNA ligase III gene products in DNA base excision repair. J Biol Chem 272:23970–23975

Chalmers AJ (2004) Poly(ADP-ribose) polymerase-1 and ionizing radiation: sensor, signaller and therapeutic target. Clin Oncol (R Coll Radiol) 16:29–39

Clark DD, Sokoloff L (1999) Circulation and energy metabolism of the brain. In: Siegel GJ, Agranoff BW, Albers RW, Fisher SK, Uhler MD (eds) Basic neurochemistry. Molecular, cellular and medical aspects, 6th edn. Lippincott-Raven, Philadelphia, pp. 637–670

Collins AR (2009) Investigating oxidative DNA damage and its repair using the comet assay. Mutat Res 681:24–32

Cooke MS, Evans MD, Dizdaroglu M, Lunec J (2003) Oxidative DNA damage: mechanisms, mutation, and disease. FASEB J 17:1195–1214

Date T, Yamaguchi M, Hirose F, Nishimoto Y, Tanihara K, Matsukage A (1988) Expression of active rat DNA polymerase beta in Escherichia coli. Biochemistry (Mosc) 27:2983–2990

Demple B, Harrison L (1994) Repair of oxidative damage to DNA: enzymology and biology. Annu Rev Biochem 63:915–948

Demple B, Sung JS (2005) Molecular and biological roles of Ape1 protein in mammalian base excision repair. DNA Repair (Amst) 4:1442–1449

Demple B, Herman T, Chen DS (1991) Cloning and expression of APE, the cDNA encoding the major human apurinic endonuclease: definition of a family of DNA repair enzymes. Proc Natl Acad Sci USA 88:11450–11454

DeRose EF, Kirby TW, Mueller GA, Bebenek K, Garcia-Diaz M, Blanco L, Kunkel TA, London RE (2003) Solution structure of the lyase domain of human DNA polymerase lambda. Biochemistry (Mosc) 42:9564–9574

Dianova II, Sleeth KM, Allinson SL, Parsons JL, Breslin C, Caldecott KW, Dianov GL (2004) XRCC1–DNA polymerase β interaction is required for efficient base excision repair. Nucleic Acids Res 32:2550–2555

Dobson CJ, Allinson SL (2006) The phosphatase activity of mammalian polynucleotide kinase takes precedence over its kinase activity in repair of single strand breaks. Nucleic Acids Res 34:2230–2237

Dou H, Mitra S, Hazra TK (2003) Repair of oxidized bases in DNA bubble structures by human DNA glycosylases NEIL1 and NEIL2. J Biol Chem 278:49679–49684

Duncan BK, Miller JH (1980) Mutagenic deamination of cytosine residues in DNA. Nature 287:560–561

Ehrlich M, Zhang XY, Inamdar NM (1990) Spontaneous deamination of cytosine and 5-methylcytosine residues in DNA and replacement of 5-methylcytosine residues with cytosine residues. Mutat Res 238:277–286

Evans MD, Dizdaroglu M, Cooke MS (2004) Oxidative DNA damage and disease: induction, repair and significance. Mutat Res 567:1–61

Fishel ML, Vasko MR, Kelley MR (2007) DNA repair in neurons: so if they don't divide what's to repair? Mutat Res 614:24–36

Fortini P (2003) The base excision repair: mechanisms and its relevance for cancer susceptibility. Biochimie 85:1053–1071

Fortini P, Pascucci B, Parlanti E, Sobol RW, Wilson SH, Dogliotti E (1998) Different DNA polymerases are involved in the short- and long-patch base excision repair in mammalian cells. Biochemistry (Mosc) 37:3575–3580

Fortini P, Parlanti E, Sidorkina OM, Laval J, Dogliotti E (1999) The type of DNA glycosylase determines the base excision repair pathway in mammalian cells. J Biol Chem 274:15230–15236

Garcia-Diaz M, Dominguez O, Lopez-Fernandez LA, de Lera LT, Saniger ML, Ruiz JF, Parraga M, Garcia-Ortiz MJ, Kirchhoff T, del Mazo J, Bernad A, Blanco L (2000) DNA polymerase lambda (Pol lambda), a novel eukaryotic DNA polymerase with a potential role in meiosis. J Mol Biol 301:851–867

Garcia-Diaz M, Bebenek K, Kunkel TA, Blanco L (2001) Identification of an intrinsic 5′-deoxyribose-5-phosphate lyase activity in human DNA polymerase lambda: a possible role in base excision repair. J Biol Chem 276:34659–34663

Garcia-Diaz M, Bebenek K, Gao G, Pedersen LC, London RE, Kunkel TA (2005) Structure-function studies of DNA polymerase lambda. DNA Repair (Amst) 4:1358–1367

Gary R, Kim K, Cornelius HL, Park MS, Matsumoto Y (1999) Proliferating cell nuclear antigen facilitates excision in long-patch base excision repair. J biol chem 274:4354–4363

Halliwell B (1992) Reactive oxygen species and the central nervous system. J Neurochem 59:1609–1623

Harrigan JA, Opresko PL, von Kobbe C, Kedar PS, Prasad R, Wilson SH, Bohr VA (2003) The Werner syndrome protein stimulates DNA polymerase beta strand displacement synthesis via its helicase activity. J Biol Chem 278:22686–22695

Hazra TK, Izumi T, Boldogh I, Imhoff B, Kow YW, Jaruga P, Dizdaroglu M, Mitra S (2002) Identification and characterization of a human DNA glycosylase for repair of modified bases in oxidatively damaged DNA. Proc Natl Acad Sci U S A 99:3523–3528

Hazra TK, Das A, Das S, Choudhury S, Kow YW, Roy R (2007) Oxidative DNA damage repair in mammalian cells: a new perspective. DNA Repair (Amst) 6:470–480

Hegde ML, Hazra TK, Mitra S (2008) Early steps in the DNA base excision/single-strand interruption repair pathway in mammalian cells. Cell Res 18:27–47

Hubscher U, Maga G, Spadari S (2002) Eukaryotic DNA polymerases. Annu Rev Biochem 71:133–163

Idriss HT, Al-Assar O, Wilson SH (2002) DNA polymerase beta. Int J Biochem Cell Biol 34:321–324

Izumi T, Hazra TK, Boldogh I, Tomkinson AE, Park MS, Ikeda S, Mitra S (2000) Requirement for human AP endonuclease 1 for repair of 3′-blocking damage at DNA single-strand breaks induced by reactive oxygen species. Carcinogenesis 21:1329–1334

Jeppesen DK, Bohr VA, Stevnsner T (2011) DNA repair deficiency in neurodegeneration. Prog Neurobiol 94:166–200

Jilani A, Ramotar D, Slack C, Ong C, Yang XM, Scherer SW, Lasko DD (1999) Molecular cloning of the human gene, PNKP, encoding a polynucleotide kinase 3′-phosphatase and evidence for its role in repair of DNA strand breaks caused by oxidative damage. J Biol Chem 274:24176–24186

Klungland A, Lindahl T (1997) Second pathway for completion of human DNA base excision-repair: reconstitution with purified proteins and requirement for DNase IV (FEN1). EMBO J 16:3341–3348

Krishna TH, Mahipal S, Sudhakar A, Sugimoto H, Kalluri R, Rao KS (2005) Reduced DNA gap repair in aging rat neuronal extracts and its restoration by DNA polymerase beta and DNA-ligase. J Neurochem 92:818–823

Kubota Y, Nash RA, Klungland A, Schar P, Barnes DE, Lindahl T (1996) Reconstitution of DNA base excision-repair with purified human proteins: Interaction between DNA polymerase beta and the XRCC1 protein. EMBO J 15:6662–6670

Le Rhun Y, Kirkland JB, Shah GM (1998) Cellular responses to DNA damage in the absence of Poly(ADP-ribose) polymerase. Biochem Biophys Res Commun 245:1–10

Lemay M, Wood KA (1999) Detection of DNA damage and identification of UV-induced photoproducts using the CometAssay kit. Biotechniques 27:846–851

Levin DS, McKenna AE, Motycka TA, Matsumoto Y, Tomkinson AE (2000) Interaction between PCNA and DNA ligase I is critical for joining of Okazaki fragments and long-patch base-excision repair. Curr Biol 10:919–922

Lindahl T (1993) Instability and decay of the primary structure of DNA. Nature 362:709–715

Lindahl T, Nyberg B (1972) Rate of depurination of native deoxyribonucleic acid. Biochemistry (Mosc) 11:3610–3618

Lindahl T, Karlstrom O (1973) Heat-induced depyrimidination of deoxyribonucleic acid in neutral solution. Biochemistry (Mosc) 12:5151–5154

Lindahl T, Nyberg B (1974) Heat-induced deamination of cytosine residues in deoxyribonucleic acid. Biochemistry (Mosc) 13:3405–3410
Loeb LA (1989) Endogenous carcinogenesis: molecular oncology into the twenty-first century—presidential address. Cancer Res 49:5489–5496
Loeb LA, Kunkel TA (1982) Fidelity of DNA synthesis. Annu Rev Biochem 51:429–457
Mackey ZB, Niedergang C, Ménissier-de Murcia J, Leppard J, Au K, Chen J, de Murcia G, Tomkinson AE (1999) DNA ligase III is recruited to DNA strand breaks by a zinc finger motif homologous to that of poly (ADP-ribose) polymerase. J Biol Chem 274:21679–21687
Mandavilli BS, Rao KS (1996a) Accumulation of DNA damage in aging neurons occurs through a mechanism other than apoptosis. J Neurochem 67:1559–1565
Mandavilli BS, Rao KS (1996b) Neurons in the cerebral cortex are most susceptible to DNA-damage in aging rat brain. Biochem Mol Biol Int 40:507–514
Matsumoto Y, Kim K (1995) Excision of deoxyribose phosphate residues by DNA polymerase beta during DNA repair. Science 269:699–702
Ostling O, Johanson KJ (1984) Microelectrophoretic study of radiation-induced DNA damages in individual mammalian cells. Biochem Biophys Res Commun 123:291–298
Pascucci B, Maga G, Hubscher U, Bjoras M, Seeberg E, Hickson ID, Villani G, Giordano C, Cellai L, Dogliotti E (2002) Reconstitution of the base excision repair pathway for 7,8-dihydro-8-oxoguanine with purified human proteins. Nucleic Acids Res 30:2124–2130
Podlutsky AJ, Dianova, II, Podust VN, Bohr VA, Dianov GL (2001) Human DNA polymerase beta initiates DNA synthesis during long-patch repair of reduced AP sites in DNA. EMBO J 20:1477–1482
Prasad R, Beard WA, Strauss PR, Wilson SH (1998) Human DNA polymerase β deoxyribose phosphate lyase. J Biol Chem 273:15263–15270
Prasad R, Lavrik OI, Kim SJ, Kedar P, Yang XP, Vande Berg BJ, Wilson SH (2001) DNA polymerase beta -mediated long patch base excision repair. Poly(ADP-ribose) polymerase-1 stimulates strand displacement DNA synthesis. J Biol Chem 276:32411–32414
Price GB, Modak SP, Makinodan T (1971) Age-associated changes in the DNA of mouse tissue. Science 171:917–920
Rao KS (1993) Genomic damage and its repair in young and aging brain. Mol Neurobiol 7:23–48
Rao KS (2007) DNA repair in aging rat neurons. Neuroscience 145:1330–1340
Richter C, Park JW, Ames BN (1988) Normal Oxidative Damage to Mitochondrial and Nuclear-DNA Is Extensive. Proc Natl Acad Sci U S A 85:6465–6467
Riley PA (1994) Free radicals in biology: oxidative stress and the effects of ionizing radiation. Int J Radiat Biol 65:27–33
Robson CN, Hochhauser D, Craig R, Rack K, Buckle VJ, Hickson ID (1992) Structure of the human DNA repair gene HAP1 and its localisation to chromosome 14q 11.2–12. Nucleic Acids Res 20:4417–4421
Seki S, Hatsushika M, Watanabe S, Akiyama K, Nagao K, Tsutsui K (1992) cDNA cloning, sequencing, expression and possible domain structure of human APEX nuclease homologous to Escherichia coli exonuclease III. Biochim Biophys Acta 1131:287–299
SenGupta D, Zmudzka B, Kumar P, Cobianchi F, Skowronski J, Wilson S (1986) Sequence of human DNA polymerase [beta] mRNA obtained through cDNA cloning. Biochem Biophys Res Commun 136:341–347
Singh NP, McCoy MT, Tice RR, Schneider EL (1988) A simple technique for quantitation of low levels of DNA damage in individual cells. Exp Cell Res 175:184–191
Sobol RW, Horton JK, Kühn R, Gu H, Singhal RK, Prasad R, Rajewsky K, Wilson SH (1996) Requirement of mammalian DNA polymerase-β in base-excision repair. Nature 379:183–186
Stucki M, Pascucci B, Parlanti E, Fortini P, Wilson SH, Hubscher U, Dogliotti E (1998) Mammalian base excision repair by DNA polymerases delta and epsilon. Oncogene 17:835–843
Subbarao K, Loeb L (1992) DNA damage and repair in brain: relationship to aging. Mutation Research/DNAging 275:317–329
Suh D, Wilson DM, Povirk LF (1997) 3′-Phosphodiesterase activity of human apurinic/apyrimidinic endonuclease at DNA double-strand break ends. Nucleic Acids Res 25:2495–2500

Swain U, Subba Rao K (2011) Study of DNA damage via the comet assay and base excision repair activities in rat brain neurons and astrocytes during aging. Mech Aging Dev 132:374–381

Tice RR, Agurell E, Anderson D, Burlinson B, Hartmann A, Kobayashi H, Miyamae Y, Rojas E, Ryu JC, Sasaki YF (2000) Single cell gel/comet assay: guidelines for in vitro and in vivo genetic toxicology testing. Environ Mol Mutagen 35:206–221

Tom S, Henricksen LA, Park MS, Bambara RA (2001) DNA ligase I and proliferating cell nuclear antigen form a functional complex. J Biol Chem 276:24817–24825

Tomkinson AE, Chen L, Dong Z, Leppard JB, Levin DS, Mackey ZB, Motycka TA (2001) Completion of base excision repair by mammalian DNA ligases. Prog Nucleic Acid Res Mol Biol 68:151–164

Whitehouse CJ, Taylor RM, Thistlethwaite A, Zhang H, Karimi-Busheri F, Lasko DD, Weinfeld M, Caldecott KW (2001) XRCC1 stimulates human polynucleotide kinase activity at damaged DNA termini and accelerates DNA single-strand break repair. Cell 104:107–117

Wilson SH (1998) Mammalian base excision repair and DNA polymerase beta. Mutat Res 407:203–215

Wilson DM, 3rd (2003) Properties of and substrate determinants for the exonuclease activity of human apurinic endonuclease Ape1. J Mol Biol 330:1027–1037

Wilson DM, 3rd, Sofinowski TM, McNeill DR (2003) Repair mechanisms for oxidative DNA damage. Front Biosci 8:d963–981

Wilson DM, 3rd, Bohr VA (2007) The mechanics of base excision repair, and its relationship to aging and disease. DNA Repair (Amst) 6:544–559

Ziegler M, Oei SL (2001) A cellular survival switch: poly(ADP-ribosyl)ation stimulates DNA repair and silences transcription. Bioessays 23:543–548

Chapter 3
Role of Brain-derived Neurotrophic Factor as a Modulator of Synaptic Plasticity

Yasuyuki Ishikawa and Masami Kojima

Abstract Brain-derived neurotrophic factor (BDNF) is one of the most active members of the neurotrophin family. BDNF not only regulates neuronal survival and differentiation, but also functions in activity-dependent plasticity processes such as long-term potentiation (LTP), long-term depression (LTD), learning and memory. BDNF is synthesized as a precursor protein (proBDNF) that is proteolytically cleaved to form the mature protein. BDNF mediates its effects via two distinct receptors: the high-affinity tropomyosin-related kinase B (TrkB) receptor, which displays specificity for BDNF and other neurotrophin family members (e.g., neurotrophin-4/5 (NT-4/5)), and the low-affinity p75 neurotrophin receptor (p75NTR), which binds to BDNF, neurotrophin-3 (NT-3), NT-4/5, and nerve growth factor (NGF). This review addresses various roles of BDNF in neuronal activity, with special emphasis on its role in mechanisms of activity-dependent synaptic plasticity. Activity-dependent synaptic plasticity, as exemplified by LTP and LTD, is widely accepted as the cellular correlate of learning and memory. LTP and LTD, each requires input specificity and occurs in two temporally distinct phases: early-LTP/LTD (E-LTP/LTD) and late-LTP/LTD (L-LTP/LTD). L-LTP and L-LTD persist for many hours and require new protein synthesis. This review discusses the impact of BDNF on translation-dependent synaptic plasticity. Increasing data indicate that

M. Kojima (✉)
Bio-interface Research Group, Health Research Inst., National Institute of Advanced Industrial Science and Technology (AIST), 1-8-31, Midorioka, Ikeda, Osaka, 563-8577, Japan
e-mail: m-kojima@aist.go.jp

Core Research for Evolutional Science and Technology (CREST), Japan Science and Technology Agency (JST), Kawaguchi, 332-0012, Japan

Y. Ishikawa
Laboratory of Functional Neuroscience, Nara Institute of Science and Technology, 8916-5, Takayama, Ikoma, Nara 630-0192, Japan

Core Research for Evolutional Science and Technology (CREST), Japan Science and Technology Agency (JST), Kawaguchi, 332-0012, Japan

M. K. Thakur, S. I. S. Rattan (eds.), *Brain Aging and Therapeutic Interventions*,
DOI 10.1007/978-94-007-5237-5_3,

the function of BDNF in synaptic plasticity requires a tight relationship between extracellular neurotrophin release, synaptic activity-dependent local protein synthesis, and BDNF polymorphism. This article also addresses the cellular and molecular mechanisms underlying the functional changes of hippocampal synapses during neuronal plasticity, including our findings in regard to the post-translational processing of proBDNF.

Keywords BDNF • TrkB • Synaptic plasticity • Polymorphism • Aging • LTP • LTD

3.1 The Neurotrophin Family

In 1950s, Levi-Montalcini and Hamburger (1953) discovered that a mouse sarcoma tumor implanted near the spinal cord of the developing chicken secreted a soluble factor, which elicited neurite outgrowth from sympathetic neurons (Levi-Montalcini and Hamburger 1953). This factor was identified as nerve growth factor (NGF) (Cohen and Levi-Montalcini 1956; Cohen 1960; Bocchini and Angeletti 1969). The discovery of NGF opened a new field in neurobiology, leading to the identification and elucidation of the cellular functions of the so-called neurotrophic factors. Neurotrophic factors include growth factors, such as epidermal growth factor (EGF) and fibroblast growth factor (FGF), and the crucially important neurotrophins (NTs). NTs are widely expressed in nearly all neuronal populations in both the central and the peripheral nervous system, and their physiological roles extend to neuronal survival, process outgrowth, and the regulation of synaptic plasticity (Bibel and Barde 2000; Poo 2001; Reichardt 2006).

Over 20 years after the discovery of NGF, Barde et al. (1982) isolated a neuronal survival-promoting factor from pig brain, namely brain-derived neurotrophic factor (BDNF) (Barde et al. 1982). In 1989, Barde and colleagues successfully achieved the molecular cloning of BDNF cDNA (Leibrock et al. 1989). Interestingly, BDNF was found to be highly homologous to NGF in terms of its amino acid sequence. This finding resulted in the identification of two additional NTs, neurotrophin-3 (NT-3) and neurotrophin-4/5 (NT-4/5) (Lessmann et al. 2003; Reichardt 2006).

3.2 Precursor and Polymorphism of Neurotrophins

The discovery of four NTs and their genes indicate marked homology to each other in terms of sequence and structure (Lessmann et al. 2003). The protein product of all NTs consists of a signal sequence, a prodomain, and the mature domain. To produce the mature protein, each NT is cleaved by intracellular and/or extracellular proteolytic enzymes (e.g., furin, pro-hormone convertase, and plasmin) (Barco et al. 2005). A surprising report demonstrated that the maturation of NTs is an important aspect of their post-transcriptional regulation and in fact determines their specificity of action. For example, Lee et al. (2001) showed that precursor NGF (proNGF) promotes neuronal death, whereas mature NGF promotes neuronal survival (Bath and Lee 2006). Furthermore, proBDNF, but not mature BDNF, enhances rat hippocampal long-term depression (LTD) through the activation of the N-methyl-D-aspartate (NMDA) receptor subunit, NR2B (Lu et al. 2005).

Another notable finding was from the study of a human single nucleotide polymorphism (SNP) in the *bdnf* gene, which converts a valine to a methionine at codon 66 (Val66Met) in the pro-region of human BDNF. The Val66Met mutation affects human memory retention, as well as the activity-dependent secretion of BDNF (Egan et al. 2003; Chen et al. 2004). This indicates that the BDNF pro-region (and/or the BDNF pro-peptide) plays a functional role beyond its traditional role as a molecular chaperone to assist in the folding of BDNF (Kolbeck et al. 1994). Since this report, accumulating evidence has suggested that the Val66Met genetic variant increases susceptibility to a variety of brain disorders, including Alzheimer's disease (Bath and Lee 2006).

3.3 Neurotrophin Receptors

The NTs interact with two distinct classes of receptors. The first receptor, the p75 neurotrophin receptor ($p75^{NTR}$), is a member of the tumor necrosis factor (TNF) receptor family (Chao 2003). $p75^{NTR}$ was originally identified as a low-affinity receptor for NGF but was subsequently shown to bind to BDNF, NT-3, and NT-4/5 with a similar low affinity (Chao 2003). The extracellular domain of $p75^{NTR}$ is characterized by the presence of cysteine-rich motifs. The cytoplasmic domain includes a 'death' domain, which is also found in the cytoplasmic domain of other members of TNF receptor family (Liepinsh et al. 1997; Bailey et al. 2004). Although $p75^{NTR}$ does not contain a catalytic kinase motif, it interacts with several proteins that transmit signals important for the regulation of neuronal survival and differentiation (Hempstead 2002).

The second receptor class corresponds to the tropomyosin-related kinase (Trk) family of receptor tyrosine kinases (TrkA, TrkB, and TrkC) (Reichardt 2006). The four mammalian NTs have been shown to activate one or more of the three members of the Trk receptor family. The extracellular domain of each Trk receptor consists of a cysteine-rich cluster, followed by a series of leucine-rich repeats, another cysteine-rich cluster, and two immunoglobulin-like domains. The Trk receptors have a transmembrane domain that spans the plasma membrane and a cytoplasmic domain that has tyrosine kinase activity. Through Trk receptors, NTs activate Ras, phosphatidylinositol 3-kinase (PI3K), and phospholipase C-1. These signaling pathways control the activity of downstream molecules, such as the mitogen-activated protein (MAP) kinases (Reichardt 2006).

Information about the two types of NT receptors and their signaling mechanisms has been extensively reviewed by others (see Reichardt 2006) and will not be further discussed in this article.

3.4 Activity-Dependent Processing and Local Synthesis of BDNF

As mentioned previously, BDNF is initially synthesized as a precursor protein (proBDNF) that is post-translationally cleaved by intracellular proteases to yield the mature BDNF protein (Seidah et al. 1996; Matsumoto et al. 2008). The proBDNF protein can also be cleaved in the extracellular space (Pang et al. 2004). This processing mechanism plays a key role in determining the cellular functions of the neurotrophin (Barker 2009; Greenberg et al. 2009). Curiously enough, the processing of BDNF is controlled in a neuronal activity-dependent manner. The mature form of BDNF binds to the TrkB tyrosine kinase receptor, promotes cell survival, and facilitates some forms of long-term potentiation (LTP). Unexpectedly, proBDNF binds preferentially to the pan-neurotrophin receptor $p75^{NTR}$ to activate apoptosis-related signaling pathways in the hippocampus and thereby facilitate LTD.

Learning, training and memory formation change the amount of BDNF mRNA and protein in the hippocampus. For example, the induction of LTP in the rat hippocampus rapidly and selectively increases the level of BDNF mRNA (Patterson et al. 1992; Castren et al. 1993), and learning increases hippocampal BDNF, proBDNF, and TrkB protein content (Silhol et al. 2007). Tongiorgi and colleagues (1997) also reported that BDNF mRNA is transported into the dendrites of rat hippocampal neurons by neuronal depolarization in vitro (Tongiorgi et al. 1997) and by epileptogenic stimulation in vivo (Simonato et al. 2002; Tongiorgi et al. 2004; Chiaruttini et al. 2008). These findings suggest that the dendritic movement of BDNF mRNA and the local translation of BDNF may contribute significantly to activity-dependent synaptic plasticity.

3.5 BDNF and Synaptic Plasticity

Synaptic plasticity in the central nervous system is thought to be critical for the processing and encoding of information by neuronal circuits, which is central to learning and memory. Alterations in synaptic plasticity are associated with aging and several diseases, including Alzheimer's disease and schizophrenia, as well as pain and addiction. LTP and LTD are forms of activity-dependent synaptic plasticity that increase or decrease the strength of synaptic transmission, respectively. LTP and LTD can be divided into at least two temporally distinct phases: early-LTP/LTD (E-LTP/LTD) and late-LTP/LTD (L-LTP/LTD). E-LTP and L-LTP parallel the two forms of memory, short-term memory (STM) and long-term memory (LTM). E-LTP occurs during the first hour or two of LTP and can be induced by a high frequency tetanus stimulation (100 pulses at 100 Hz), increasing the strength of synaptic transmission and activating signaling molecules such as protein kinases. L-LTP persists for many hours and requires *de novo* synthesis of plasticity-related proteins (PRPs). L-LTP can be induced in rat acute hippocampal slice preparations by the use of multiple-spaced electrical tetani (Frey et al. 1988; Huang and Kandel 1994).

Mature BDNF and proBDNF are both released from cultured rat hippocampal neurons. A substantial body of work indicates that mature BDNF is necessary and sufficient for the regulation of E-LTP and the maintenance of L-LTP through the TrkB receptor, whereas proBDNF promotes LTD through the activation of $p75^{NTR}$ at the rat hippocampus and *Xenopus* neuromuscular synapses. High-frequency stimulation favors BDNF release and TrkB-dependent LTP in the CA1 zone of the rat hippocampus, while low-frequency stimulation stimulates proBDNF release (Nagappan et al. 2009; Yang et al. 2009).

The relationship between BDNF action and the balance of excitatory-inhibitory synaptic activity is an important issue in the field of synaptic plasticity (Lessmann and Brigadski 2009). Glutamate receptors, including NMDA and non-NMDA receptors, play distinct roles in synaptic plasticity. BDNF phosphorylates the NR1 and NR2B subunits of the NMDA receptor and upregulates the GluR1 subunit of the α-amino-3-hydroxy-5-methyl-4-isoxazolepropionic acid (AMPA) receptor, as well as GluR2/3 subunits. Of particular interest, mature BDNF decreases the excitability of GABAergic inter-neurons through the activation of TrkB, while proBDNF does not affect GABAergic activity in the mouse dentate gyrus (Holm et al. 2009). GABAergic function, at least in some conditions, exerts a crucial role in the regulation of the induction of LTP and LTD in rat hippocampal slices (Chevaleyre and Castillo 2003).

3.5.1 Regulation of LTP by BDNF

Regulation of hippocampal E-LTP by BDNF has been shown in experiments using BDNF gene knockout mice and BDNF-scavenging proteins. For example, E-LTP is markedly impaired in BDNF knockout mice (Korte et al. 1995; Patterson et al. 1996). Furthermore, the in vitro scavenging of endogenous BDNF by a TrkB-IgG fusion protein (Figurov et al. 1996) has been shown to reduce the magnitude of E-LTP. Appreciable evidence now indicates that BDNF acutely enhances E-LTP by increasing synaptic responses to tetanic stimulation and by enhancing the docking of synaptic vesicles, possibly through changes in the extent of phosphorylation of several synaptic proteins (Gottschalk et al. 1999; Pozzo-Miller et al. 1999; Jovanovic et al. 2000). To this point, application of BDNF-scavenging proteins and BDNF blocking antibodies abolished E-LTP after LTP-inducing tetanic stimulation (Kang et al. 1997; Chen et al. 1999). Finally, BDNF elicits E-LTP in the dentate gyrus of the hippocampus, increasing the function of NMDA receptors (Levine et al. 1998; Kovalchuk et al. 2002).

On the other hand, L-LTP is modulated by BDNF/TrkB signaling. L-LTP was impaired in both BDNF knockout mice and in the presence of a TrkB blocking antibody (Korte et al. 1998). Moreover, the conversion of proBDNF to BDNF by tissue plasminogen activator (tPA)/plasmin was shown to be essential for L-LTP (Pang et al. 2004), and L-LTP was impaired in mice with a targeted mutation in the phospholipase C-γ (PLC-γ) docking site (but not the Shc docking site) on TrkB (Minichiello et al. 2002).

3.5.2 Regulation of Local Protein Synthesis by BDNF

BDNF-induced L-LTP has been shown to depend on local protein synthesis in rat hippocampal dendrites (Kang and Schuman 1995, 1996). Dendritic protein synthesis is also cited in other paradigms of synaptic plasticity (Huber et al. 2000; Miller et al. 2002). Accumulating biochemical data indicate that BDNF stimulates dendritic synthesis of numerous different proteins by increasing the trafficking of mRNA into the dendrites, as well as by enhancing the local translation of existing dendritic mRNA. In rodent primary neurons, BDNF induces the dendritic synthesis of synaptic proteins, which include activity-regulated cytoskeleton-associated protein (Arc/Arg3.1), Ca^{2+}/calmodulin-dependent protein kinase IIα (CaMKIIα), type 1 inositol 1,4,5-trisphosphate receptor (IP_3R1), Homer2, NR1, GluR1, and Lim kinase 1 (Limk1) (Aakalu et al. 2001; Yin et al. 2002; Schratt et al. 2004; Takei et al. 2004; Schratt et al. 2006).

3.5.3 Regulation of LTD by proBDNF

BDNF and proBDNF have opposite effects on the regulation of synaptic plasticity (Lu et al. 2005). Woo et al. (2005) demonstrated that proBDNF facilitates hippocampal LTD by the activation of $p75^{NTR}$ in mouse (Woo et al. 2005). This facilitation requires NR2B activation. Thus, mature BDNF and proBDNF exert a bidirectional modulation of synaptic plasticity through TrkB and $p75^{NTR}$, respectively. The BDNF pro-peptide is cleaved out of the precursor protein (proBDNF) to produce mature BDNF. However, the biological role of the BDNF pro-peptide is still poorly understood. Our group discovered that the BDNF pro-peptide itself facilitates hippocampal LTD and elicits the endocytosis of the AMPA-type receptor, suggesting a novel role for the BDNF pro-peptide in synaptic plasticity.

3.5.4 The Role of BDNF on Synaptic Tagging and Capture

E-LTP elicited by a weak stimulus normally fades in 1–2 h. L-LTP elicited by a strong stimulus continues for more than 3 h and necessitates new protein synthesis for its persistence. If a strong tetanus stimulus is applied to a synaptic input, a weak tetanus applied to a distinct synaptic input on the same cell can evoke persistent LTP. A synaptic molecular "tag" or "mark" that forms in response to the stimulus is hypothesized to interact with and enable the capture of newly synthesized PRPs (Frey and Morris 1997).

Recently, BDNF and TrkB were shown to be involved in synaptic tagging and capture in rodent hippocampus (Barco et al. 2005; Lu et al. 2011; Sajikumar and Korte 2011). To examine whether BDNF and TrkB can capture newly synthesized PRPs, two-pathway stimulation was done in hippocampal slices. In a weak-after-strong stimulation paradigm, TrkB-blocking reagents prevented the formation of the tag during strong stimulation. Although L-LTP was impaired in this pathway, PRP production did in fact occur (Lu et al. 2011). Therefore, TrkB may exert synaptic tagging in BDNF-dependent L-LTP.

3.5.5 BDNF and Short-term and Long-term Memory

There are two known types of memory: STM and LTM. STM, like E-LTP, is of short duration and lasts from a few minutes to a few hours. Furthermore, STM does not require *de novo* protein synthesis. In contrast, LTM, like L-LTP, lasts for several hours, days, or longer (Bailey et al. 2004; Medina et al. 2008). BDNF modulates both STM and LTM in the adult rat hippocampus (Alonso et al. 2002). Thus, BDNF might be involved in the expression and persistence of long-term synaptic plasticity in the adult brain. In addition, the BDNF-dependent phase is likely to be crucial for the persistence of LTM in the rat hippocampus (Bekinschtein et al. 2007).

Repetitive trans-cranial magnetic stimulation (rTMS) of the brain promotes lasting changes of excitatory neurotransmission and is associated with neuroplasticity and memory. The rTMS response has shown to be modulated by BDNF polymorphism (Cheeran et al. 2008), indicating that BNDF polymorphism modulates human brain function. More recently, Gersner et al. (2011) demonstrated that rTMS affected the level of BDNF and GluA1 AMPA receptor subunit in rat. Furthermore, the level of phosphorylated GluA1 was comparatively assessed in awake and anesthetized rats and was found to be lower in anesthetized animals and higher in rats that were awake. Hence, rTMS may be useful for the assessment of PRP expression in neuroplasticity and memory-related disorders (Gersner et al. 2011).

3.6 BDNF and Aging

Aging is associated with memory impairments (see Rosenzweig and Barnes 2003), such as memory loss and false memories. Deterioration in brain anatomy, physiology, plasticity and network dynamics can contribute to age-related memory impairment. The most reliable cellular system to experimentally address the effects of aging on long-term memory is hippocampal L-LTP. Recently, it was reported that deteriorations in LTP and spatial learning occurred during normal aging, without a significant loss of neurons in rodent (Pang and Lu 2004; Rex et al. 2005). A parallel decrease in the level of BDNF occurred during aging in the primate and the human. Moreover, BDNF induction by ampakine reversed the impairment of LTP in middle-aged rodents (Rex et al. 2006). Interestingly, the impact of age, weight and gender on BDNF levels in human platelets and plasma was recently investigated (Lommatzsch et al. 2005).

3.7 Conclusion

The data strongly supported a critical role for BDNF in synaptic plasticity and memory. Given them, it should be expected that BDNF has a role on the development of drug, treatment for brain disorders, in particular, aging. The ability of stimulation to modulate BDNF expression also opens up the possibility for this therapy to be used to treat these disorders, which may involve BDNF, such as Alzheimer's disease, post traumatic stress disorder, or mood disorders. Ultimately and obviously, a better understanding of therapeutic approach is essential to optimize its safety and efficacy.

Acknowledgements This work was supported by the Core Research for Evolutional Science and Technology (CREST) program of the Japan Science and Technology Agency (JST).

References

Aakalu G, Smith WB, Nguyen N, Jiang C, Schuman EM (2001) Dynamic visualization of local protein synthesis in hippocampal neurons. Neuron 30:489–502

Alonso M, Vianna MR, Depino AM et al (2002) BDNF-triggered events in the rat hippocampus are required for both short- and long-term memory formation. Hippocampus 12:551–560

Bailey CH, Kandel ER, Si K (2004) The persistence of long-term memory: a molecular approach to self-sustaining changes in learning-induced synaptic growth. Neuron 44:49–57

Barco A, Patterson SL, Alarcon JM, Gromova P, Mata-Roig M, Morozov A, Kandel ER (2005) Gene expression profiling of facilitated L-LTP in VP16-CREB mice reveals that BDNF is critical for the maintenance of LTP and its synaptic capture. Neuron 48:123–137

Barde YA, Edgar D, Thoenen H (1982) Purification of a new neurotrophic factor from mammalian brain. EMBO J 1:549–553

Barker PA (2009) Whither proBDNF? Nat Neurosci 12:105–106

Bath KG, Lee FS (2006) Variant BDNF (Val66Met) impact on brain structure and function. Cogn Affect Behav Neurosci 6:79–85

Bekinschtein P, Cammarota M, Igaz LM, Bevilaqua LR, Izquierdo I, Medina JH (2007) Persistence of long-term memory storage requires a late protein synthesis- and BDNF- dependent phase in the hippocampus. Neuron 53:261–277

Bibel M, Barde YA (2000) Neurotrophins: key regulators of cell fate and cell shape in the vertebrate nervous system. Genes Dev 14:2919–2937

Bocchini V, Angeletti PU (1969) The nerve growth factor: purification as a 30,000-molecular-weight protein. Proc Natl Acad Sci U S A 64:787–794
Castren E, Pitkanen M, Sirvio J, Parsadanian A, Lindholm D, Thoenen H, Riekkinen PJ (1993) The induction of LTP increases BDNF and NGF mRNA but decreases NT-3 mRNA in the dentate gyrus. Neuroreport 4:895–898
Chao MV (2003) Neurotrophins and their receptors: a convergence point for many signalling pathways. Nat Rev Neurosci 4:299–309
Cheeran B, Talelli P, Mori F et al (2008) A common polymorphism in the brain-derived neurotrophic factor gene (BDNF) modulates human cortical plasticity and the response to rTMS. J Physiol 586:5717–5725
Chen G, Kolbeck R, Barde YA, Bonhoeffer T, Kossel A (1999) Relative contribution of endogenous neurotrophins in hippocampal long-term potentiation. J Neurosci 19:7983–7990
Chen ZY, Patel PD, Sant G, Meng CX, Teng KK, Hempstead BL, Lee FS (2004) Variant brain-derived neurotrophic factor (BDNF) (Met66) alters the intracellular trafficking and activity-dependent secretion of wild-type BDNF in neurosecretory cells and cortical neurons. J Neurosci 24:4401–4411
Chevaleyre V, Castillo PE (2003) Heterosynaptic LTD of hippocampal GABAergic synapses: a novel role of endocannabinoids in regulating excitability. Neuron 38:461–472
Chiaruttini C, Sonego M, Baj G, Simonato M, Tongiorgi E (2008) BDNF mRNA splice variants display activity-dependent targeting to distinct hippocampal laminae. Mol Cell Neurosci 37:11–19
Cohen S (1960) Purification of a Nerve-growth promoting protein from the mouse salivary gland and its neuro-cytotoxic antiserum. Proc Natl Acad Sci U S A 46:302–311
Cohen S, Levi-Montalcini R (1956) A nerve growth-stimulating factor isolated from snake venom. Proc Natl Acad Sci U S A 42:571–574
Egan MF, Kojima M, Callicott JH et al (2003) The BDNF val66met polymorphism affects activity-dependent secretion of BDNF and human memory and hippocampal function. Cell 112:257–269
Figurov A, Pozzo-Miller LD, Olafsson P, Wang T, Lu B (1996) Regulation of synaptic responses to high-frequency stimulation and LTP by neurotrophins in the hippocampus. Nature 381:706–709
Frey U, Morris RG (1997) Synaptic tagging and long-term potentiation. Nature 385:533–536
Frey U, Krug M, Reymann KG, Matthies H (1988) Anisomycin, an inhibitor of protein synthesis, blocks late phases of LTP phenomena in the hippocampal CA1 region in vitro. Brain Res 452:57–65
Gersner R, Kravetz E, Feil J, Pell G, Zangen A (2011) Long-term effects of repetitive transcranial magnetic stimulation on markers for neuroplasticity: differential outcomes in anesthetized and awake animals. J Neurosci 31:7521–7526
Gottschalk WA, Jiang H, Tartaglia N, Feng L, Figurov A, Lu B (1999) Signaling mechanisms mediating BDNF modulation of synaptic plasticity in the hippocampus. Learn Mem 6:243–256
Greenberg ME, Xu B, Lu B, Hempstead BL (2009) New insights in the biology of BDNF synthesis and release: implications in CNS function. J Neurosci 29:12764–12767
Hempstead BL (2002) The many faces of p75NTR. Curr Opin Neurobiol 12:260–267
Holm MM, Nieto-Gonzalez JL, Vardya I, Vaegter CB, Nykjaer A, Jensen K (2009) Mature BDNF, but not proBDNF, reduces excitability of fast-spiking interneurons in mouse dentate gyrus. J Neurosci 29:12412–12418
Huang YY, Kandel ER (1994) Recruitment of long-lasting and protein kinase A-dependent long-term potentiation in the CA1 region of hippocampus requires repeated tetanization. Learn Mem 1:74–82
Huber KM, Kayser MS, Bear MF (2000) Role for rapid dendritic protein synthesis in hippocampal mGluR-dependent long-term depression. Science 288:1254–1257
Jovanovic JN, Czernik AJ, Fienberg AA, Greengard P, Sihra TS (2000) Synapsins as mediators of BDNF-enhanced neurotransmitter release. Nat Neurosci 3:323–329

Kang H, Schuman EM (1995) Long-lasting neurotrophin-induced enhancement of synaptic transmission in the adult hippocampus. Science 267:1658–1662

Kang H, Schuman EM (1996) A requirement for local protein synthesis in neurotrophin-induced hippocampal synaptic plasticity. Science 273:1402–1406

Kang H, Welcher AA, Shelton D, Schuman EM (1997) Neurotrophins and time: different roles for TrkB signaling in hippocampal long-term potentiation. Neuron 19:653–664

Kolbeck R, Jungbluth S, Barde YA (1994) Characterisation of neurotrophin dimers and monomers. Eur J Biochem 225:995–1003

Korte M, Carroll P, Wolf E, Brem G, Thoenen H, Bonhoeffer T (1995) Hippocampal long-term potentiation is impaired in mice lacking brain-derived neurotrophic factor. Proc Natl Acad Sci U S A 92:8856–8860

Korte M, Kang H, Bonhoeffer T, Schuman E (1998) A role for BDNF in the late-phase of hippocampal long-term potentiation. Neuropharmacology 37:553–559

Kovalchuk Y, Hanse E, Kafitz KW, Konnerth A (2002) Postsynaptic induction of BDNF-mediated long-term potentiation. Science 295:1729–1734

Lee R, Kermani P, Teng KK, Hempstead BL (2001) Regulation of cell survival by secreted proneurotrophins. Science 294:1945–1948

Leibrock J, Lottspeich F, Hohn A, Hofer M, Hengerer B, Masiakowski P, Thoenen H, Barde YA (1989) Molecular cloning and expression of brain-derived neurotrophic factor. Nature 341:149–152

Lessmann V, Brigadski T (2009) Mechanisms, locations, and kinetics of synaptic BDNF secretion: an update. Neurosci Res 65:11–22

Lessmann V, Gottmann K, Malcangio M (2003) Neurotrophin secretion: current facts and future prospects. Prog Neurobiol 69:341–374

Levi-Montalcini R, Hamburger V (1953) A diffusible agent of mouse sarcoma, producing hyperplasia of sympathetic-ganglia and hyperneurotization of viscera in the chick embryo. J Exp Zool 123:233–287

Levine ES, Crozier RA, Black IB, Plummer MR (1998) Brain-derived neurotrophic factor modulates hippocampal synaptic transmission by increasing N-methyl-D-aspartic acid receptor activity. Proc Natl Acad Sci U S A 95:10235–10239

Liepinsh E, Ilag LL, Otting G, Ibanez CF (1997) NMR structure of the death domain of the p75 neurotrophin receptor. EMBO J 16:4999–5005

Lommatzsch M, Zingler D, Schuhbaeck K, Schloetcke K, Zingler C, Schuff-Werner P, Virchow JC (2005) The impact of age, weight and gender on BDNF levels in human platelets and plasma. Neurobiol Aging 26:115–123

Lu B, Pang PT, Woo NH (2005) The yin and yang of neurotrophin action. Nat Rev Neurosci 6:603–614

Lu Y, Ji Y, Ganesan S et al (2011) TrkB as a potential synaptic and behavioral tag. J Neurosci 31:11762–11771

Matsumoto T, Rauskolb S, Polack M, Klose J, Kolbeck R, Korte M, Barde YA (2008) Biosynthesis and processing of endogenous BDNF: CNS neurons store and secrete BDNF, not pro-BDNF. Nat Neurosci 11:131–133

Medina JH, Bekinschtein P, Cammarota M, Izquierdo I (2008) Do memories consolidate to persist or do they persist to consolidate? Behav Brain Res 192:61–69

Miller S, Yasuda M, Coats JK, Jones Y, Martone ME, Mayford M (2002) Disruption of dendritic translation of CaMKIIalpha impairs stabilization of synaptic plasticity and memory consolidation. Neuron 36:507–519

Minichiello L, Calella AM, Medina DL, Bonhoeffer T, Klein R, Korte M (2002) Mechanism of TrkB-mediated hippocampal long-term potentiation. Neuron 36:121–137

Nagappan G, Zaitsev E, Senatorov VV Jr, Yang J, Hempstead BL, Lu B (2009) Control of extracellular cleavage of ProBDNF by high frequency neuronal activity. Proc Natl Acad Sci U S A 106:1267–1272

Pang PT, Lu B (2004) Regulation of late-phase LTP and long-term memory in normal and aging hippocampus: role of secreted proteins tPA and BDNF. Aging Res Rev 3:407–430

Pang PT, Teng HK, Zaitsev E et al (2004) Cleavage of proBDNF by tPA/plasmin is essential for long-term hippocampal plasticity. Science 306:487–491

Patterson SL, Grover LM, Schwartzkroin PA, Bothwell M (1992) Neurotrophin expression in rat hippocampal slices: a stimulus paradigm inducing LTP in CA1 evokes increases in BDNF and NT-3 mRNAs. Neuron 9:1081–1088

Patterson SL, Abel T, Deuel TA, Martin KC, Rose JC, Kandel ER (1996) Recombinant BDNF rescues deficits in basal synaptic transmission and hippocampal LTP in BDNF knockout mice. Neuron 16:1137–1145

Poo MM (2001) Neurotrophins as synaptic modulators. Nat Rev Neurosci 2:24–32

Pozzo-Miller LD, Gottschalk W, Zhang L et al (1999) Impairments in high-frequency transmission, synaptic vesicle docking, and synaptic protein distribution in the hippocampus of BDNF knockout mice. J Neurosci 19:4972–4983

Reichardt LF (2006) Neurotrophin-regulated signalling pathways. Philos Trans R Soc Lond B Biol Sci 361:1545–1564

Rex CS, Kramar EA, Colgin LL, Lin B, Gall CM, Lynch G (2005) Long-term potentiation is impaired in middle-aged rats: regional specificity and reversal by adenosine receptor antagonists. J Neurosci 25:5956–5966

Rex CS, Lauterborn JC, Lin CY, Kramar EA, Rogers GA, Gall CM, Lynch G (2006) Restoration of long-term potentiation in middle-aged hippocampus after induction of brain-derived neurotrophic factor. J Neurophysiol 96:677–685

Rosenzweig ES, Barnes CA (2003) Impact of aging on hippocampal function: plasticity, network dynamics, and cognition. Prog Neurobiol 69:143–179

Sajikumar S, Korte M (2011) Metaplasticity governs compartmentalization of synaptic tagging and capture through brain-derived neurotrophic factor (BDNF) and protein kinase Mzeta (PKMzeta). Proc Natl Acad Sci U S A 108:2551–2556

Schratt GM, Nigh EA, Chen WG, Hu L, Greenberg ME (2004) BDNF regulates the translation of a select group of mRNAs by a mammalian target of rapamycin-phosphatidylinositol 3-kinase-dependent pathway during neuronal development. J Neurosci 24:7366–7377

Schratt GM, Tuebing F, Nigh EA, Kane CG, Sabatini ME, Kiebler M, Greenberg ME (2006) A brain-specific microRNA regulates dendritic spine development. Nature 439:283–289

Seidah NG, Benjannet S, Pareek S, Chretien M, Murphy RA (1996) Cellular processing of the neurotrophin precursors of NT3 and BDNF by the mammalian proprotein convertases. FEBS Lett 379:247–250

Silhol M, Arancibia S, Maurice T, Tapia-Arancibia L (2007) Spatial memory training modifies the expression of brain-derived neurotrophic factor tyrosine kinase receptors in young and aged rats. Neuroscience 146:962–973

Simonato M, Bregola G, Armellin M, Del Piccolo P, Rodi D, Zucchini S, Tongiorgi E (2002) Dendritic targeting of mRNAs for plasticity genes in experimental models of temporal lobe epilepsy. Epilepsia 43 Suppl 5:153–158

Takei N, Inamura N, Kawamura M, Namba H, Hara K, Yonezawa K, Nawa H (2004) Brain-derived neurotrophic factor induces mammalian target of rapamycin-dependent local activation of translation machinery and protein synthesis in neuronal dendrites. J Neurosci 24:9760–9769

Tongiorgi E, Righi M, Cattaneo A (1997) Activity-dependent dendritic targeting of BDNF and TrkB mRNAs in hippocampal neurons. J Neurosci 17:9492–9505

Tongiorgi E, Armellin M, Giulianini PG et al (2004) Brain-derived neurotrophic factor mRNA and protein are targeted to discrete dendritic laminas by events that trigger epileptogenesis. J Neurosci 24:6842–6852

Woo NH, Teng HK, Siao CJ, Chiaruttini C, Pang PT, Milner TA, Hempstead BL, Lu B (2005) Activation of p75NTR by proBDNF facilitates hippocampal long-term depression. Nat Neurosci 8:1069–1077

Yang F, Je HS, Ji Y, Nagappan G, Hempstead B, Lu B (2009) Pro-BDNF-induced synaptic depression and retraction at developing neuromuscular synapses. J Cell Biol 185:727–741

Yin Y, Edelman GM, Vanderklish PW (2002) The brain-derived neurotrophic factor enhances synthesis of Arc in synaptoneurosomes. Proc Natl Acad Sci U S A 99:2368–2373

Chapter 4
Mitochondrial Dysfunction in Sporadic Alzheimer's Disease: Mechanisms, Consequences and Interventions

Sasanka Chakrabarti and Maitrayee Sinha

Abstract Mitochondrial dysfunction is a key element of sporadic Alzheimer's disease (AD) pathogenesis. This review attempts to provide a detailed account of various findings related to mitochondrial structural and functional alterations as obtained from post-mortem AD brains or transgenic animal models or cell based models of AD. The accumulated evidence indicates a significant impairment of mitochondrial bioenergetic functions with diminished cytochrome oxidase activity, distinctive structural alterations such as small fragmented mitochondria with abnormal cristae and abnormal cellular distribution of this organelle in AD. The mitochondrial defects in AD have been linked to toxic actions of amyloid beta peptide oligomers on mitochondria and this possibility has been supported by many in vitro studies utilizing isolated brain mitochondria. The entry as well as localization of amyloid precursor protein and amyloid beta peptides in mitochondria in AD brain has been the subject of intense and interesting research and the review has described this aspect in the context of mitochondrial dysfunction. The cross-talk of mitochondrial dysfunction with oxidative stress and inflammatory response in AD has been outlined and the involvement of the former with programmed cell death in the diseased brain has also been highlighted. The review ends with a few suggestions on therapeutic interventions in AD pertaining to interactions of amyloid beta peptide and mitochondria.

Keywords Mitochondria • Amyloid beta peptide • Amyloid precursor protein • Reactive oxygen species • Programmed cell death • Antioxidant

S. Chakrabarti (✉) · M. Sinha
Department of Biochemistry, Institute of Post-Graduate Medical Education and Research, Kolkata, India
e-mail: profschakrabarti95@gmail.com

M. K. Thakur, S. I. S. Rattan (eds.), *Brain Aging and Therapeutic Interventions*,
DOI 10.1007/978-94-007-5237-5_4,

4.1 Alzheimer's Disease: A Brief Summary of Essential Facts

Alzheimer's disease (AD) accounts for the majority cases of dementia in the elderly people and incidence of the disease increases twofold every 5 years after the age of 65 years. Alzheimer's disease is posing a major challenge to the socio-economic and health care support system in many countries across the world. In 2010, Alzheimer's Disease International estimated that there are 35.6 million people living with dementia worldwide of which about 26 million are afflicted with AD. The disease appears in familial and sporadic forms with the latter constituting nearly 90–95 % of AD population (Bird 2001). Mutations of several genes, e.g. Amyloid precursor protein (APP), Presenilin 1 (PS1) and Presenilin 2 (PS2) are held responsible for the familial form of the disease with an earlier onset, while sporadic AD has a multi-factorial pathogenesis with interplay of genetic predisposition and extra-genetic mechanisms (Bird 2001; Dekosky 2002). The cardinal clinical feature of AD is a progressively devastating loss of memory and cognition and the disease is diagnosed by careful neuropsychiatric tests and imaging studies but often confused with other forms of dementia including vascular dementia and Lewy body dementia. The confirmed diagnosis of AD is achieved only after autopsy when post-mortem examination of brain reveals the presence of extracellular depositions (amyloid plaques) and intraneuronal neurofibrillary tangles associated with diffused atrophy of brain and neuronal loss in regions like hippocampus, parahippocampal gyrus, amygdala, frontal, parietal, temporal cortices and certain subcortical nuclei (Dekosky 2002). The amyloid plaques which contain depositions of amyloid β peptide in the form of insoluble fibrils are surrounded by degenerating axons and dendrites, while neurofibrillary tangles are formed by paired helical filaments composed of hyperphosphorylated tau protein (Yates and McLoughlin 2008). The typical AD pathology is, however, often complicated by various other features like the presence of vascular pathology characteristic of vascular dementia, but a detailed analysis of this is not within the purview of the present article.

The etiopathogenesis of sporadic AD remains elusive despite intensive research in various experimental models and studies in disease biomarkers and risk factors as also biochemical and molecular biological analysis of post-mortem brain samples of AD (Selkoe 2001; LaFerla et al. 2007; Lin and Beal 2006). The dominant hypothesis of AD pathogenesis (amyloid cascade hypothesis) circles around the cascade of toxic effects of amyloid β which is a peptide of 39–42 amino acids derived from the precursor protein APP by the sequential actions of β and γ secretases (LaFerla et al. 2007). Human APP gene is located on chromosome 21 and several mRNA species are generated by alternate splicing giving rise to proteins of different chain lengths which further undergo post-translational modifications like N- and O- linked glycosylations, phosphorylation, and sulphation (Zheng and Koo 2006). Three major varieties of APP with amino acid residues of 695, 751 and 770 contain Aβ. APP 695 which lacks KPI domain is predominantly found in neurons while APP 751 and APP 770 are more ubiquitously distributed (Cam and Bu 2006; Zheng and Koo 2006).

APP is a type of class I integral membrane protein belonging to a family whose members are distributed in diverse species from *Drosophila* and *C. elegans* to mammals and these members share several common domains (Zheng and Koo 2006). In mammals, three members of APP family, e.g. APP, APP like protein 1 (APLP1) and APP like protein 2 (APLP2) exist (Reinhard et al. 2005; Zheng and Koo 2006). The actual physiological function of APP is not clearly established, but various domains of the molecule interact with a range of proteins and many potential functions have been attributed to this molecule which includes cell adhesion, cell-cell interaction, synaptogenesis, neurite outgrowth, axonal transport, cell survival and death, cell signalling, etc. (Reinhard et al. 2005; Zheng and Koo 2006). The processing of APP in amyloidogenic and non-amyloidogenic pathways is now well-established which involves three different proteolytic enzymes e.g. α-, β- and γ- secretases (Zheng and Koo 2006). Although several forms of amyloid β peptide are present in AD brains, the one consisting of 42 amino acids (Aβ 42) is considered as the most toxic species and this protein has the propensity for oligomerization and aggregation forming initially the soluble oligomers and later the insoluble fibrils where the peptide attains a characteristic crossed β strand conformation (Hung et al. 2008; Nichols et al. 2005). The accumulating body of evidence suggests that the soluble oligomers of Aβ 42 and not the monomers or the insoluble fibrils are responsible for the toxicity of amyloid β peptide (Hung et al. 2008; de Felice et al. 2004). It is suggested that soluble oligomers of amyloid β peptide trigger and/or reinforce a network of interdependent damage pathways that include mitochondrial dysfunction, oxidative stress and inflammatory reactions in AD brain, leading to wide spread neuronal death and degeneration of the processes.

4.2 Mitochondrial Dysfunction in Sporadic AD

4.2.1 Mitochondria: Bioenergetics and Physiology

Mitochondria occupied the centre stage of biochemical research for decades when the magnificent machinery of energy metabolism known as oxidative phosphorylation system (OX-PHOS) was identified and the details of the system worked out within this organelle. Embedded in the inner membrane of mitochondria, the OX-PHOS consists of a series of supra-molecular assemblies of proteins (complex I to IV) containing various cytochromes and iron-sulphur centres through which electrons flow as the reducing equivalents NADH and FADH2 get oxidized and the energy released during this process is utilized by the complex V (F_0 F_1 ATP synthase) to synthesize ATP (Brand and Nicholls 2011; Nicholls and Ferguson 2001). The process of oxidation is coupled to phosphorylation through the development of an electro-chemical gradient which is generated by the transfer of H^+ ions through different complexes from the matrix side to the intermembrane space. The magnitude of the electrochemical gradient 180–220 mV is contributed both by membrane potential (140–180 mV) and the pH gradient of 1.4 units. Apart from providing the energy currency of the cell through OX–PHOS, mitochondria also play crucial roles in Ca^{2+}homeostasis, maintenance of intracellular pH and ROS (reactive oxygen species) metabolism and mitochondrial output of ROS forms the major component of total ROS load of the cells (Brand and Nicholls 2011; Murphy 2009; Nicholls and Ferguson 2001; Halliwell and Gutteridge 2007). The damaging actions of ROS on cells and their organelles have been known for quite some time, but the involvement of the former in regulation of intracellular signalling pathways and gene expression profile is gradually being revealed and thus mitochondrial involvement in these processes is becoming an important research issue (Halliwell and Gutteridge 2007). The redox responsive transcription factors like NF-κβ, AP 1, etc., link mitochondrial ROS generation with alterations of gene expression (Mauro et al. 2011; Higuchi et al. 2002). Thus the bioenergetic and ROS production functions of mitochondria are the major determinants of cell physiology and both these aspects have been explored very intensively in the context of AD pathology.

The other important processes that regulate mitochondrial physiology, morphology and dynamics are fusion, fission and biogenesis and the pathways and proteins involved in these processes are being established (Scarpulla 2008; Chen and Chan 2009). Mitochondria are now considered as dynamic networks rather than discrete rigid organelles that divide and again fuse with each other and get distributed to different parts of the cells and the phenomena of fusion and fission in mitochondria regulate mitochondrial turnover, metabolic efficiency, shape and motility and probably also the processes like mitophagy and apoptosis (Chen and Chan 2009; Twig et al. 2008). For mitochondrial fusion, several proteins like Mfn 1, Mfn 2 and OPA 1 have been identified, while for the fission process Drp 1, Fis 1 and Mff are thought to play critical roles (Chen and Chan 2009). On the other hand, a plethora of information is already available on mitochondrial biogenesis that regulates mitochondrial size and number in the tissue and requires concerted expressions of many nuclear and mtDNA genes (Scarpulla 2008; Hock and Kralli 2009). The biogenesis programme of mitochondria is under the control of PGC1 (Peroxisome proliferator-activated receptor-gamma coactivator 1) family of coactivators of which the major regulator is PGC 1α and this protein controls the biogenesis through several transcription factors like Nuclear respiratory factor (NRF) 1, NRF 2 and Mitochondrial transcription factor A (Tfam) (Scarpulla 2008; Hock and Kralli 2009). In various physiological conditions, mitochondrial biogenesis is altered through modulation of PGC 1α activity presumably through the action of 5′ AMP-activated protein kinase (AMP kinase), calcium/calmodulin dependent protein kinase type IV (CAMK IV), endothelial nitric oxide synthase (eNOS) and other mediators (Scarpulla 2008; Hock and Kralli 2009; Kelly and Scarpula 2004). The accumulation of information on these newer aspects of mitochondrial functions and physiology has also led to investigations to determine if these processes are altered in neurodegenerative disorders. Further, the molecular details of the involvement of this organelle in programmed cell death pathways like apoptosis and necrosis have been firmly established, which also explains why the dysfunction of this organelle is so often linked with AD which is characterized by extensive neuronal death.

4.2.2 Evidence of Mitochondrial Involvement of AD

Evidence accrued from the analysis of post-mortem AD brains indicates both structural and functional mitochondrial impairment as a central mechanism underlying AD pathogenesis and the studies in transgenic animal models and cell based models indicate that mitochondrial structural and functional alterations are linked to toxic actions of oligomers of Aβ42 and further this possibility gains support from a number of in vitro studies (Cassarino and Bennett Jr. 1999).

4.2.3 Post-mortem Evidence

In AD brain, a consistent decrease in cytochrome oxidase activity has been reported by several groups, but decreased activities of other enzyme complexes of brain mitochondria, e.g., pyruvate dehydrogenase, α-ketoglutarate dehydrogenase, isocitrate dehydrogenase, thiolase, ATP citrate lyase, etc. have also been demonstrated in this disease condition (Cassarino and Bennett Jr. 1999; Pagani and Eckert 2011). On the other hand, two TCA-cycle enzymes succinate dehydrogenase and malate dehydrogenase have been shown to be increased in AD brain, whereas other enzymes of this pathway like aconitase, citrate synthase, etc. remain unaffected (Bubber et al. 2005; Atamna and Frey 2007). The decreased level of complex III core protein I has been reported in temporal cortex of AD brains using a proteomics based analysis, while complex I subunits (24 kDa, 75 kDa) are also reported to decrease in different brain regions of this disease condition (Kim et al. 2000). However, other studies have indicated increased levels of cytochrome oxidase and mtDNA in AD brain by using immunocytochemistry and in situ hybridization (Hirai et al. 2001). Quantitative RT–PCR has been used to study the expression pattern of mitochondrial genes. It shows a downregulation of mtDNA genes coding for complex I, while the expression levels of complex III and complex IV are increased in AD brain (Gibson and Shi 2010; Reddy and Beal 2008). In AD brain, oxidative damage marker of DNA, 8-hydroxy 2-deoxy guanosine, accumulates in mtDNA in much higher proportion compared to that in age-matched control and further mtDNA is much more affected than nDNA (Wang et al. 2005; Mecocci et al. 1994). On the other hand, no conclusive evidence of occurrence of heritable common mutation of mtDNA has been obtained so far in AD. However, in cybrids created with mtDNA obtained from platelets of AD patients, very significant impairment of mitochondrial functions has been observed (Cassarino and Bennet Jr. 1999).

Mitochondrial ultrastructural alterations have been reported in AD brains which include smaller sizes of mitochondria and abnormal or broken cristae and such mitochondrial changes are most conspicuous in neurons showing loss of dendritic spines and arborizations (Baloyannis et al. 2004; Hirai et al. 2001). The distribution of mitochondria in neurons in AD affected brains is perinuclear and very few organelles are seen in the terminals of the processes (Manczak et al. 2006; Wang et al. 2008).

The altered structure and dynamics of mitochondria in AD is because of an alteration in the balance of mitochondrial fusion and fission with a shift towards fission (Calkins et al. 2011). Using qRT-PCR and immunoblotting techniques, an increased expression of Fis1 and Drp1 fission related proteins and decreased levels of fusion regulating proteins like Mfn1, Mfn2 and Opa1 have been noticed in post-mortem AD brain (Manczak et al. 2006; Wang et al. 2008). Immunofluorescence studies have shown co-localization of Drp1 with intraneuronal Aβ oligomers and further increased S-nitrosylated Drp1 has been seen in AD brains (Manczak et al. 2006; Chen and Chan 2009). Studies in post-mortem brains of AD have also revealed that both APP and Aβ42 localize within mitochondria and the entry of the peptides into mitochondria presumably takes place through translocase of outer membrane (TOM) and translocase of inner membrane (TIM) (Devi et al. 2006; Hansson Petersen et al. 2008). Mitochondrial biogenesis has also been shown to be impaired in hippocampal neurons from AD with a decrease in the levels of transcription factors and co-activators related to mitochondrial biogenesis like PGC 1α, NRF 1, NRF 2 and Tfam (Sheng et al. 2011).

4.2.4 Evidence from AD Models

A surfeit of interesting studies in transgenic animals or organisms or in cells over expressing wild or mutant APP and other studies with pharmacological cell–based models have demonstrated several types of mitochondrial dysfunctions which could be related to toxic actions of oligomeric Aβ42 or other amyloid beta peptides on mitochondria or to abnormal accumulation of phosphorylated tau and these have clear implications in AD pathology. In double Swedish and London mutant APP transgenic mice, a loss of transmembrane potential, decreased ATP synthesis, increased ROS formation and decreased cytochrome oxidase activity have been reported in brain mitochondria (Hauptmann et al. 2009). In Tg2576 transgenic model, the expression profile of many genes concerned with mitochondrial energy metabolism is altered at 2, 5 and 18 months of age (Manczak et al. 2006). In triple transgenic AD mice, decreased mitochondrial respiration and inhibition of pyruvate dehydrogenase complex with evidence of excess ROS formation and oxidative damage have been reported (Yao et al. 2009). In another study with triple transgenic AD mice (pR5/APP/PS2), the levels of complex I and complex IV have been found to be diminished using mass spectrometry based proteomics study (Eckert et al. 2010). In transgenic AD mice carrying 3 mutated human transgenes (APP/PS1/Tau), proteomic analysis has shown that upregulation or downregulation occurs in 23 different mitochondrial proteins (Chou et al. 2011). Altered expressions of mtDNA genes have been reported in the brains of AD transgenic mice in some other studies (Reddy et al. 2004).

In M17 cells over expressing APPwt or APPswe, mitochondrial structural abnormalities and altered distributions have been observed compared to control M17 cells and further such mitochondrial anomalies are more extensive in M17 cells with APPswe (Wang et al. 2008). The mitochondria in M17 cells over expressing APP in this study have been seen as fragmented with elongated net like structure and mitochondrial fission protein Fis 1 is elevated, while Drp1 and OPA 1 are decreased (Wang et al. 2008). The functional alterations observed in mitochondria in such APP over expressing cells include a decreased membrane potential with ATP depletion and enhanced ROS production (Anandatheerthavarada et al. 2003). In another study with M17 cell containing APPswe, decreased mitochondrial biogenesis is accompanied by decreased mtDNA/nDNA ratio, decreased ATP content and decreased activity of cytochrome oxidase (Sheng et al. 2011).

A popular model to study the etiopathogenesis of AD uses cultured cell lines like SHSY5Y, PC12, NT2, Neuro2a, etc. as also primary cultures of hippocampal neurons exposed to different amyloid β peptides, e.g. Aβ42, Aβ40, Aβ25–35 etc. for varying periods of time. Such models have demonstrated a range of toxic actions of oligomeric Aβ42 which also include extensive impairment of mitochondrial functions and structural alterations (Jin et al. 2010). Alterations in mitochondrial membrane potential, release of cytochrome c in the cytosol, decreased mitochondrial respiration, inhibition of respiratory chain complexes, enhanced ROS formation and inhibition of key enzymes of TCA cycle have all been reported as possible consequences of Aβ42 toxicity in cultured cells which have provided important clues in understanding AD pathogenesis (Qiao et al. 2005; Rhein et al. 2009; Casley et al. 2002; Gao and Tang 2006).

4.2.5 Evidence from In Vitro Studies with Isolated Mitochondria

Although varied forms of mitochondrial dysfunctions have been identified in postmortem brain of AD patients as well as AD experimental models, the involvement of Aβ42 or its oligomeric form in this process has been inferred somewhat obliquely. On the other hand, in vitro experiments with isolated brain mitochondria exposed to oligomeric Aβ42 or other amyloid peptides have not only provided direct evidence of Aβ peptide interaction with mitochondria, but also indicated the possible mechanisms underlying this phenomenon. Such studies have shown that Aβ42 and other amyloid peptides cause mitochondrial membrane depolarization, depletion of ATP, mitochondrial swelling, decreased state 3 respiration and release of cytochrome c in isolated mitochondria (Rodrigues et al. 2001; Kim et al. 2002). Although several studies have indicated that Aβ peptide can inhibit cytochrome oxidase activity, a recent publication has shown that in isolated rat brain mitochondria Aβ42 fails to inhibit complex IV activity and further the toxic effects of oligomeric Aβ42 are more severe in aged brain mitochondria (Sinha et al. 2011). The mechanisms of mitochondrial bioenergetic impairment induced by Aβ42 or other similar amyloid peptides are not clearly worked out, but specific interactions with mitochondrial proteins like cycophilin D, ANT or UCP or ABAD (Aβ-binding alcohol dehydrogenase) could be a distinct possibility (Moreira et al. 2002; Sinha et al. 2011). On the other hand, several groups have documented the pore-forming ability of oligomers of Aβ peptides in synthetic lipid vesicles or biomembranes allowing cations to pass through these channels, which could also explain some of the toxic effects of these peptides on mitochondria (Lal et al. 2007). Some rather elaborate structural studies have been carried out to define the membrane spanning channels produced by Aβ oligomers which could be important as potential therapeutic targets (Arispe et al. 2007; Lal et al. 2007).

4.2.6 Mitochondrial Localization of Aβ Peptide: Mechanisms and Significance

The above description clearly brings out the central importance of Aβ peptide toxicity on mitochondria in AD pathogenesis, but at the same time raises certain issues related to intracellular trafficking of APP and Aβ and their localization in mitochondria. Although the major localization of APP is on plasma membrane from where Aβ is released extracellularly by the action of secretases, there is compelling evidence that in AD brain intracellular build up of Aβ takes place and it progressively accumulates in mitochondria in this disease condition (Chen and Yan 2010; Pagani and Eckert 2011; LaFerla et al. 2007; Devi et al. 2006; Hansson Petersen et al. 2008). Such accumulation of intracellular Aβ also occurs in the brain of transgenic AD mice models as also in cells overexpressing wild or mutant APP (Chen and Yan 2010; Pagani and Eckert 2011). It is now known that apart from the plasma membrane, APP is also localized in trans Golgi network, endoplasmic reticulum and endosomal—lysosomal vesicles and it is conceivable that from such sources, intracellular Aβ42 pool is created through actions of β and γ secretases (LaFerla et al. 2007; Pagani and Eckert 2011). The intracellular pool of Aβ peptide is further enriched by re-uptake of extra-cellular Aβ through receptor-mediated processes and NMDA receptors, nicotinic cholinergic receptors, APOE receptors, RAGE (Receptor for Advanced Glycation End Products), members of LDL receptor family, FPRL 1(formyl peptide receptor-like 1) etc. have all been shown as candidate receptors for Aβ (Bu et al. 2006; Pagani and Eckert 2011; LaFerla et al. 2007). The entry and localization of Aβ peptides within mitochondria have been analyzed in several studies and the involvement of translocase of outer membrane (TOM) has been documented in this process (Hansson Petersen et al. 2008). Such specific mechanisms of mitochondrial entry of amyloid peptides, however, do not exclude other mechanisms of entry of Aβ peptides such as direct embedding in lipid bilayer of mitochondria as has been shown in case of synthetic lipid vesicles (Arispe et al. 2007). Based on some extensive studies in post-mortem AD brains, one group has proposed that APP contains target signals and gains entry within mitochondria through import channels and they have shown that APP forms stable 480 kDa complex with translocase of outer membrane 40 (TOM 40) and a super complex of 620 kDa with both TOM 40 and TIM 23 (translocase of inner membrane 23) (Devi et al. 2006; Anandatheerthavarada et al. 2003). Whether Aβ peptides including Aβ42 are generated in mitochondria in situ from mitochondria—associated APP is not conclusively established

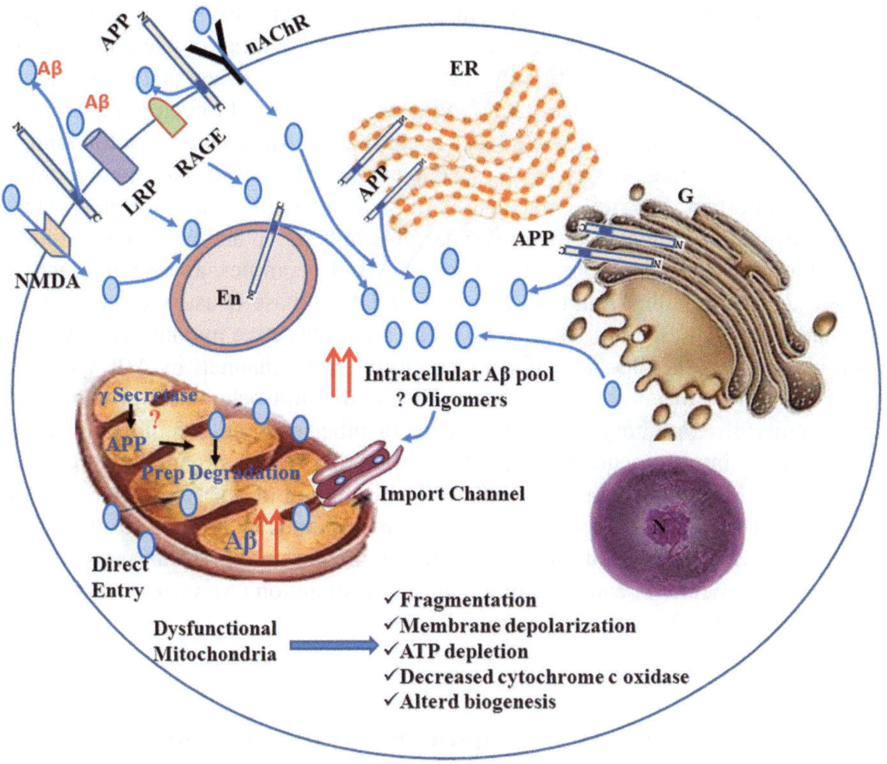

Fig. 4.1 Trafficking of amyloid beta peptide en route to mitochondria: scenario in AD brain. The distribution of APP is shown on the plasma membrane and in other membranous compartments of the cell including mitochondria, although the trafficking pathways of APP are not clearly defined. Aβ is generated extracellularly from plasma membrane bound APP and re-enters the cell through diverse receptors. Intracellularly, Aβ may be generated from APP in one or more of the membranous compartments. Aβ enters the mitochondria, but probably not synthesized within the organelle, through import channels or directly by embedding in lipid bilayer and localizes on the inner membrane. Accumulated Aβ within mitochondria leads to dysfunction of the organelle. The sites where oligomerization of Aβ begins intracellularly are not known. *ER* Endoplasmic reticulum, *En* Endosome, *G* Galgi Body, *N* Nucleus. (This is a hypothetical diagram based on available information and inputs from similar diagrams presented in reference. (LaFerla et al. 2007; Pagani and Eckert 2011))

and even though the presence of γ secretase in mitochondria has been documented, β secretase has so far not been identified within mitochondria (Chen and Yan 2010). However, evidence has also been provided indicating the potential formation of Aβ peptides from mitochondria-associated APP as also degradation of amyloid peptides through the action of novel peptidase (Prep) (Pavlov et al. 2011; Falkevall et al. 2006). A schematic view of Aβ peptide trafficking and the entry of the peptide into mitochondria is shown in Fig. 4.1.

The accumulation of Aβ42 within mitochondria in AD brain offers several possibilities that may underlie the phenomenon of mitochondrial dysfunction so conspicuous in this disease condition. As stated earlier in this review that interaction of oligomerized Aβ peptide with mitochondrial target proteins like cyclophilin D, ANT, UCP etc. could explain the toxic effects of aggregated Aβ protein on mitochondria, but other targets like ABAD, F_0 F_1 ATP synthase, TCA cycle enzymes could be equally important, but molecular details of such interactions are not clear. However, recent studies reveal some molecular of details of Aβ and ABAD interactions including the crystallographic structure Aβ-ABAD complex as also interactions of Aβ and cyclophilin D and Aβ and F_0 F_1 ATP synthase (Lustbader et al. 2004; Du and Yan 2010; Schmidt et al. 2008). The other attractive hypothesis forwarded in this context is the blockage of mitochondrial import channels by APP with consequent failures of entry of bonafide nDNA coded mitrochondrial proteins such as subunits of respiratory chain complexes or other enzyme complexes or transport proteins into mitochondria causing dysfunction of this organelle (Devi et al. 2006; Anandateerthavarada et al. 2003). The formation of aberrant cation-specific ion channels in synthetic lipid vesicles or biomembranes by oligomerized Aβ42 or ROS mediated damage caused by the latter on membrane lipids and proteins may also be instrumental in causing mitochondrial dysfunction (Arispe et al. 2007; Rodrigues et al. 2001).

4.3 Consequences of Mitochondrial Dysfunction in AD

The obvious implications of mitochondrial dysfunction in AD include cross–talk among different pathologic mechanisms of this disease and also the phenomenon of programmed cell death (Fig. 4.2). The important pathogenic processes in AD brain other than Aβ accumulation and mitochondrial dysfunction are oxidative stress and inflammatory response through microglial activation (Smith et al. 2000; Akiyama et al. 2000). The oxidative stress in AD brain presumably has multiple contributors such as metal dysregulation, ROS formation from transition metals bound to Aβ peptide and ROS release from activated microglia and there is overwhelming evidence of accumulation of oxidative damage markers in post-mortem AD brain (Smith et al. 2000; Smith et al. 2007; Abranov and Duchen 2005; Akiyama et al. 2000). Mitochondrial dysfunction especially an inhibited respiratory chain activity can significantly contribute to oxidative stress existing in AD brain by enhanced production of ROS which in turn may further damage the mitochondrial respiratory chain complexes as well as mtDNA leading to further generation of ROS and creation of a vicious cycle (Cassarino et al. 1999; Szeto 2006). Moreover, ROS can activate the microglia and promote the formation of pro-inflammatory cytokines and contribute to inflammatory response which is an important element of AD pathogenesis (Akiyama et al. 2000). It is also important to note that ROS from dysfunctional mitochondria or elsewhere could also enhance the expression of APP as has been shown in some studies and this mechanism would lead to further forma-

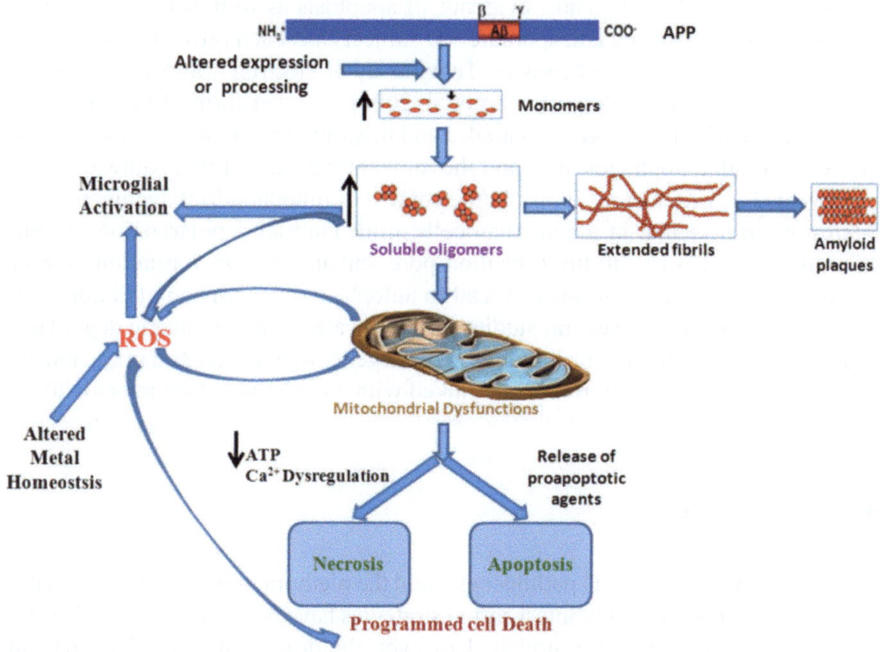

Fig. 4.2 Mitochondrial dysfunction and other pathologic mechanisms in AD brain. Mitochondrial dysfunction re-inforces other damage pathways like oxidative stress, inflammatory response and Aβ accumulation and finally triggers programmed cell death in AD brain

tion of Aβ42 and worsening of the disease condition (Tamagno et al. 2002). Finally, mitochondrial dysfunction and ROS formation can activate the programmed cell death pathways in AD brain.

Two major cell death pathways of apoptosis and necrosis are considered as two types of Programmed Cell Death (PCD) based on characteristic morphological alterations, nature of initiating death signals, involvement of caspases, availability of ATP, involvement of Ca^{2+} dysregulation and proteolytic enzymes and other molecular details, although the pathways are not neatly separated and distinctions tend to blur in many cases (Syntichaki and Travernarakis 2002; Bras et al. 2005). For example, the initiating death agent may lead to apoptosis in one system, but necrosis in another, or apoptosis in a lower concentration but necrosis at a higher dose (Syntichaki and Travernarakis 2002; Bras et al. 2005). Further, a continuum of apoptosis and necrosis may co-exist in some cases of cell death (Bras et al. 2005). The centrality of mitochondrial involvement, however, in both these cell death pathways is clearly established. The release of cytochrome c, apoptogenic factors (Smac/Diablo, Omi/Htr 2, APF etc.), from depolarized mitochondria could initiate and propagate apoptosis while an excessive ROS production or a severe depletion of ATP synthesis or Ca^{2+} dysregulation caused by damaged mitochondria may lead to necrosis and therefore, it is unlikely that one exclusive pathway of cell death will be operative in AD brain. Thus, evidence of apoptosis as well as necrosis in post-mortem brains of familial and sporadic AD subjects has been presented by different groups using immunohistochemistry, Tunel assay or electron microscopy (Su et al. 1994; Velez-Pardo et al. 2001; Eckert et al. 2003). Another form of PCD is termed autophagy by which damaged organelles and misfolded proteins are removed from the cell through autophagosomes and the molecular details of this pathway are being revealed (Moreira et al. 2010). In the context of mitochondrial dysfunction, it is interesting to note that in mammalian cells mitochondrial depolarization, opening of mitochondrial permeability transition pore, enhanced ROS formation or accumulation of mtDNA mutations can lead to autophagy or mitophagy (Elmore et al. 2001; Kim et al. 2007). Several studies have indicated that autophagic degradation pathway is an important contributor to neurodegeneration in AD and mitochondrial dysfunction and Aβ accumulation are linked with autophagy (Moreira et al. 2010).

4.4 Intervention

Given the complexity of AD pathogenesis and the plethora of information available, it is not surprising that many intervention strategies have been suggested and proved to be useful in experimental models. However, the drug treatment of AD patients continues to be extremely inadequate and the disease progresses relentlessly with the patients usually succumbing to the illness within 5–10 years after the diagnosis. Acetylcholinesterase inhibitors are probably the most commonly used drugs for AD which brings about some improvement in cognition, while others like selegeline, vitamin E, non-steroidal anti-inflammatory drugs are of doubtful benefit. Therefore, it is imperative to identify new therapeutic targets and potential drugs for AD and in fact a long list of such drugs in different phases of clinical trial exists (Alzheimer Research Forum, Drugs in Clinical Trials, www.alzforum.org). We would mention the therapeutic targets in the context of the present article primarily restricted to toxic interactions of Aβ peptide and mitochondria.

From the perspective of what has so far been stated in this review, the intervention strategies can be adopted at several levels e.g. oligomerisation of Aβ peptide and its interaction with mitochondria, the mitochondrial bioenergetic failure and structural alterations and the cross-talk between oxidative stress and mitochondrial dysfunction. The compounds that can inhibit Aβ peptide over production (inhibitors of β and γ secretases) or oligomerisation in experimental systems (nano-particle conjugated metal chelator, melatonin, etc.) would prevent the formation of toxic species capable of causing mitochondrial dysfunction and might be beneficial for the treatment of AD (Bonda et al. 2010). Mitochondrial stabilizing agents and also those which can impact fusion/fission process are likely to prevent Aβ induced mitochondrial dysfunction and would be potential drugs for AD. The compounds (e.g. latrepirdine) which can inhibit opening of permeability transition pore in mitochondria may prove to be important in this context (Bonda et al. 2010). Since mitochondrial dysfunction and ROS formation reinforce each other forming a vicious cycle in AD brain, it is expected that natural anti-oxidants and specially mitochondria targeted anti-oxidants (Q10, acetyl–L-carnitine, α-lpoic acid, Mito-Q, SS peptides etc.) would retard the progress of AD pathogenesis (Palacios et al. 2011; Szeto 2006; Bonda et al. 2010). Lastly compounds interacting or blocking the so called 'amyloid channels' in lipid bilayer could be another group of potential drugs for AD (Arispe et al. 2007). Many of these potential drugs for AD have been tested in various in vitro systems or in transgenic AD models or cell based models where promising results are obtained, but they have to pass rigorous clinical trials before introduction in the market. If these drugs could produce clinical benefit to the patients, not only this will be a great help to the clinicians and AD patients, but this will indirectly validate also the 'models' so extensively used by the bio-medical researchers without knowing how far from the reality these 'models' are.

References

Abramov AY, Duchen MR (2005) The role of an astrocytic NADPH oxidase in the neurotoxicity of amyloid beta peptides. Philos Trans R Soc Lond B Biol Sci 360:2309–2314

Akiyama H, Barger S, Barnum S, Bradt B, Bauer J, Cole GM, Cooper NR, Eikelenboom P, Emmerling M, Fiebich BL, Finch CE, Frautschy S, Griffin WS, Hampel H, Hull M, Landreth G, Lue L, Mrak R, Mackenzie IR, McGeer PL, O'Banion MK, Pachter J, Pasinetti G, Plata-Salaman C, Rogers J, Rydel R, Shen Y, Streit W, Strohmeyer R, Tooyoma I, Van Muiswinkel FL, Veerhuis R, Walker D, Webster S, Wegrzyniak B, Wenk G, Wyss-Coray T (2000) Inflammation and Alzheimer's disease. Neurobiol Aging 21:383–421

Anandatheerthavarada HK, Biswas G, Robin MA, Avadhani NG (2003) Mitochondrial targeting and a novel transmembrane arrest of Alzheimer's amyloid precursor protein impairs mitochondrial function in neuronal cells. J Cell Biol 161:41–54

Arispe N, Diaz JC, Simakova O (2007) Aβ ion channels prospects for treating Alzheimer's disease with Aβ channel blockers. Biochim Biophys Acta 1768:1952–1965

Atamna H, Frey WH (2007) Mechanisms of mitochondrial dysfunction and energy deficiency in Alzheimer's disease. Mitochondrion 7:297–310

Baloyannis SJ, Costa V, Michmizos D (2004) Mitochondrial alterations in Alzheimer's disease. Am J Alzheimers Dis Other Demen 19:89–93

Bird TD (2001) Alzheimer's disease and other primary dementias. In: Braunwald E, Fauci AS, Kasper DL, Hauser SL, Longo D, Jameson JL (eds) Harrison's Principles of Internal Medicine. McGraw-Hill, New York, p 2391–2399

Bonda DJ, Lee HP, Lee H, Friedlich AL, Perry G, Zhu X, Smith MA (2010) Novel therapeutics for Alzheimer's disease: an update. Curr Opin Drug Discov Devel 13:235–246

Brand MD, Nicholls DG (2011) Assessing mitochondrial dysfunction in cells. Biochem J 435:297–312

Bras M, Queenan B, Susin SA (2005) Programmed cell death via mitochondria: different modes of dying. Biochemistry (Moscow) 70:231–239

Bubber P, Haroutunian V, Fisch G, Blass JP, Gibson GE (2005) Mitochondrial abnormalities in Alzheimer brain: mechanistic implications. Ann Neurol 57:695–703

Bu G, Cam J, Zerbinatti C (2006) LRP in amyloid-beta production and metabolism. Ann N Y Acad Sci 1086:35–53

Calkins MJ, Manczak M, Mao P, Shirendeb U, Reddy PH (2011) Impaired mitochondrial biogenesis, defective axonal transport of mitochondria, abnormal mitochondrial dynamics and synaptic degeneration in a mouse model of Alzheimer's disease. Hum Mol Genet 20:4515–4529

Cam JA, Bu G (2006) Modulation of β-amyloid precursor protein trafficking and processing by the low density lipoprotein receptor family. Molecular Neurodegeneration 1:8 doi:10.1186/1750-1326-1-8

Casley CS, Canevari L, Land JM, Clark JB, Sharpe MA (2002) Beta-amyloid inhibits integrated mitochondrial respiration and key enzyme activities. J Neurochem 80:91–100

Cassarino DS, Bennett JP Jr (1999) An evaluation of the role of mitochondria in neurodegenerative diseases: mitochondrial mutations and oxidative pathology, protective nuclear responses, and cell death in neurodegeneration. Brain Res Brain Res Rev 29:1–25

Chen H, Chan DC (2009) Mitochondrial dynamics—fusion, fission, movement, and mitophagy—in neurodegenerative diseases. Hum Mol Genet 18:169–176

Chen JX, Yan SS (2010) Role of mitochondrial amyloid-β in Alzheimer's disease. J Alzheimers Dis 20:S569–S578

Chou JL, Shenoy DV, Thomas N, Choudhary PK, Laferla FM, Goodman SR, Breen GA (2011) Early dysregulation of the mitochondrial proteome in a mouse model of Alzheimer's disease. J Proteomics 74:466–479

De Felice FG, Vieira MNN, Saraiva LMM, Villar JDF, Abreu JG, Liu R, Chang L, Klein WL, Ferreiral SRT (2004) Targeting the neurotoxic species in Alzheimer's disease: inhibitors of Aβ oligomerization. FASEB J 18:1366–1372

Dekosky ST (2002) Neurobiology and molecular biology of Alzheimer's disease. Rev Neurol 35:752–760

Devi L, Prabhu BM, Galati DF, Avadhani NG, Anandatheerthavarada HK (2006) Accumulation of amyloid precursor protein in the mitochondrial import channels of human Alzheimer's disease brain is associated with mitochondrial dysfunction. J Neurosci 35:9057–9068

Du H, Yan SS (2010) Mitochondrial permeability transition pore in Alzheimer's disease: cyclophilin D and amyloid beta. Biochim Biophys Acta 1802:198–204

Eckert A, Marques CA, Keil U, Schüssel K, Müller WE (2003) Increased apoptotic cell death in sporadic and genetic Alzheimer's disease. Ann NY Acad Sci 1010:604–609

Eckert A, Schulz KL, Rhein V, Götz J (2010) Convergence of amyloid-β and tau pathologies on mitochondria in vivo. Mol Neurobiol 41:107–114

Elmore SP, Qian T, Grissom SF, Lemasters JJ (2001) The mitochondrial permeability transition initiates autophagy in rat hepatocytes. FASEB J 15:2286–2297

Falkevall A, Alikhani N, Bhushan S, Pavlov PF, Busch K, Johnson KA, Eneqvist T, Tjernberg L, Ankarcrona M, Glaser E (2006) Degradation of the amyloid beta-protein by the novel mitochondrial peptidasome, PreP. J Biol Chem 281:29096–29104

Gao X, Tang XC (2006) Huperzine attenuates mitochondrial dysfunction in β-amyloid-treated PC12 cells by reducing oxygen free radicals accumulation and improving mitochondrial energy metabolism. J Neurosci Res 83:1048–1057

Gibson GE, Shi Q (2010) A mitocentric view of Alzheimer's disease suggests multi-faceted treatments. J Alzheimers Dis 20:S591–S607

Halliwell B, Gutteridge JMC (2007) Free radicals in biology and medicine, 4th edn. Clarendon Press, Oxford

Hansson Petersen CA, Alikhani N, Behbahani H, Wiehager B, Pavlov PF, Alafuzoff I, Leinonen V, Ito A, Winblad B, Glaser E, Ankarcrona M (2008) The amyloid peptide is imported into mitochondria via the TOM import machinery and localized to mitochondrial cristae. Proc Natl Acad Sci USA 105:13145–13150

Hauptmann S, Scherping I, Dröse S, Brandt U, Schulz KL, Jendrach M, Leuner K, Eckert A, Müller WE (2009) Mitochondrial dysfunction: an early event in Alzheimer pathology accumulates with age in AD transgenic mice. Neurobiol Aging 30:1574–1586

Higuchi M, Manna SK, Sasaki R, Aggarwal BB (2002) Regulation of the activation of nuclear factor kappaB by mitochondrial respiratory function: evidence for the reactive oxygen species-dependent and -independent pathways. Antioxid Redox Signal 6:945–955

Hirai K, Aliev G, Nunomura A, Fujioka H, Russell RL, Atwood CS, Johnson AB, Kress Y, Vinters HV, Tabaton M, Shimohama S, Cash AD, Siedlak SL, Harris PL, Jones PK, Petersen RB,

Perry G, Smith MA (2001) Mitochondrial abnormalities, in Alzheimer's disease. J Neurosci 21:3017–3023

Hock MB, Kralli A (2009) Transcriptional control of mitochondrial biogenesis and function. Annu Rev Physiol 71:177–203

Hung LW, Ciccotosto GD, Giannakis E, Tew JD, Perez K, Masters CL, Cappai R, Wade JD, Barnham KJ (2008) Amyloid-β peptide (Aβ) neurotoxicity is modulated by the rate of peptide aggregation: a dimers and trimers correlate with neurotoxicity. J Neurosci 28:11950–11958

Jin H, Liu T, Wang WX, Xu JH, Yang PB, Lu HX, Sun QR, Hu HT (2010) Protective effects of [Gly14]-humanin on beta-amyloid-induced PC12 cell death by preventing mitochondrial dysfunction. Neurochem Int 56:417–423

Kelly DP, Scarpulla RC (2004) Transcriptional regulatory circuits controlling mitochondrial biogenesis and function. Genes Dev 18:357–368.

Kim HS, Lee JH, Lee JP, Kim EM, Chang KA, Park HC, Jeong SJ, Wittendorp MC, Seo JE, Choi SH, Suh YH (2002) Amyloid β peptide induces cytochrome c release from isolated mitochondria. Neuroreport 13:1989–1993

Kim I, Rodriguez-Enriquez S, Lemasters JJ (2007) Selective degradation of mitochondria by mitophagy. Arch Biochem Biophys 462:245–253

Kim SH, Vlkolinsky R, Cairns N, Lubec G (2000) Decreased levels of complex III core protein 1 and complex V beta chain in brains from patients with Alzheimer's disease and Down syndrome. Cell Mol Life Sci. 57:1810–1816

LaFerla FM, Green KN, Oddo S (2007) Intracellular amyloid-β in Alzheimer's disease. Nat Rev Neurosci 8:499–509

Lal R, Lin H, Quist AP (2007) Amyloid beta ion channel: 3D structure and relevance to amyloid channel paradigm. Biochim Biophys Acta 1768:1966–1975

Lin MT, Beal MF (2006) Mitochondrial dysfunction and oxidative stress in neurodegenerative diseases. Nature 443:787–795

Lustbader JW, Cirilli M, Lin C, Xu HW, Takuma K, Wang N, Caspersen C, Chen X, Pollak S, Chaney M, Trinchese F, Liu S, Moore FG, Lue LF, Walker DG, Kuppusamy P, Zewier JL, Arancio O, Stern D, Yan SS, Wu H (2004) ABAD directly links Aβ to mitochondrial toxicity in Alzheimer's disease. Science 304:448–452

Manczak M, Anekondam TS, Henson E, Park BS, Quinn J, Reddy PH (2006) Mitochondria are a direct site of A beta accumulation in Alzheimer's disease neurons: implications for free radical generation and oxidative damage in disease progression. Hum Mol Genet 15:1437–1449

Mauro C, Leo SC, Anso E, Rocha S, Thotakura AK, Trnatore L, Moretti M, Smaele ED, Beg AA, Tergaonkar V, Chandel NS, Franzoso G (2011) NF-κB controls energy homeostasis and metabolic adaptation by upregulating mitochondrial respiration. Nat Cell Biol 13:1272–1279

Mecocci P, MacGarvey U, Beal MF (1994) Oxidative damage to mitochondrial DNA is increased in Alzheimer's disease. Ann Neuro 36:747–751

Moreira PI, Santos MS, Moreno A, Rego AC, Oliveira C (2002) Effect of amyloid beta-peptide on permeability transition pore: a comparative study. J Neurosci Res 69:257–267

Moreira PI, Santos RX, Zhu X, Lee HG, Smith MA, Casadesus G, Perry G (2010) Autophagy in Alzheimer's disease. Expert Rev Neurother 10:1209–1218

Murphy MP (2009) How mitochondria produce reactive oxygen species. Biochem J 417:1–13

Nicholls DG, Ferguson SJ (2001) Bioenergetics 3, 3rd eds Academic, California, USA

Nichols MR, Moss MA, Reed DK, Daniel SCM, Hoh JH, Rosenberry TT (2005) Amyloid-β protofibrils differ from amyloid-β aggregates induced in dilute hexafluoroisopropanol in stability and morphology. J Biol Chem 280:2471–2480

Pagani L, Eckert A (2011) Amyloid-beta interaction with mitochondria. Int J Alzheimers Dis. doi:10.4061, 925050

Palacios HH, Yendluri BB, Parvathaneni K, Shadlinski VB, Obrenovich ME, Leszek J, Gokhman D, Gasiorowski K, Bragin V, Aliev G (2011) Mitochondrion-specific antioxidants as drug treatments for Alzheimer disease. CNS Neurol Disord Drug Targets 10:149–162

Pavlov PF, Wiehager B, Sakai J, Frykman S, Behbahani H, Winblad B, Ankarcrona M (2011) Mitochondrial γ-secretase participates in the metabolism of mitochondria-associated amyloid precursor protein. FASEB J 25:78–88

Qiao H, Koya RC, Nakagawa K, Tanaka H, Fujita H, Takimoto M, Kuzumaki N (2005) Inhibition of Alzheimer's amyloid-beta peptide-induced reduction of mitochondrial membrane potential and neurotoxicity by gelsolin. Neurobiol Aging 26:849–855

Reddy PH, Beal MF (2008) Amyloid beta, mitochondrial dysfunction and synaptic damage: implications for cognitive decline in aging and Alzheimer's disease. Cell 14:45–53

Reddy PH, McWeeney S, Park BS, Manczak M, Gutala RV, Partovi D, Jung Y, Yau V, Searles R, Mori M, Quinn J (2004) Gene expression profiles of transcripts in amyloid precursor protein transgenic mice: upregulation of mitochondrial metabolism and apoptotic genes is an early cellular change in Alzheimer's disease. Hum Mol Genet 13:1225–1240

Reinhard C, Hébert SS, De Strooper B (2005) The amyloid-β precursor protein: integrating structure with biological function. EMBO J 24:3996–4006

Rhein V, Baysang G, Rao S, Meier F, Bonert A, Müller-Spahn F, Eckert A (2009) Amyloid-beta leads to impaired cellular respiration, energy production and mitochondrial electron chain complex activities in human neuroblastoma cells. Cell Mol Neurobiol 29:1063–1071

Rodrigues CM, Sola S, Brito MA, Brondino CD, Brites D, Moura JJ (2001) Amyloid beta-peptide disrupts mitochondrial membrane, lipid and protein structure: protective role of tauroursodeoxycholate. Biochem Biophys Res Commun 281:468–474

Scarpulla RC (2008) Transcriptional paradigms in mammalian mitochondrial biogenesis and function. Physiol Rev 88:611–638.

Schmidt C, Lepsverdize E, Chi SL, Das AM, Pizzo SV, Dityatev A, Schachner M (2008) Amyloid precursor protein and amyloid β-peptide bind to ATP synthase and regulate its activity at the surface of neural cells APP, Aβ and regulation of ATP synthase activity. Mo Psychiatry 13:953–969

Selkoe DJ (2001) Alzheimer's disease: genes, proteins, and therapy. Physiol Rev 81:741–766

Sheng B, Wang X, Su B, Lee HG, Casadesus G, Perry G, Zhu X (2011) Impaired mitochondrial biogenesis contributes to mitochondrial dysfunction in Alzheimer's disease. J Neurochem. doi:10.1111/j.1471-4159.2011.07581.x

Sinha M, Behera P, Bhowmick P, Banerjee K, Basu S, Chakrabarti S (2011) Aging promotes amyloid beta peptide induced mitochondrial dysfunctions in rat brain: a molecular link between aging and Alzheimer's disease. J Alzheimers Dis (in press)

Smith MA, Rottkamp CA, Nunomura A, Raina AK, Perry G (2000) Oxidative stress in Alzheimer's disease. Biochim Biophys Acta 1502:139–144

Smith DG, Cappai R, Barnham KJ (2007) The redox chemistry of the Alzheimer's disease amyloid β peptide. Biochim Biophys Acta 1768:1976–1990

Su JH, Anderson AJ, Cummings BJ, Cotman CW (1994) Immunohistochemical evidence for apoptosis in Alzheimer's disease. Neuroreport 5:2529–2533

Syntichaki P, Tavernarakis N (2002) Uncontrollable catastrophe, or is there order behind the chaos? EMBO Reports 3:604–609

Szeto HH (2006) Mitochondria-targeted peptide antioxidants: novel neuroprotective agents. AAPS J 8:619–642

Tamagno E, Bardini P, Obbili A, Vitali A, Borghi R, Zaccheo D, Pronzato MA, Danni O, Smith MA, Perry G, Tabaton M (2002) Oxidative stress increases expression and activity of BACE in NT2 neurons. Neurobiol Dis 10:279–288

Twig G, Elorza A, Molina AJ, Mohamed H, Wikstrom JD, Walzer G, Stiles L, Haigh SE, Katz S, Las G, Alroy J, Wu M, Py BF, Yuan J, Deeney JT, Corkey BE, Shirihai OS (2008) Fission and selective fusion govern mitochondrial segregation and elimination by autophagy. EMBO J 27:433–446

Velez-Pardo C, Arroyave ST, Lopera F, Castaño AD, Jimenez Del Rio M (2001) Ultrastructure evidence of necrotic neural cell death in familial Alzheimer's disease brains bearing presenilin-1 E280A mutation. J Alzheimers Dis 3:409–415

Wang J, Xiong S, Xie C, Markesbery WR, Lovell MA (2005) Increased oxidative damage in nuclear and mitochondrial DNA in Alzheimer's disease. J Neurochem 93:953–962

Wang X, Sua B, Siedlaka SL, Moreirab PI, Fujiokac H, Wang Y, Casadesus G, Zhu X (2008) Amyloid-β overproduction causes abnormal mitochondrial dynamics via differential modulation of mitochondrial fission/fusion proteins. Proc Natl Acad Sci 105:19318–19323

Yao J, Irwin RW, Zhao L, Nilsen J, Hamilton RT, Brinton RD (2009) Mitochondrial bioenergetic deficit precedes Alzheimer's pathology in female mouse model of Alzheimer's disease. Proc Natl Acad Sci 106:14670–14675

Yates D, McLoughlin DM (2008) The molecular pathology of Alzheimer's disease. Psychiatry 7:1–5

Zheng H, Koo EH (2006) The amyloid precursor protein: beyond amyloid. Molecular Neurodegeneration 1:5. doi:10.1186/1750-1326-1-5

Wang J, Xiong S, Xie C, Markesbery WR, Lovell MA (2005) Increased oxidative damage in nuclear and mitochondrial DNA in Alzheimer's disease. J Neurochem 93:953–962
Wang X, Su B, Siedlak SL, Moreira PI, Fujioka H, Wang Y, Casadesus G, Zhu X (2008) Amyloid-β overproduction causes abnormal mitochondrial dynamics via differential modulation of mitochondrial fission/fusion proteins. Proc Natl Acad Sci USA 105:19318–19323
Yao J, Irwin RW, Zhao L, Nilsen J, Hamilton RT, Brinton RD (2009) Mitochondrial bioenergetic deficit precedes Alzheimer's pathology in female mouse model of Alzheimer's disease. Proc Natl Acad Sci USA 106:14670–14675
Yates D, McLoughlin DM (2008) The molecular pathology of Alzheimer's disease. Psychiatry 7:1–5
Zheng H, Koo EH (2006) The amyloid precursor protein: beyond amyloid. Mol Neurodegener 1:5. doi:10.1186/1750-1326-1-5

Chapter 5
Brain Aging: Influence of Early-Life Events on Late-Life Brain Disorders

Debomoy K. Lahiri

Abstract The prominent symptoms of Alzheimer's disease (AD) include severe loss of memory, failure of cognition and reasoning, and overall deficit of other intellectual abilities. AD usually appears late in adult life, but when the disease initiates and how long the disease processes take to develop are presently unknown. To address this issue, the "Latent Early–life Associated Regulation" (LEARn) model has been proposed. This model explains the etiology of AD and integrates both the neuropathological features (e.g., amyloid-beta plaques and hyperphosphorylated tau tangles) and environmental conditions (e.g., dietary imbalance, metal exposure, and pestichemicals) associated with AD. As per the LEARn model, environmental agents could perturb gene regulation in a long–term fashion, beginning at early developmental stages, but these perturbations would not have pathological results until significantly later in life, if an additional perturbation were to occur. The LEARn model postulates latent expression of specific genes triggered at an early stage of life. The LEARn model operates via the regulatory region (promoter) of the gene, specifically through changes in methylation and oxidation status within the promoter of specific genes. Thus, the LEARn model unifies genetic and environmental risk factors to explain the etiology of the most common, sporadic form of AD. Finally, the possible medical remediation is discussed with reference to the relatively long term of latency under the LEARn model.

Keywords Aging • Dementia • Diet • Environment • Epigenome • Epigenetics • Gene-environment • Idiopathic disorders • Metals • Latency • Neurodegenerative disorders

D. K. Lahiri (✉)
Department of Psychiatry, Institute of Psychiatric Research, Indiana University School of Medicine, 791 Union Drive, Indianapolis, IN 46202, USA
e-mail: dlahiri@iupui.edu

M. K. Thakur, S. I. S. Rattan (eds.), *Brain Aging and Therapeutic Interventions*,
DOI 10.1007/978-94-007-5237-5_5,

5.1 Introduction: Major Neuropathochemical Features of Alzheimer's Disease

Alzheimer's disease (AD) is the most common form of dementia among the elderly, and age is the greatest risk factor for AD and other neurodegenerative disorders. The major symptoms of AD include severe loss of memory, failure of cognition and reasoning, and overall deficit of other intellectual abilities. Epidemiologically AD is the most common form of dementia among the elderly in Western countries (Hebert et al. 2003). AD is estimated to comprise up to 70 % of all dementia in the United States (Plassman et al. 2007) afflicting approximately 5.4 million individuals (Alzheimer's Association 2012). Particularly, AD is a heterogeneous disease with unknown etiology. Currently there is no medication that can fully treat AD or halt the progression of the disease. These age-related disorders, such as AD and Parkinson's disease, usually appear late in adult life, but when they start and how long the disease processes precede to manifest are presently unknown. Thus, it is important to address the timing and nature of triggers that lead to AD in late-life. This review discusses the influence of early–life events on late-life brain disorders under the recently proposed conceptual framework of the "Latent Early–life Associated Regulation" (LEARn) model, and provides ways of medical remediation. Indeed, the proposed mechanisms of LEARn, changes in methylation and/or oxidative damage to DNA, should provide potential solutions to a LEARn–type environmental exposure.

Neuropathological examination reveals excessive deposition of two major proteinaceous aggregates in AD. Neurochemically, they are hyperphosphorylated microtubule associated protein τ "tangles" and senile plaques formed mostly of the amyloid–β peptide (Aβ). Aβ is proteolytically derived from the large β–amyloid precursor protein (APP). Indeed, the amyloid plaques and τ tangles form the basis for the two currently–dominant models in the AD field—the "amyloid hypothesis" and the "τ hypothesis" (Sambamurti et al. 2006). According to the amyloid hypothesis, the neurotoxicity of Aβ dimers and oligomers and/or damage caused by Aβ plaque aggregation is the primary cause of AD. According to the τ hypothesis, the aggregation of hyperphosphorylated τ leads to neuronal cell death and resulting neuropathology, and Aβ aggregation would be a result of cellular damage imposed by τ aggregation. However, both these models fail to fully explain the etiology and the role of environment of sporadic form of the disease. Herein, I discuss the role of early–life events on late-life brain disorders, such as AD, and propose an effective strategy for the prevention of AD.

5.2 Genetics and Major Risk Factors of AD

Recent studies from different laboratories suggest that AD is a disorder of complex etiology, combining environmental, genetic and epigenetic factors (Table 5.1). A minority of AD cases can be attributed to autosomal familial AD (FAD) mutations in the coding sequences of AD–associated genes, such as APP and presenilin 1

Table 5.1 Different forms of Alzheimer's disease, their causes and possible remedies

Major forms	Major driver	Major causes	Possible remedies
FAD-Familial AD	Genotype	Mutation in particular genes such as APP718 V/M	Difficult/non-existent (future gene therapy technique?)
SAD-Sporadic AD	Environment, and other unknown factors	Head trauma, nutritional imbalance, metals, pestichemicals	Restore healthy environment
LAD-LEARn AD	Gene × environment interaction	Somatic epitype? G_{SE} epigenetic markers via the promoter sequences	Proper dietary supplements (e.g., folate) during developmental period

(PSEN1). However, this form of AD does not explain the far more prevalent sporadic late–onset AD (LOAD), which results from a combination of various factors. The known risk factors for sporadic LOAD include age, limited education, high dietary cholesterol, head trauma and the presence of APOEε4 genotype. There are further associations with protein expression in addition to APP or PSEN1 such as the insulin degrading enzyme (IDE), α2–macroglobulin and endothelin converting enzyme 2 (ECE2) (Lahiri et al. 2003). Furthermore, AD risk has been associated with promoter polymorphisms that are located in the 5′-flanking region of the APOE and APP genes (Ge et al. 2007; Lahiri et al. 2005). It should be mentioned that other studies have shown no association between APOEε4 allele status and AD in a population that differs from the typical sample from Western industrialized populations (Hall et al. 2006), suggesting the role of environmental factors. Oxidative stress and abnormal metal levels in the brain and inflammatory factors are, likewise, linked to AD (Bellingham et al. 2004). Notably, age poses the greatest risk for LOAD of all known risk factors. No single LOAD risk factor is necessary and sufficient for AD to appear. None of the current etiological models have so far explained the sporadic nature of AD and the low penetrance of known risk factors, and this review is meant to bridge this gap of knowledge and prose a remedial intervention.

5.3 Necessity of a Unifying Framework, the "LEARn Model", to Explain the Etiology of AD

Most work presumes that AD is a late phenomenon, i.e., AD follows quickly after whatever stimulus triggers it, but current evidence does not reasonably exclude AD from being early/developmental in nature. Although AD manifests late in adult life, it is not clearly understood when the disease actually starts, nor how long it takes for the associated events and processes to develop into disease. The factors that trigger the cascade of pathobiochemical processes of the disease are unclear. The main unresolved questions concern the timing and nature of AD triggering. That is to say, any unifying hypothesis for the etiology of AD must take into account not only neuropathological features but also the multiple environmental factors associated with AD, including dietary imbalance, hormonal factors, inflammation after head injury and toxicological exposure. In order to address the interaction of environment and genes that is in play with AD, Lahiri and colleagues have proposed a "Latent Early-life Associated Regulation" (LEARn) model, which may explain the etiology of AD and other neuropsychiatric and developmental disorders (Lahiri et al. 2007). Conceptually, the LEARn model begins with environmental agents (e.g., heavy metals), intrinsic factors (e.g., inflammatory cytokines), and dietary factors (e.g., folate and cholesterol) acting to alter gene regulation in a latent, long–term fashion (Fig. 5.1). This initiates at early developmental stages, but these perturbations do not yield pathological results until significantly later in life (Lahiri et al. 2007; Basha et al. 2005). One such pathological result would be development of AD–like pathology in aged monkeys after infantile exposure to environmental lead (Pb) (Wu et al. 2008). Although similar hypotheses were developed in the 1980s by Barker and colleagues (Barker et al. 2002), their model is incomplete and based on low birth weight and rapid childhood weight gain without proposing any underlying molecular mechanism. Notably, the LEARn model is based on the regulatory structure common to eukaryotic genes and epigenetic processes operating at certain specific sites within the promoter (regulatory) region of specific genes. In other words, while the LEARn model is not inconsistent with the classic "Barker model" of fetal origins of adult disease, it enlarges upon that model by providing specific biochemical and molecular biological pathways that can be directly tested.

5.4 Main Biochemical Features of the LEARn Model

As per the LEARn model, the foundation of latent early regulation is epigenetic modification of gene regulatory sequences with delayed, latent, changes in gene expression levels. In fact, the LEARn pathway does not reject the already present variation of the genetic substrate, but combines it with long–term response to differences in environmental stresses. At the genome level, human DNA is commonly modified by DNA oxidation and by methylation, which involves the addition of a methyl group to cytosine residues at CpG dinucleotides. The methylation reaction is catalyzed by DNA methyltransferase (DNMT) enzymes. In the DNA sequence, CpG dinucleotides are often found in clusters called CpG islands. In normal tissues, CpG islands are primarily unmethylated, and the aberrant methylation of CpG islands has been related to disease (Levenson 2010). Importantly, changing the methylation status of a gene, for example, hypomethylation in the promoter region leads to elevated gene expression, whereas hypermethylation results in decreased gene expression. How does environment act in this process? It is suggested experimentally that environmental factors, including exposure to metals and dietary variation, may operate by interfering with the (de)methylation of CpG clusters, thus altering affinity with potential transcription factors proteins, such as MeCP2 and SP1. Further, the activity of DNMT is reduced by heavy metal (cadmium) exposure (Takigu-

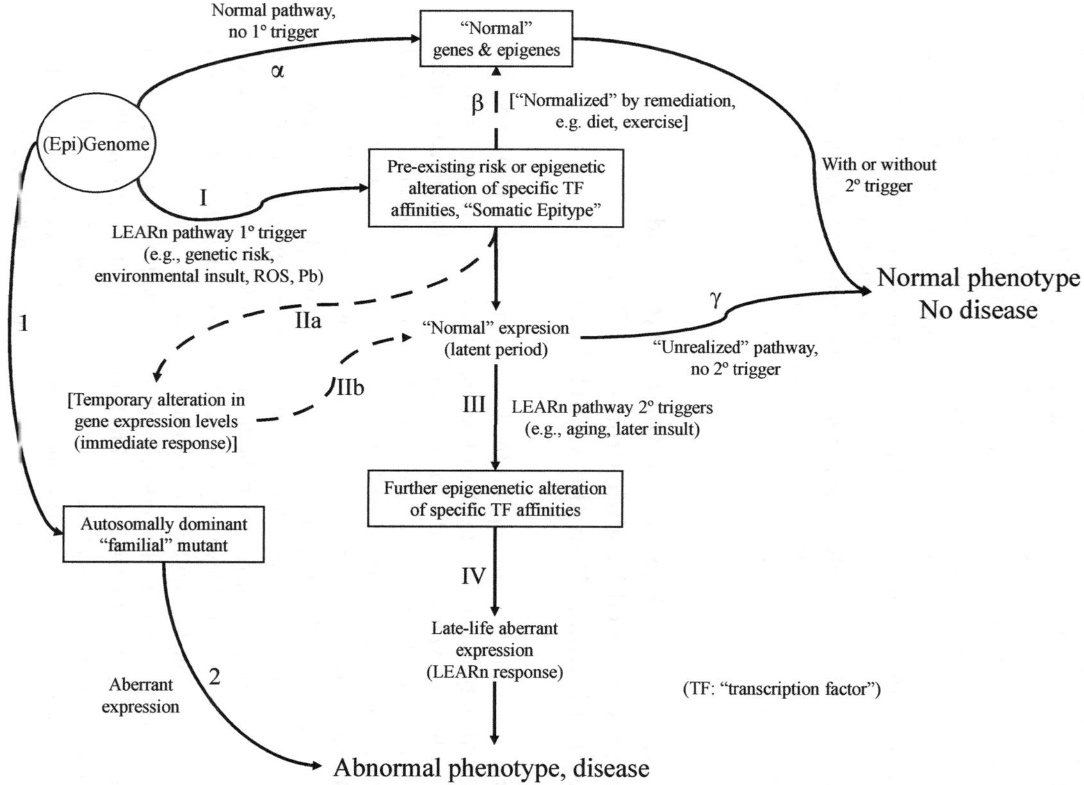

Fig. 5.1 Diagrammatic representation of the LEARn model. Elements are discussed throughout the text. The sequence of a gene or genes obtains changes in methylation or oxidation via environmental stress (1° trigger "I"). These changes may have a short term effect that quickly returns to normal expression (IIa, IIb). Later, a "triggering hit" (2° trigger, III) would affect genes epigenetically altered by the 1° trigger. Gene expression would reach (IV) the disease state. Intermediate hits/triggers may be necessary. This is in contrast to conventional autosomally dominant "genetic" disorders, in which a mutant gene (1) leads to aberrant expression (2) and disease. Non-disease outcomes can take more than one pathway. In the "normal" pathway (α), no 1° trigger occurs. The "normalized" pathway (β) would follow a 1° trigger, but environmental remediation, including diet, exercise, or possible drug treatments, would result in resumption of a non-pathogenic epigenetic state. The "unrealized" pathway (γ) would follow a 1° trigger but lack 2° trigger(s). No disease would occur, but the primary epigenetic alteration would still exist.

chi et al. 2003). It is noteworthy that viral and bacterial infection can result in persistent changes in host chromosomal DNA methylation (Zhang et al. 2010; Paschos et al. 2009; Nakajima et al. 2010). Moreover, heavy metals such as Pb are known to induce oxidative stress (Fowler et al. 2004), and oxidative stress modulates DNA methylation during malignant transformation (Campos et al. 2007). In addition, the oxidation of d–guanosine to 8–oxo–d–guanine interferes with the DNA–binding capacity of MeCP to a methylated cytosine (Valinluck et al. 2004) generating an "effective demethylation" due to oxidative damage of DNA. At the chromatin site, histone acetylation may also function in this process, with differences in acetylation occurring in response to DNA methylation or demethylation (Dobosy and Selker 2001). Consequently, this leads to chromatin remodeling, another level of gene regulation. Several studies suggest that changes in DNA oxidation and methylation are the fundamental means through which epigenetic differences arise in response to the environment, and importantly these acquired epigenetic changes can persist for an indefinite time and even stably transmitted to offspring (Nakajima et al. 2010; Hughes et al. 2009; Zeh and Zeh 2008).

5.5 Main Operational Features of the LEARn Model: Latent and Delayed Modification of APP Gene Expression Explain How the Model Work

Several recent experimental results support the LEARn model. One of the specific examples of LEARn–type activity involves the response of both rat and monkey APP genes to early–life exposure to Pb. In an elegant study, Basha and colleagues reported that when they added Pb acetate into the drinking water of dams of infant rats, levels of APP mRNA rose and then fell back to normal levels when Pb was taken away from their diet. Surprisingly, they noticed that at the age of 20 months, these early-exposed rats' APP expression levels and levels of Aβ peptide increased both beyond control rats and beyond levels founding in rats exposed to Pb at 20 months of age. This change occurred even though levels of Pb in the early-exposed rats had returned to background levels by this time (Basha et al. 2005), suggesting that it was not due to some hidden Pb reservoir in these rats.

To address species specificity, the rodent work was extended to primates when cynomolgus monkeys that had been exposed to Pb for the first month of life were sacrificed for brain tissue analysis at the age of 26 years. Comparative analysis of their brains with control (non–exposed) monkeys revealed that levels of both APP and Aβ were significantly elevated, but Pb levels were the same between exposed and non–exposed monkeys. Moreover, exposed monkeys showed greater brain amyloid aggregation than did non–exposed monkeys (Wu et al. 2008). At the human level, it has recently been shown that methylation levels for an individual person can change over lifespan in a significant portion of a human population (Bjornsson et al. 2008).

The LEARn pathway can be viewed at different levels with positive confirmatory conclusions. For example, a different delayed neurological response has also been shown in rats subjected to postnatal inflammation. The treatment resulted in increased susceptibility to seizure in adulthood (Galic et al. 2008). In humans, a pair of monozygotic twins had been raised together but was discordant for AD, and interestingly, they had differential DNA methylation in temporal neocortical neurons (Mastroeni et al. 2009a, b). Connecting the dots with stress and age, it is revealed that DNA methylation changes in response to stress persist late into life (Murgatroyd et al. 2009; Hamilton et al. 2001). DNA oxidation changes with age (Gmitterova et al. 2009), and these changes can be environmentally modified (Hamilton et al. 2001).

Notably, differences in guanine oxidation that correlate with symptoms have been found in Parkinson's disease models (Kikuchi et al. 2010). Apart from AD and other neurodegenerative disorders, significant differences in methylation between healthy and diseased individuals have been found in several disorders, including schizophrenia, bipolar disorder, suicide following abuse during childhood, and AD, among others (Lahiri et al. 2009).

5.6 Relevance of the LEARn Model in AD

Recent work suggests that the APP protein, Aβ peptide, and τ protein are physiologically important, and all appear in healthy individuals. In that case, their mere presence is not a sign of active or incipient AD. Therefore, some kinds of triggers to the disease must exist, which are independent of the simple presence of these proteins. In this context, the LEARn model would explain developmental triggering and latent expression of the APP gene at pathological levels. Results of knockout animals have shown that APP has necessary functions, although there is redundancy with other APP protein family members (Herms et al. 2004). Then, what would provoke APP and Aβ peptides to be overproduced in sporadic cases of AD? According to the LEARn model, the initial APP triggering mechanism activates early in life, at developmental stages, and sites of action would be within the promoter or regulatory region of APP and associated genes. The trigger would be sustained through epigenetic means, such as DNA methylation. It is also possible that genes with products shown to be protective against AD will have altered methylation patterns due to environmental stress. It is important to acknowledge that a long–latent condition such as LEARn–induced predisposition to AD is likely to function as a "two–hit" disorder, similarly to those found in currently accepted models of cancer etiology (Knudson 1971). For AD, this second hit could be a broad spectrum of changes in gene expression, especially upregulation of inflammatory factors, which has been shown to be a function of normal aging (Lu et al. 2004). Whether the broad changes in DNA methylation recently reported (Bjornsson et al. 2008) would reflect a first or later hits is not yet fully known. It should be emphasized that these environmental insults do not "intentionally" target AD–related genes in the brain, rather certain genes, by juxtaposition of CpG sites with important active/inactive transcription factor sites, would be particularly vulnerable to the effects of environmental stresses that alter CpG methylation patterns. I propose that testing these changes could, in part, be performed by microarray analysis of sporadic and familial AD, if these assays were longitudinal, tracing individual expression profiles across a lifetime and permitting comparison of the same AD and non–AD individuals at multiple life stages. We propose, therefore, that a large proportion, perhaps the majority of sporadic AD is actually "LEARn AD", a result of specific, and mechanistic environment/epigenome interaction (Table 5.1).

5.7 Epigenetics Drive the LEARn Pathway

The LEARn model is the result of an expression of the larger concepts of epigenetics and the epigenome, specifically adapted to the etiology of sporadic disorders of long latency. The epigenome can be defined as the collection of epigenetic markers associated with a specific individual organism's genome (Whitelaw and Whitelaw 2006). This epigenome, similar to its underlying genome, has specific epigenotypes, which are generated by modification of DNA methylation or oxidation, by changes in histone acetylation patterns, and by variations in the physical arrangement of chromosomal material (van Vliet et al. 2007). Thus, it is the expression of these epigenotypes, whether they be inherited by imprintation or acquired during life as somatic epitypes (Lahiri and Maloney 2006) that specifically contribute to development of sporadic psychobiological diseases.

From a medical standpoint, one may say that the epigenome is inherently less stable than is the genome because the epigenome is subject to epigenetic drift, which is a change in epigenetic markers over time within an individual lifespan. It is true that on a population level, this has been difficult to measure, but epigenetic drift, specifically in the methylation of an individual person's genome, has recently been demonstrated in the well–characterized Icelandic sample set and in a cohort of families in Utah (Bjornsson et al. 2008). Notably, the function of LEARn mediation of disease rests upon not only the presence of epigenetic variation but also its location. Indeed, the LEARn–susceptible gene promoters are predicted to have regions of CpG doublets overlapping critical transcription factor binding sites. Mechanistically, modification of the methylation status of these sites is the basis of modification of LEARn–vulnerable gene expression. Should such a gene happens to code for a transcription factor or DNA methylation pathway protein, this could result in a LEARn feedback loop, in which local and short–term environmental stress sets up a self-perpetuating cascade that could significantly modify the entire epigenome.

5.8 The LEARn Model Differs from the "Acute Toxic" Model

The biological effects and physiological consequences from the LEARn model differ from the acute toxic model. As per the LEARn model described above, environmentally–induced changes in methylation and oxidative damage as the physical mechanism that perturbs gene expression (Bolin et al. 2006), and the effects of these perturbations would be latent. Lack of an acute response or cessation of acute response would be followed some time later, after an additional trigger or triggers occurred, and they are not always immediately apparent in the same manner found in conventional toxic responses. Notably, apparent reversal of the symptoms of acute exposure to environmental stressors, such as Pb or poor nutrition, does not mean that there will be no long–lasting repercussions of an environmental insult. Under the LEARn model, conventional anti–toxicity treatments would be insufficient, as removing the cause does not remove the effect. For instance, bans enacted upon lead (Pb) in gasoline in previous decades would significantly reduce levels of Pb in urban dwellers. Nevertheless, the LEARn model would suggest that incidence of AD would not be likely to reduce in response until 50–60 years after the bans were enacted, when individuals would begin to reach ages at risk of LOAD but would not have suffered high levels of childhood Pb exposure. Importantly, the possibility of "latent sequelae" to asymptomatic exposure to Pb was raised over 30 years ago, albeit without proposing a specific mechanism of activity (De la Burde and Choat 1972).

Biologically–based medical remediation is possible due to the relatively long term of latency under the LEARn model. Indeed, the proposed mechanisms of LEARn, changes in methylation and/or oxidative damage to DNA, should provide potential solutions to a LEARn–type environmental exposure. For instance, fruit juices, such as concentrated apple juice, were reported to reverse acute oxidative damage and be a useful source of S–adenosyl methionine, reversing hypomethylation in mice (Chan and Shea 2006). Similarly, dietary melatonin supplementation reduced levels of Aβ in mouse cerebral cortex (Lahiri et al. 2004). These results justify an investigation of the use of appropriate dietary supplementation early in life, as a prophylactic or treatment measure against possible latent response to environmental insult. Furthermore, exercise in rats has been found to modulate the activity of mucosal betaine–homocysteine methyltransferase 2, potentially reducing aberrant methylation (Buehlmeyer et al. 2008). This indicates the possibility that lifestyle habits believed to protect against AD, such as physical exercise (Kivipelto and Solomon 2008) may work through remediation of early–life aberrant DNA methylation. In addition, we may not have fully insulated ourselves from significant future threats of exposures to toxic and epitoxic materials such as Pb. Recent events have shown that post-industrial societies cannot consider themselves to be safe from exposures, regardless of what regulations might be imposed (Notice of Violation 2010). Thus, the LEARn model presented here has far–reaching implications in personal health practices and public policy.

Acknowledgements This work was supported by grants from the Alzheimer's association (11-206418), and NIH (AG18379 and AG18884) to DKL, and Indiana Alzheimer's Disease Center grant (IADC) to Dr. B. Ghetti.

References

Barker DJ, Eriksson JG, Forsen T, Osmond C (2002) Fetal origins of adult disease: strength of effects and biological basis. Int J Epidemiol 31(6):1235–1239

Basha MR, Wei W, Bakheet SA, Benitez N, Siddiqi HK, Ge YW, Lahiri DK, Zawia NH (2005) The fetal basis of amyloidogenesis: exposure to lead and latent overexpression of amyloid precursor protein and beta-amyloid in the aging brain. J Neurosci 25(4):823–829

Bellingham SA, Lahiri DK, Maloney B, La Fontaine S, Multhaup G, Camakaris J (2004) Copper depletion down-regulates expression of the Alzheimer's disease amyloid-beta precursor protein gene. J Biol Chem 279(19):20378–20386

Bjornsson HT, Sigurdsson MI, Fallin MD, Irizarry RA, Aspelund T, Cui H, Yu W, Rongione MA, Ekstrom TJ, Harris TB, Launer LJ, Eiriksdottir G, Leppert MF, Sapienza C, Gudnason V, Feinberg AP (2008) Intra-individual change over time in DNA methylation with familial clustering. JAMA 299(24):2877–2883

Bolin CM, Basha R, Cox D, Zawia NH, Maloney B, Lahiri DK, Cardozo-Pelaez F (2006) Exposure to lead and the developmental origin of oxidative DNA damage in the aging brain. FASEB J 20(6):788–790

Buehlmeyer K, Doering F, Daniel H, Kindermann B, Schulz T, Michna H (2008) Alteration of gene expression in rat colon mucosa after exercise. Ann Anat 190(1):71–80

Campos AC, Molognoni F, Melo FH, Galdieri LC, Carneiro CR, D'Almeida V, Correa M, Jasiulionis MG (2007) Oxidative stress modulates DNA methylation during melanocyte anchorage blockade associated with malignant transformation. Neoplasia 9(12):1111–1121

Chan A and Shea TB (2006) Supplementation with apple juice attenuates presenilin-1 overexpression during dietary and genetically-induced oxidative stress. J Alzheimers Dis 10(4):353–358

De la Burde B and Choat MS (1972) Does asymptomatic lead exposure in children have latent sequelae? J Pediatrics 81(6):1088–1091

Dobosy JR and Selker EU (2001) Emerging connections between DNA methylation and histone acetylation. Cell Mol Life Sci 58:721–727

Fowler BA, Whittaker MH, Lipsky M, Wang G, Chen XQ (2004) Oxidative stress induced by lead, cadmium and arsenic mixtures: 30-day, 90-day, and 180-day drinking water studies in rats: an overview. Biometals 17(5–6):567–568

Galic MA, Riazi K, Heida JG, Mouihate A, Fournier NM, Spencer SJ, Kalynchuk LE, Teskey GC, Pittman QJ (2008) Postnatal inflammation increases seizure susceptibility in adult rats. J Neurosci 28(27):6904–6913

Ge Y-W, Maloney B, Alley GM, Lahiri DK (2007) Important differences between human and mouse APOE gene promoters: implications in Alzheimer's Disease. J Neurochem 103(3):1237–1257

Gmitterova K, Heinemann U, Gawinecka J, Varges D, Ciesielczyk B, Valkovic P, Benetin J, Zerr I (2009) 8-OHdG in cerebrospinal fluid as a marker of oxidative stress in various neurodegenerative diseases. Neurodegener Dis 6(5–6):263–269

Hall K, Murrell J, Ogunniyi A, Deeg M, Baiyewu O, Gao S, Gureje O, Dickens J, Evans R, Smith-Gamble V, Unverzagt FW, Shen J, Hendrie H (2006) Cholesterol, APOE genotype, and Alzheimer disease: an epidemiologic study of Nigerian Yoruba. Neurology 66(2):223–227

Hamilton ML, Van Remmen H, Drake JA, Yang H, Guo ZM, Kewitt K, Walter CA, Richardson A (2001) Does oxidative damage to DNA increase with age? Proc Natl Acad Sci U S A 98(18):10469–10474

Hebert LE, Scherr PA, Bienias JL, Bennett DA, Evans DA (2003) Alzheimer disease in the US population: prevalence estimates using the 2000 census. Arch Neurol 60(8):1119–1122

Herms J, Anliker B, Heber S, Ring S, Fuhrmann M, Kretzschmar H, Sisodia S, Muller U (2004) Cortical dysplasia resembling human type 2 lissencephaly in mice lacking all three APP family members. EMBO J 23(20):4106–4115
Hughes LA, Van Den Brandt PA, de Bruine AP, Wouters KA, Hulsmans S, Spiertz A, Goldbohm RA, de Goeij AF, Herman JG, Weijenberg MP, van Engeland M (2009) Early life exposure to famine and colorectal cancer risk: a role for epigenetic mechanisms. PLoS One 4(11):e7951
Kikuchi Y, Yasuhara T, Agari T, Kondo A, Kuramoto S, Kameda M, Kadota T, Baba T, Tajiri N, Wang F, Tayra JT, Hanbai L, Miyoshi Y, Borlongan CV, Date I (2010) Urinary 8-OHdG elevations in a partial lesion rat model of Parkinson's disease correlate with behavioral symptoms and nigrostriatal dopaminergic depletion. J Cell Physiol. doi:10.1002/jcp.22467
Kivipelto M and Solomon A (2008) Alzheimer's disease—the ways of prevention. J Nutr Health Aging 12(1):89S–94S
Knudson AG Jr (1971) Mutation and cancer: statistical study of retinoblastoma. Proc Natl Acad Sci U S A 68(4):820–823
Lahiri DK, Chen D, Ge YW, Bondy SC, Sharman EH (2004) Dietary supplementation with melatonin reduces levels of amyloid beta-peptides in the murine cerebral cortex. J Pineal Res 36(4):224–231
Lahiri DK, Farlow MR, Sambamurti K, Greig NH, Giacobini E, Schneider LS (2003) A critical analysis of new molecular targets and strategies for drug developments in Alzheimer's disease. Curr Drug Targets 4(2):97–112
Lahiri DK and Maloney B (2006) Genes are not our destiny: the somatic epitype bridges between the genotype and the phenotype. Nat Rev Neurosci 7. doi:10.1038/nrn2022-c1
Lahiri DK, Maloney B, Basha MR, Ge YW, Zawia NH (2007) How and when environmental agents and dietary factors affect the course of Alzheimer's disease: the "LEARn" model (Latent Early Associated Regulation) may explain the triggering of AD. Curr Alzheimer Res 4(2):219–228
Lahiri DK, Maloney B, Zawia NH (2009) The LEARn model: an epigenetic explanation for idiopathic neurobiological diseases. Mol Psychiatry 14(11):992–1003. doi:mp200982 [pii] 10.1038/mp.2009.82
Lahiri DK, Wavrant De-Vrieze F, Ge Y-W, Maloney B, Hardy J (2005) Characterization of two APP gene promoter polymorphisms that appear to influence risk of late-onset Alzheimer's disease. Neurobiol Aging 26(10):1329–1341
Levenson VV (2010) DNA methylation as a universal biomarker. Expert Rev Mol Diagn 10(4):481–488
Lu T, Pan Y, Kao SY, Li C, Kohane I, Chan J, Yankner BA (2004) Gene regulation and DNA damage in the ageing human brain. Nature 429(6994):883–891
Mastroeni D, Coleman PD, Grover A, Sue L, McKee A, Rogers J (2009a) Differential DNA methylation in neurons of identical twins discordant for Alzheimer's disease. Alzheimers Dement 5:p 145
Mastroeni D, McKee A, Grover A, Rogers J, Coleman PD (2009b) Epigenetic differences in cortical neurons from a pair of monozygotic twins discordant for Alzheimer's disease. PLoS One 4(8):e6617
Murgatroyd C, Patchev AV, Wu Y, Micale V, Bockmuhl Y, Fischer D, Holsboer F, Wotjak CT, Almeida OF, Spengler D (2009) Dynamic DNA methylation programs persistent adverse effects of early-life stress. Nat Neurosci 12(12):1559–1566
Nakajima T, Enomoto S, Yamashita S, Ando T, Nakanishi Y, Nakazawa K, Oda I, Gotoda T, Ushijima T (2010) Persistence of a component of DNA methylation in gastric mucosa after Helicobacter pylori eradication. J Gastroenterol 45(1):37–44
Paschos K, Smith P, Anderton E, Middeldorp JM, White RE, Allday MJ (2009) Epstein-barr virus latency in B cells leads to epigenetic repression and CpG methylation of the tumour suppressor gene Bim. PLoS Pathog 5(6):e1000492
Plassman BL, Langa KM, Fisher GG, Heeringa SG, Weir DR, Ofstedal MB, Burke JR, Hurd MD, Potter GG, Rodgers WL, Steffens DC, Willis RJ, Wallace RB (2007) Prevalence of dementia in the United States: the aging, demographics, and memory study. Neuroepidemiology 29(1–2):125–132

Sambamurti K, Suram A, Venugopal C, Prakasam A, Zhou Y, Lahiri DK, Greig NH (2006) A partial failure of membrane protein turnover may cause Alzheimer's disease: a new hypothesis. Curr Alzheimer Res 3(1):81–90

Takiguchi M, Achanzar WE, Qu W, Li G, Waalkes MP (2003) Effects of cadmium on DNA-(Cytosine-5) methyltransferase activity and DNA methylation status during cadmium-induced cellular transformation. Exp Cell Res 286(2):355–365

Valinluck V, Tsai HH, Rogstad DK, Burdzy A, Bird A, Sowers LC (2004) Oxidative damage to methyl-CpG sequences inhibits the binding of the methyl-CpG binding domain (MBD) of methyl-CpG binding protein 2 (MeCP2). Nucl Acids Res 32(14):4100–4108

Van Vliet J, Oates NA, Whitelaw E (2007) Epigenetic mechanisms in the context of complex diseases. Cell Mol Life Sci 64(12):1531–1538

Whitelaw NC, Whitelaw E (2006) How lifetimes shape epigenotype within and across generations. Hum Mol Genet 15(1):R131–137

Wu J, Basha MR, Brock B, Cox DP, Cardozo-Pelaez F, McPherson CA, Harry J, Rice DC, Maloney B, Chen D, Lahiri DK, Zawia NH (2008) Alzheimer's disease (AD)-like pathology in aged monkeys after infantile exposure to environmental metal lead (Pb): evidence for a developmental origin and environmental link for AD. J Neurosci 28(1):3–9

Zeh JA, Zeh DW (2008) Maternal inheritance, epigenetics and the evolution of polyandry. Genetica 134:45–54

Zhang S, Barros SP, Niculescu MD, Moretti AJ, Preisser JS, Offenbacher S (2010) Alteration of PTGS2 promoter methylation in chronic periodontitis. J Dent Res 89(2):133–137

Alzheimer's Association (2012) Alzheimer's disease facts and figures. Alzheimer's & Dementia 8(2):14-15

Notice of Violation (2010) Notice of violation of the safe drinking water and toxic enforcement act of 1986 (proposition 65), section 25249.6 of the California health and safety code, for exposing consumers of apple juice, grape juice, packaged peaches, packaged pears, and fruit cocktail to lead. http://www.envirolaw.org/documents/100609-NoticeLetterwithExhibits.PDF. Accessed 11 June 2010

Chapter 6
The Importance of the Environment in Brain Aging: Be Happy, Live Longer!

Mónica De la Fuente and Lorena Arranz

Abstract The prevalence of age-related neurodegenerative disorders in the elderly has dramatically increased in parallel to life expectancy and social aging. This demands development of effective therapeutic/preventive interventions aimed to slow down the negative effects of aging and extend health-span. Here, we overview the mechanisms underlying brain aging in the context of the oxi-inflamm-aging theory, and discuss cutting edge promising findings opening up the possibility to reverse brain and physiological aging based on environmental enrichment. The enriched environment (EE) represents an experimental approach in animal models to an active social, mental and physical life-style in humans. Interaction with the EE provides the animals with a diversion from the monotonous and thus stressful cage life. Most important, maintenance of life-long "diversion" by means of EE extends lifespan in mice. This sighting confirms the great influence of life-style upon brain aging, and suggests that the "happier" we are, the longer we might live in good health.

Keywords Aging • Brain • Environmental enrichment • Longevity extension • Neuro-immune-endocrine communication

6.1 Introduction—Why does the Brain Age?

According to the World Health Organization projections, life expectancy in western countries will continue its increasing trend of three months per year during the next years. The news that we are living longer is indeed positive. However, nowadays advanced age is often accompanied by chronic disease and neurodegenerative disorders that limit quality of life. Taking this into consideration, longer disabled life might not be such good news after all. Therefore, interventions that can either slow

---

M. De la Fuente (✉) · L. Arranz
Departamento de Fisiología (Fisiología Animal II), Facultad de Ciencias Biológicas, Universidad Complutense, 28040 Madrid, España
e-mail: mondelaf@bio.ucm.es

M. K. Thakur, S. I. S. Rattan (eds.), *Brain Aging and Therapeutic Interventions*,
DOI 10.1007/978-94-007-5237-5_6,

or reverse the negative effects of aging would have major benefits for individuals and societies, as they promise to open the way for increasing health-span—that is, the number of years in healthy, active life.

Aging is associated with progressive loss of function across multiple systems, remarkably the regulatory systems namely the nervous, endocrine and immune systems. Functions of the nervous system especially affected by aging are sensation, cognition, memory and motor activity. Notably, cognitive decline has emerged as one of the greatest health threats of old age, with nearly 50 % of adults over the age of 85 afflicted with Alzheimer's disease (AD) (Hebert et al. 2003). In this scenario, the oldest-old humans represent by contrast a population relatively resistant to degenerative brain processes (von Gunten et al. 2010). Moreover, brain functionality, in terms of cognition and behavior, is also better preserved in mice that achieve exceptional longevity (Kinney-Forshee et al. 2004; Sun and Bartke 2007).

In an attempt to understand the neuronal mechanisms underlying normal and pathological brain aging, the neurobiology of aging has been one of the most rapidly expanding areas of scientific endeavor over the past two decades. Now, it is widely believed that the cause of brain aging is that underlying the overall process of aging—that is, the chronic oxidative stress leading to progressive damage of biomolecules (Rattan 2008; De la Fuente and Miquel 2009). Accumulation of damage ultimately gives rise to the age-related decline in physiological functions, including the nervous function (Muller et al. 2007; De la Fuente 2008). Thus, oxidative stress plays a crucial role in the age-associated cognitive decline as well as in the neuronal loss occurring in neurodegenerative diseases like AD (Markesbery 1997).

The hippocampus, structure of the central nervous system (CNS) with high degree of flexibility and adaptation as regards neurogenesis, is clearly affected by this age-related oxidative stress. Thereby neurogenesis is impaired and this explains the learning and cognitive deterioration in aged subjects (Couillard-Despres et al. 2011). Moreover, hippocampal neurogenesis alterations may contribute to increasing stress-related disorders in old age (Kozorovitskiy and Gould 2004; Sairanen et al. 2005). However, in contrast to neurodegenerative diseases, the cognitive decline in 'normal aging' seems not to be associated with a significant loss of neurons (Gallagher et al. 1996), suggesting that the only difference between healthy and pathological aging might be the rate/degree of oxidation. Importantly, several strategies have been shown to be effective for slowing down this degree of oxidation and thereby extend longevity in experimental animals, for instance caloric restriction (Barja 2002), and more recently, maintained exposure to environmental enrichment (Arranz et al. 2010a).

6.2 Oxidative Stress as a Basis of Brain Aging

The age-related damage caused by oxidative stress is due to a progressive imbalance between endogenous antioxidant and oxidant compounds (De la Fuente 2008; De la Fuente and Miquel 2009). As regards antioxidant defenses, a variety of studies show decreased content and/or activity in the aging brain. Glutathione (GSH) is the principal intracellular non-protein thiol and plays a major role in preservation of the intracellular redox state in most cells, tissues and organs, including brain (Dröge 2002). Low GSH content, GSH : GSSG (oxidized form) ratio and/or GSH-related enzymes have been described with increasing age in all mammalian brain regions studied, including the hippocampus (Calabrese et al. 2004; Balu et al. 2005; Donahue et al. 2006; Zhu et al. 2006; Singh et al. 2011). Superoxide dismutase (SOD) and catalase (CAT) are two protective enzymes that function in close association for detoxification of highly reactive free radicals (Barber and Harris 1994). SOD provides the first line of defense against reactive oxygen species by scavenging superoxide radicals to H_2O_2. Subsequently, CAT catalyzes the conversion of H_2O_2 into H_2O and O_2. Both SOD and CAT activities diminish with aging in the brain (Navarro and Boveris 2004; Singh et al. 2011).

Additionally, neuronal membranes are especially sensitive to damage by hydroxyl radicals, given that they are densely packed with proteins and polyunsaturated fatty acids. Ultimately, this could lead to reduction in the number of nerve cells (Morrison and Hof 1997) and increase of pigment lipofuscin, free radicals, and oxidative damage markers in neuronal and glial cells (Mark et al. 1997). Indeed, the age-related increase in oxidative brain damage is best exemplified by products of lipid peroxidation (Calabrese et al. 2004; Zhu et al. 2006) and protein oxidation (Sigueira et al. 2005; Poon et al. 2006). For instance, an increase in protein carbonyl levels has been demonstrated for several brain regions including the hippocampus (Sigueira et al. 2005). In contrast, we found lower double bound and peroxidizability indexes in the brain of long-lived animals when compared to old specimens, whereas protein oxidative markers of damage in brain from adult and long-lived animals showed similar levels (Arranz et al. 2012).

Age-related oxidative modifications have also been found in nuclear and mitochondrial DNA (Hamilton et al. 2001). Gene expression studies of brain aging in mice, rats, chimpanzees and humans confirm an age-dependent upregulation of oxidative stress-response genes (Hasty et al. 2003; Longo and Finch 2003; Yankner et al. 2008). Moreover, genes that mediate oxidative stress responses constitute the largest class of genes upregulated in the aging human prefrontal cortex (Lu et al. 2004). In this regard, Lu et al. (2004) showed that aging of the human cortex is characterised by reduced expression of genes that mediate synaptic plasticity, including NMDA and AMPA receptor function, calcium-mediated signaling, and synaptic vesicle release and recycling. This gene silencing was correlated with age-dependent DNA damage to the promoters of these genes. Of note, the young adult and extreme aged human populations are relatively homogeneous in their gene expression patterns in the prefrontal cortex. However, the middle age population between 40 and 70 years of age exhibits much greater heterogeneity. Thus, individuals may diverge in their rates of aging as they transit through middle age, approaching a state of 'old age' at different rates (Lu et al. 2004). Furthermore, recent studies show that DNA damage can induce changes in histone modification patterns and thereby in gene expression through SIRT1 (Oberdoerffer et al. 2008; O'Hagan et al. 2008), a conserved lifespan regulatory gene linking oxidative stress and epigenomics.

Mitochondria play a key role in aging, given that they are main sources of oxygen radicals and presumably the major targets of ROS (Miquel et al. 1980). Mitochondrial DNA is particularly vulnerable to oxidative damage, showing a more than tenfold greater mutation rate than nuclear DNA (Dröge and Schipper 2007). Mutated mitochondrial DNA may code for abnormal cytochromes and cause infidelity of the electron transport chain associated with increased superoxide radical production. Additionally, a decrease in the activity of cytochrome c oxidase and glutathione in synaptic mitochondria has been observed in the brain of aged mice (Ferrandiz et al. 1994). Ultimately, this would give rise to a vicious cycle of progressively increasing oxidative stress (Sastre et al. 2003; Viña et al. 2003). Moreover, accumulation of peroxidation products in mitochondria leads to a decrease in ATP production and compromises the maintenance of cellular homeodynamics (Chance et al. 1979). Mitochondrial dysfunction and mitochondria-derived ROS have been involved in both normal brain aging and neurodegenerative diseases (Toescu and Verkhratsky 2003; Lin and Beal 2006). In the mammalian CNS, cellular senescence is often associated with the accumulation of mitochondria-derived cytoplasmic inclusions such as Gomori-positive glial granules and corpora amylacea (Brunk and Terman 2002; Schipper 2004).

Taken together, oxidative damage accumulates in the aging brain and in areas such as the hippocampus is crucial for the age-related impairment in cognition and memory, both essential for preservation of life-quality in humans. Moreover, the brain does not function in isolation but closely related to other regulatory systems, such as the immune and endocrine systems (De la Fuente 2008).

6.3 Homedynamic Decay: Neuro-Immune-Endocrine Disruption During Aging

As mentioned by Rattan (2008), senescence and death are the final manifestations of age-related failure of the homeodynamic machinery. Age-related changes occur not only in the nervous function but also affect the other regulatory systems involved in homeodynamics, i.e. the endocrine and the immune systems, as well as the communication among them. This is responsible for homeodynamic capacity loss and results ultimately in age-related increased morbidity and mortality (De la Fuente and Miquel 2009).

Now we know that the three regulatory systems are intimately linked and interdependent. There is a "neuroendocrine-immune" system that coordinates homeodynamics and thereby preserves health (Besedovsky and Del Rey 2007). The communication among these systems allows understanding of why depression, emotional stress and anxiety are accompanied by greater vulnerability to infections, cancers and autoimmune diseases in humans (Arranz et al. 2007, 2009; Costa-Pinto and Palermo-Nieto 2010). In mice, our research group has shown that animals exhibiting excess reactivity to stress and chronic anxiety suffer accelerated immune senescence and also die prematurely (Guayerbas et al. 2002a, b; Guayerbas and De la Fuente 2003).

Consequences of the aging immune system are decreased resistance to infections and increased autoimmune processes and cancer. These features are indicative of a less competent immune system and exert a great influence on the age-related morbidity and mortality as mentioned above (Wayne et al. 1990; High 2004; De la Fuente and Miquel 2009). In fact, the increased death rate found in older adult humans is due, at least in part, to an increase in the incidence of infections (Castle et al. 2007). Although there are contradictory results on the impact of aging upon the immune response, it is presently accepted that almost every component of the immune system undergoes striking age-associated re-structuring, leading to changes that may include enhanced as well as diminished functions (De la Fuente and Miquel 2009). This process is overall termed immunosenescence (Pawelec et al. 2002).

Nowadays it is becoming clear that these alterations to the immune system can interfere in the function of the nervous system. Age-related peripheral chronic inflammation has been described to influence central glial cells, leading to neuroinflammation, which in areas such as the hippocampus plays a key role in the cognitive decline associated to the aging process and age-related diseases such as AD (von Bernhardi 2007). Interestingly, both humans and mice who achieve longevity have been shown to preserve a low peripheral chronic inflammatory status (De Martinis et al. 2005, 2006; Arranz et al. 2010b).

Moreover, peripheral T and B cells enter the normal brain in low numbers and carry out functional activities, whereas recent data from our research group point to a differential affectation of both cell types in old and long-lived mice (Arranz et al. 2010c, d). T cells are also thought to contribute to the pathogenesis of AD (Marx et al. 1998). More recently, Stichel and Luebbert (2007) have suggested that progressive accumulation of T lymphocytes during normal aging in brain areas such as the hippocampus might have a great impact on the progressive cognitive impairment that occurs with aging. T cells locate preferably in perivascular areas, indicative of recruitment from systemic sources, and the T cell load is different depending on the brain area considered, which suggests a selective entry (Stichel and Luebbert 2007).

Several changes accompany aging of the endocrine system, including for example decrease of growth hormone/insulin-like factor-1 axis (somatopause) and sexual hormones, i.e. estradiol (menopause), testosterone (andropause) and dehydroepiandrosterone (adrenopause) (Makrantonaki et al. 2010). Moreover, age-related disturbances of the hypothalamic-pituitary-adrenal (HPA) axis are responsible for decreased stress adaptability in old subjects, which contributes importantly to health impairment (Lupien et al. 2009).

It is obviously difficult to determine whether this age-related deterioration of the nervous, endocrine and immune systems occurs simultaneously or starts in one of them and thereby spreads to the others. In the past, the age-related changes in the communication among the homeodynamic systems were proposed as the main cause for physiological senescence (Fabris 1990). Although this is still an open question, more recently we have proposed that the age-related impairment of the immune system could affect the functions of the other regulatory systems through increased oxidative and inflammatory stress (De la Fuente and Miquel 2009). Whatsoever, another key question arises: could we take advantage of this strong communication among regulatory systems to reverse aging damage?

6.4 The Environment Counts! Beneficial Effects of Enriched Environment on Brain and Neuro-Immune-Endocrine Aging

Environmental enrichment (EE) is a good experimental approach in animal models to understand the effect of maintenance of an active social, mental and physical life in humans. The most common EE protocol in rodents is grouped housing using large cages with a variety of objects (running wheels, tunnels, ladders, etc) and spatial configurations, which are changed frequently. This more complex housing induces sensory, cognitive, motor and social stimulation (Nithianantharajan and Hannan 2006). The continual exposure to new objects enables the animals to acquire sensory and cognitive experiences (van Praag et al. 2000). Notably, when facing novel stressful situations, animals living under enriched conditions show reduced escape-related behaviors (Zambrana et al. 2007), which could be considered adaptive and indicative of improved ability to cope with stress. From this point of view, the EE could be interpreted as a hormetic intervention, in which animals are constantly exposed to novelty, abundant sensorial stimulation, and thus mild-stress. Indeed, hormesis stimulates maintenance and repair systems and strengthens the homeodynamic space of organisms (Rattan 2010), improving adaptation and thereby slowing down the effects of aging. Availability of running wheels, ropes, ladders, tunnels or bridges allows exercising, and housing in relatively large cages in groups of typically 6–12 animals facilitates social interaction (Pham et al. 2002). The EE represents thus a joyful and stimulating habitat as opposed to the regular monotonous housing.

These environments enriched in intellectual and/or physical activities have been reported to reverse many of the adverse effects of the aging process on the nervous system at the neural, cognitive and behavioral level (Mattson et al. 2001; Segovia et al. 2006, 2009; Zambrana et al. 2007). Moreover, EE reduces brain pathology and improves cognition and behavioral responses in a variety of murine models for age-related neurodegenerative diseases such as AD (Arendash et al. 2004; Lazarov et al. 2005; Görtz et al. 2008).

Animals exposed to EE show numerous differences when compared to animals living in standard housing (van Praag et al. 2000) such as upregulation of adult neurogenesis specific to the hippocampus (Brown et al. 2003), the brain structure critical for learning and affectivity. Among the reported behavioral effects of EE, improvements in learning and memory are remarkable (Nilsson et al. 1999; Bruel-

Jungerman et al. 2005), in addition to decreased emotional reactivity by means of anxiety-like behaviors (Roy et al. 2001). However, Meshi et al. (2006) demonstrated that the effects of EE on spatial learning, habituation to an unfamiliar environment, and conflict-based anxiety do not require adult hippocampal neurogenesis. The authors proposed upregulation of growth factors such as brain-derived neurotrophic factor, as well as morphological changes such as increased dendritic branching and synaptogenesis (van Praag et al. 2000) as plausible candidate mechanisms.

In this regard, a more recent study demonstrated the importance of the epigenetic status in the control of brain neuronal gene expression underlying synaptic plasticity and memory. Fischer et al. (2007) used a mouse model in which inducible expression of p25, regulator of cyclin-dependent kinase 5, elicits neurodegeneration. Transient expression of p25 in adult mice resulted in certain degree of neurodegeneration and synapse loss in the hippocampus, together with memory loss. EE promoted the recovery of lost memories, accompanied by increased synaptic plasticity and the induction of activating histone acetylation marks. These findings highlight the role of epigenetic changes in memory loss associated with neurodegeneration, and suggest that loss of memory storage is distinct from loss of neural pathways that access stored memory (Fisher et al. 2007). Given that human brain aging is characterised by memory loss and reduced synaptic connectivity but no significant neuronal loss, it is likely that loss of ability to access stored memories underlies age-dependent memory deficits (Bishop et al. 2010). If this is so, life-style strategies affecting the epigenetic landscape could ameliorate the cognitive deficits associated with aging and neurodegenerative disorders.

As mentioned above, research on stress in older adults has shown that chronic stress mimics, exacerbates, and possibly accelerates the effects of aging on immunity (Hawkley and Cacioppo 2004). Additionally stress-related emotional responses are exacerbated in aged subjects (Zambrana et al. 2007). Interaction with the EE provides animals with a diversion from the monotonous and thus stressful cage life, resulting in lower HPA axis activity, in terms of adrenocorticotropic hormone and corticosterone levels, both in baseline conditions and after mild stress (Belz et al. 2003). Our group has confirmed that the improvement of emotional responses after short-term (5–8 weeks) EE exposure reported by several authors (Benaroya-Milshtein et al. 2004) is more marked in aged subjects (Zambrana et al. 2007). In parallel, we have shown that short-term (8–16 weeks) exposure to EE exerts a great influence on immunity, leading to a striking improvement of leukocyte functions and decreased oxidative stress affecting immune cells, especially in animals at older ages, in which the age-related immune deterioration is more marked (Arranz et al. 2010a). This scenario strongly supports the proposal that EE-related neuroendocrine improvements underlie improvement of the age-related immune changes exerted by EE exposure. Thus, basic research on experimental animals demonstrates the importance of maintaining active mental and/or physical activity to preserve health and life quality in terms of immunity and neuroendocrine responses with aging. EE might be providing a clue for healthy overall aging: "happiness". In humans, negative emotions are intimately linked to the initiation and/or progression of cancer, HIV, cardiovascular disease, and autoimmune disorders (Barak 2006).

However, effects of positive emotions, especially "happiness", on physiological parameters and immunity have received very little attention. The specific physiological responses induced by pleasant stimuli were recently investigated with the immune and endocrine systems being monitored when pleasant stimuli such as odors and emotional pictures were presented to subjects. The results revealed that pleasant emotions induce changes such as increase in secretory immunoglobulin A and decrease in salivary cortisol (Barak 2006). Then, could positive emotions delay or even avoid the onset of disease in humans? Could "happiness" help us preserve our health during aging and extend our lifespan?

6.5 A Magnetic Resonance Imaging Study of Enriched Environment and the Aging Brain

Magnetic resonance imaging (MRI) is a non-invasive method that allows the characterisation and evaluation of neuropathological lesions that are involved in human and other species, brain aging and diseases such as AD. In humans, MRI can help discriminate between AD and normal aging based on the degree of cerebral atrophy (Murphy et al. 1992; Tien et al. 1993). When using T2-weighted images (T2WI) on a high-field MR unit, low signal intensity in the nuclei of the extra pyramidal system has been described in humans. In adults, prominently low signal intensity has been reported in the substantia nigra, pallidum, red nucleus, and dentate nucleus. The putamen shows intermediate intensity levels, whereas the thalamus and caudate nucleus exhibit the highest intensities (Drayer et al. 1986; Chen et al. 1989; Schenker et al. 1993). In the elderly brain, the hypointense structures are the same, but their intensities are lower than in young adults (Drayer et al. 1986). Moreover, variations of the normal intensity pattern of the brain measured by MRI are sometimes associated with degenerative disorders (Bartzokis et al. 1994).

We have recently studied the age-related changes in brain morphology by MRI in mice, including animals that had achieved exceptional longevity, and determined the effects of EE on those changes. ICR (CD1) female mice of different ages at the time of the study, namely adult (44±4 weeks), old (69±4 weeks), very old (92 ±4 weeks) and extreme long-lived (125±4 weeks), were used. They were housed in cages under standard or EE conditions (16–18 weeks) (Arranz et al. 2010a). The animals were subjected to MRI for the study of the T2WI signal intensity and T2 relaxation times of relevant brain areas, and cerebrospinal fluid was also evaluated.

Hyperintense areas in the T2WI images, which represent brain atrophy, were more pronounced in animals at older ages, including long-lived mice (Fig. 6.1). These hyperintense areas were less evident in enriched than in control animals. Among all brain regions studied, entorhinal cortex was found to be primarily affected in very old mice ($p<0.01$ vs. old controls), whereas cerebral deterioration in the long-lived seemed to initiate in somatosensory cortex ($p=0.061$ vs. adult controls). Both brain areas were better preserved in the enriched groups. Thus, very old en-

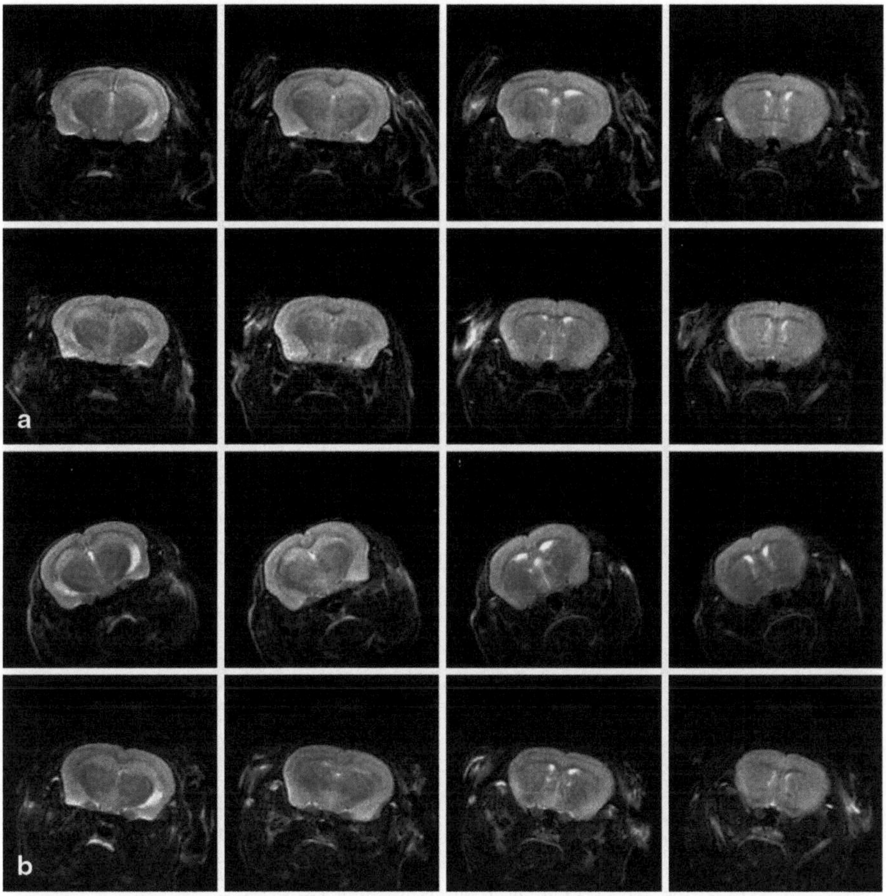

Fig. 6.1 Hyper intense areas are more pronounced in animals at older ages than in the adults. T2-weighted with fat suppression coronal images for four contiguous brain slices of two adult (**a**) and two long-lived (**b**) ICR/CD1 female mice. Bright areas of high intensity signal correspond to cerebrospinal fluid and represent brain atrophy

riched mice showed similar T2 relaxation times in entorhinal cortex to old controls and a trend towards higher T2 values as compared to adult controls ($p=0.098$) in somatosensory cortex (Table 6.1).

In view of these results, mice that naturally achieve longevity exhibit brain morphological changes in different areas in comparison with younger old animals. Although this is a preliminary study which should be confirmed in future work increasing the sample numbers to improve the statistical power of the present data, it is of great interest considering that, using a similar technique, entorhinal cortex has been described to be the most affected area within the hippocampal formation in patients of AD as compared to healthy humans (Small et al. 2000). Taken together, generally old but not the long-lived would suffer from a decline in memory abilities

Table 6.1 T2 relaxation times (ms) in several brain areas of control and environmentally enriched (EE) adult, old, very old and long-lived ICR/CD1 female mice

T2 (ms)	Adult		Old		Very old		Long-lived
	Control	EE	Control	EE	Control	EE	Control
CC	66.18±1.70	68.72±1.68	64.69±2.12	66.63±0.32	65.48±0.97	69.60±1.83	62.37±4.34
Amg	72.61±1.55	71.38±2.00	75.78±1.69	68.44±1.61	72.33±1.76	70.02±5.41	71.33±4.28
Hip1	63.82±1.22	67.36±1.87	67.80±1.71	67.71±3.10	61.07±2.66	68.30±1.50	64.30±4.81
Hip2	64.74±1.43	67.64±3.24	70.10±1.65	71.91±3.02	67.27±1.39	72.24±1.76	69.55±7.49
Hip3	67.03±1.09	68.70±1.71	67.79±1.76	65.97±1.97	69.19±0.83	70.46±3.96	61.61±4.66
EtrC	69.14±2.03	72.81±1.81	76.99±1.30**	70.26±2.22	65.51±1.22**	78.05±3.41	72.32±3.14
SSC	67.09±1.08*†	68.35±2.19	65.52±2.06	65.71±1.73	65.63±0.76	74.79±1.32†	60.64±3.33*
MC	68.12±1.13	70.24±1.90	67.64±2.69	68.14±1.07	68.23±0.97	73.78±2.07	62.39±4.38

The mean±standard error of 4–16 values corresponding to that number of animals is shown (14–16 adults; 5 old; 4–5 very old; 6 long-lived). Very old controls showed significant lower T2 values than old controls in EtrC ($^{**}p<0.01$), whereas long-lived mice showed a trend towards decreased T2 values in SSC as compared to the adults ($^{*}p=0.061$). By contrast, very old enriched animals had similar T2 values to old controls in EtrC and a trend towards higher T2 values than the adults in SSC ($^{\dagger}p=0.098$). *CC* cingulate cortex, *Amg* amygdala, *Hip1, 2, 3* hippocampus (slice1, 2, 3), *EtrC* entorhinal cortex, *SSC* somatosensory cortex, and *MC* motor cortex and proneness to AD-like dementia. Long-lived mice would in contrast be primarily affected in learning behaviors, which are integrated in the somatosensory cortex.

In addition, the present results suggest that T2WI hyperintense areas (high T2 relaxation time areas), which correspond to cerebrospinal fluid and indicate cerebral atrophy (Murphy et al. 1992), are more pronounced in aged than in adult mice, which confirm previous work in humans and mouse lemurs (Murphy et al. 1992; Dhenain et al. 1997). Moreover, according to our data, accumulation of cerebrospinal fluid also occurs in the brain of long-lived mice, suggesting that moderate cerebral atrophy accompanies both normal and healthy aging. Similar results have been described for healthy humans of 66–96 years of age (Coffey et al. 1998). The physiological consequences of this atrophy deserve future research, but should not be major given that they do not prevent achieving longevity. Besides, our results show a trend towards lower atrophy in enriched animals than in non-enriched controls, especially as regards the most affected areas in old and long-lived mice, this is the hippocampus and the somatosensory cortex, respectively. The T2 decline in entorhinal cortex from very old mice as compared to younger mice is reversed by the enriched environment. These data are in agreement with previous published work on the improvement in the age-related impairment in cognition when animals are exposed to EE (Mattson et al. 2001; Segovia et al. 2006, 2009; Mora et al. 2007), since the most benefitted cerebral areas seem to be those associated to learning and memory abilities.

In conclusion, differential age-related brain morphological changes in old and long-lived mice could contribute to different susceptibility and/or development of age-related brain dysfunction. EE stands out as a useful strategy to improve these age-related changes in brain morphology.

6.6 Conclusions: Be Happy, Live Longer?

Indeed, the positive effects of the EE are manifested by many molecular, cellular and functional modifications, leading to an overall improvement in the physiological and physical well being of experimental animals even under short-term exposure. Most important, our research group has shown that long-term exposure of mice to EE significantly extends their lifespan (Arranz et al. 2010a). Moreover, we have demonstrated that the only strategy efficient in improving longevity is exposure to the EE from adulthood and prolonged until natural death.

Importantly, longitudinal studies in human centenarians have shown lifelong preserved immunity as a marker of longevity (De la Rosa et al. 2006; Alonso-Fernández et al. 2008; Alonso-Fernández and De la Fuente 2011) and cross-sectional studies in naturally long-living mice have reproduced these results (Puerto et al. 2005; De la Fuente and Miquel 2009; Arranz et al. 2010c). Likewise, as mentioned above, our research group has shown that mice exhibiting intrinsic excess reactivity to stress and chronic anxiety suffer accelerated immune senescence and die prematurely (Guayerbas et al. 2002a, b; Guayerbas and De la Fuente 2003; Viveros et al.

2007). Similarly, negative emotions, depression, emotional stress and anxiety are intimately linked to the initiation and/or progression of cancer, infections, cardiovascular disease, and autoimmune disorders in humans (Barak 2006; Arranz et al. 2007, 2009; Costa-Pinto and Palermo-Nieto 2010).

Taken together, although short-term EE is enough for health and life quality improvements, the active life should be initiated at early stages of the aging process and preserved until death to improve lifespan. Lifelong well-preserved immunity as well as emotional responses are likely to underlie lifespan extension by long-term EE exposure. This sighting confirms the great influence of life-style upon brain and physiological aging, and suggests that the "happier" we are, the longer we might live in good health.

Acknowledgments This work was supported by the Spanish Ministry of Science and Innovation (BFU2008–04336, BFU2011–30336) and Ministry of Health (RETICEF, RD06/0013/003), and Research Group of UCM (910379). The authors would like to thank the CAI of Nuclear Magnetic Resonance and Electron Spin of the UCM, especially to Mª Encarnación Fernández and David Castejón for their technical support. Additional thanks to Nuria M. De Castro and Ianire Maté for helpful assistance, and José Regidor for technical advice.

References

Alonso-Fernández P, Puerto M, Maté I, Ribera JM, De la Fuente M (2008) Neutrophils of centenarians show function levels similar to those of young adults. J Am Geriatr Soc 56:2244–2251

Alonso-Fernández P, De la Fuente M (2011) Role of the immune system in aging and longevity. Curr Aging Sci 4:78–100

Arendash GW, Garcia MF, Costa DA, Cracchiolo JR, Wefes IM, Potter H (2004) Environmental enrichment improves cognition in aged Alzheimer's transgenic mice despite stable beta-amyloid deposition. Neuroreport 15:1751–1754

Arranz L, Guayerbas N, De la Fuente M (2007) Impairment of several immune functions in anxious women. J Psychosom Res 62:1–8

Arranz L, De Vicente A, Muñoz M, De la Fuente M (2009) Impairment of immune function in the social excluded homeless population. Neuroimmunomodulation 16:251–260

Arranz L, De Castro NM, Baeza I, Maté I, Viveros MP, De la Fuente M (2010a) Environmental enrichment improves age-related immune system impairment. Long-term exposure since adulthood increases life span in mice. Rejuvenation Res 13:415–428

Arranz L, Lord JM, De la Fuente M (2010b) Preserved ex vivo inflammatory status and cytokine responses in naturally long-lived mice. Age (Dordr) 32:451–466

Arranz L, Caamaño JH, Lord JM, De la Fuente M (2010c) Preserved immune functions and controlled leukocyte oxidative stress in naturally long-lived mice: possible role of nuclear factor kappa B. J Gerontol A Biol Sci Med Sci 65:941–950

Arranz L, De Castro NM, Baeza I, De la Fuente M (2010d) Differential expression of Toll-like receptor 2 and 4 on peritoneal leukocyte populations from long-lived and non-selected old female mice. Biogerontology 11:475–482

Arranz L, Naudí A, De la Fuente M, Pamplona R (2012) Exceptionally old mice are highly resistant to lipoxidation-derived molecular damage. Age (Dordr). doi: 10.1007/s11357–012-9391–0

Balu M, Sangeetha P, Murali G, Panneerselvam C (2005) Age-related oxidative protein damages in central nervous system of rats: modulatory role of grape seed extract. Int J Dev Neuroscience 23:501–507

Barak Y (2006) The immune system and happiness. Autoimmun Rev 5:523–527

Barber DA, Harris SR (1994) Oxygen free radicals and antioxidants: a review. Am Pharm 34:26–35

Barja G (2002) Endogenous oxidative stress: relationship to aging, longevity and caloric restriction. Aging Res Rev 1:397–411

Bartzokis G, Sultzer D, Mintz J, Holt LE, Marx P, Phelan CK, Marder SR (1994) In vivo evaluation of brain iron in Alzheimer's disease and normal subjects using MRI. Biol Psychiatry 35:480–487

Belz EE, Kennell JS, Czambel RK, Rubin RT, Rhodes ME (2003) Environmental enrichment lowers stress-responsive hormones in singly housed male and female rats. Pharmacol Biochem Behav 76:481–486

Benaroya-Milshtein N, Hollander N, Apter A, Kukulansky T, Raz N, Wilf A, Yaniv I, Pick CG (2004) Environmental enrichment in mice decreases anxiety, attenuates stress responses and enhances natural killer cell activity. Eur J Neurosci 20:1341–1347

Besedovsky HO, Del Rey A (2007) Physiology of psychoneuroimmunology: a personal view. Brain Behav Immun 21:34–44

Bishop NA, Lu T, Yankner BA (2010) Neural mechanisms of aging and cognitive decline. Nature 464:529–535

Brown J, Cooper-Kuhn CM, Kempermann G, Van Praag H, Winkler J, Gage FH, Kuhn HG (2003) Enriched environment and physical activity stimulate hippocampal but not olfactory bulb neurogenesis. Eur J Neurosci 17:2042–2046

Bruel-Jungerman E, Laroche S, Rampon C (2005) New neurons in the dentate gyrus are involved in the expression of enhanced long-term memory following environmental enrichment. Eur J Neurosci 21:513–521

Brunk UT, Terman A (2002) The mitochondrial-lysosomal axis theory of aging: accumulation of damaged mitrochondria as a result of imperfect autophagocytosis. Eur J Biochem 269:1996–2002

Calabrese V, Scapagnini G, Ravagna A, Colombrita C, Spadaro F, Butterfield DA, Guffrida Stella AM (2004) Increased expression of heat shock proteins in rat brain during aging: relationship with mitochondrial function and glutathione redox state. Mech Aging Dev 125:325–335

Castle SC, Uyemura K, Fulop T, Makinodan T (2007) Host resistance and immune responses in advanced age. Clin Geriatr Med 23:463–79

Chance B, Sies H, Boveris A (1979) Hydroperoxide metabolism in mammalian organs. Physiol Rev 59:527–605

Chen JC, Hardy PA, Clauberg M, Joshi JG, Parravano J, Deck JH, Henkelman RM, Becker LE, Kucharczyk W (1989) T2 values in the human brain: comparison with quantitative assays of iron and ferritin. Radiology 173:521–526

Coffey CE, Lucke JF, Saxton JA, Ratcliff G, Unitas LJ, Billig B, Bryan RN (1998) Sex differences in brain aging: a quantitative magnetic resonance imaging study. Arch Neurol 55:169–179

Costa-Pinto FA, Palermo-Nieto J (2010) Neuroimmune interactions in stress. Neuroimmunomodulation 17:196–199

Couillard-Despres S, Iglseder B, Aigner L (2011) Neurogenesis, cellular plasticity and cognition: the impact of stem cells in the adult and aging brain. Gerontology 57:559–564

De la Fuente M (2008) Role of neuroimmunomodulation in aging. Neuroimmunomodulation 15:213–223

De la Fuente M, Miquel J (2009) An update of the oxidation-inflammation theory of aging: the involvement of the immune systemin oxi-inflamm-aging. Curr Pharm Des 15:3003–3026

De Martinis M, Franceschi C, Monti D, Ginaldi L (2005) Inflamm-aging and lifelong antigenic load as major determinants of aging rate and longevity. FEBS Lett 579:2035–2039

De Martinis M, Franceschi C, Monti D, Ginaldi L (2006) Inflammation markers predicting frailty and mortality in the elderly. Exp Mol Pathol 80:219–227

De la Rosa O, Pawelec G, Peralbo E, Wikby A, Mariani E, Mocchegiani E, Tarazona R, Solana R (2006) Immunological biomarkers of aging in man: changes in both innate and adaptive immunity are associated with health and longevity. Biogerontology 7:471–481

Dhenain M, Michot JL, Volk A, Picq JL, Boller F (1997) T2-weighted MRI studies of mouse lemurs: a primate model of brain aging. Neurobiol Aging 18:517–521
Donahue AN, Aschner M, Lash LH, Syversen T, Sonntag WE (2006) Growth hormone administration to aged animals reduces disulfideglutathione levels in hippocampus. Mech Aging Dev 127:57–63
Drayer B, Burger P, Darwin R, Riederer S, Herfkens R, Johnson GA (1986) MRI of brain iron. AJR Am J Roentgenol 147:103–110
Dröge W (2002) Aging-related changes in the thiol/disulfide redox state: implications for the use of thiol antioxidants. Exp Gerontol 37:1333–1345
Dröge W, Schipper HM (2007) Oxidative stress and aberrant signaling in aging and cognitive decline. Aging Cell 6:361–370
Fabris N (1990) A neuroendocrine-immune theory of aging. Int J Neurosci 51:373–375
Ferrandiz ML, Martínez M, De Juan E, Diez A, Bustos G, Miquel J (1994) Impairment of mitochondrial oxidative phosphorylation in the brain of aged mice. Brain Res 644:335–338
Fischer A, Sananbenesi F, Wang X, Dobbin M, Tsai LH (2007) Recovery of learning and memory is associated with chromatin remodelling. Nature 447:178–182
Gallagher M, Landfield PW, McEwen B (1996) Hippocampal neurodegeneration in aging. Science 274:484–485
Görtz N, Lewejohann L, Tomm M, Ambrée O, Keyvani K, Paulus W, Sachser N (2008) Effects of environmental enrichment on exploration, anxiety, and memory in female TgCRND8 Alzheimer mice. Behav Brain Res 191:43–48
Guayerbas N, De la Fuente M (2003) An impairment of phagocytic function is linked to a shorter life span in two strains of prematurely aging mice. Dev Comp Immunol 27:339–350
Guayerbas N, Catalán M, Víctor VM, Miquel J, De la Fuente M (2002a) Relation of behaviour and macrophage function to life span in a murine model of premature immunosenescence. Behav Brain Res 134(1–2):41–48
Guayerbas N, Puerto M, Víctor VM, Miquel J, De la Fuente M (2002b) Leukocyte function and life span in a murine model of premature immunosenescence. Exp Gerontol 37(2–3):249–256
Hamilton ML, Van Remmen H, Drake JA, Yang H, Guo ZM, Kewitt K, Walter CA, Richardson A (2001) Does oxidative damage to DNA increase with age? Proc Natl Acad Sci U S A 98:10469–10474
Hasty P, Campisi J, Hoeijmakers J, van Steeg H, Vijg J (2003) Aging and genome maintenance: lessons from the mouse? Science 299(5611):1355–1359
Hawkley LC, Cacioppo JT (2004) Stress and the aging immune system. Brain Behav Immun 18:114–119
Hebert LE, Scherr PA, Bienias JL, Bennett DA, Evans DA (2003) Alzheimer disease in the US population: prevalence estimates using the 2000 census. Arch Neurol 60:1119–1122
High KP (2004) Infection as a cause of age-related morbidity and mortality. Aging Res Rev 3:1–14
Kinney-Forshee BA, Kinney NE, Steger RW, Bartke A (2004) Could a deficiency in growth hormone signaling be beneficial to the aging brain? Physiol Behav 80:589–594
Kozorovitskiy Y, Gould E (2004) Dominance hieraechy influences adult neurogenesis in the dentate gyrus. J Neurosci 24:6755–6759
Lazarov O, Robinson J, Tang YP, Hairston IS, Korade-Mirnics Z, Lee VM, Hersh LB, Sapolsky RM, Mirnics K, Sisodia SS (2005) Environmental enrichment reduces Abeta levels and amyloid deposition in transgenic mice. Cell 120:701–713
Lin MT, Beal MF (2006) Mitochondrial dysfunction and oxidative stress in neurodegenerative diseases. Nature 443:787–795
Longo VD, Finch CE (2003) Evolutionary medicine: from dwarf model to healthy centenarians? Science 299:1342–1346
Lu T, Pan Y, Kao SY, Li C, Kohane I, Chan J, Yankner BA (2004) Gene regulation and DNA damage in the aging human brain. Nature 429:883–891
Lupien SJ, McEwen BS, Gunnar MR, Heim C (2009) Effects of stress throughout the lifespan on the brain, behaviour and cognition. Nature Rev Neurosci 10:434–445

Makrantonaki E, Schonknecht P, Hossini AM, Kaiser E, Katsouli MM, Adjaye J, Schröder J, Zouboulis CC (2010) Skin and brain age together: the role of hormones in the aging process. Exp Gerontol 45:801–813

Mark RE, Griffin ST, Graham DI (1997) Aging associated changes in human brain. J Neuropathol Exp Neurol 56:1269–1275

Markesbery WR (1997) Oxidative stress hypothesis in Alzheimer's disease. Free Radic Biol Med 23:134–147

Marx F, Blasko I, Pavelka M, Grubeck-Loebenstein B (1998) The possible role of the immune system in Alzheimer's disease. Exp Gerontol 33:871–881

Mattson MP, Duan W, Lee J, Guo Z (2001) Suppression of brain aging and neurodegenerative disorders by dietary restriction and environmental enrichment: molecular mechanisms. Mech Aging Dev 122:757–778

Meshi D, Drew MR, Saxe M, Ansorge MS, David D, Santarelli L, Malapani C, Moore H, Hen R (2006) Hippocampal neurogenesis is not required for behavioral effects of environmental enrichment. Nat Neurosci 9:729–731

Miquel J, Economos AC, Fleming J, Johnson JE Jr (1980) Mitochondrial role in cell aging. Exp Gerontol 15:575–591

Mora F, Segovia G, del Arco A (2007) Aging, plasticity and environmental enrichment: structural changes and neurotransmitter dynamics in several areas of the brain. Brain Res Rev 55:78–88

Morrison JH, Hof PR (1997) Life and death of neurons in the aging brain. Science 278:412–419

Muller FL, Lustgarten MS, Jang Y, Richardson A, Van Remmen H (2007) Trends in oxidative aging theories. Free Radic Biol Med 43:477–503

Murphy DG, DeCarli C, Schapiro MB, Rapoport SI, Horwitz B (1992) Age-related differences in volumes of subcortical nuclei, brain matter, and cerebrospinal fluid in healthy men as measured with magnetic resonance imaging. Arch Neurol 49:839–845

Navarro A, Boveris A (2004) Rat brain and liver mitochondria develop oxidative stress and lose enzymatic activities on aging. Am J Physiol Regul Integr Comp Physiol 287:R1244–R1249

Nilsson M, Perfilieva E, Johansson U, Orwar O, Eriksson PS (1999) Enriched environment increases neurogenesis in the adult rat dentate gyrus and improves spatial memory. J Neurobiol 39:569–578

Nithianantharajan J, Hannan AJ (2006) Enriched environments, experience-dependent plasticity and disorders of nervous system. Nat Rev Neurosci 7:697–709

Oberdoerffer P, Michan S, McVay M, Mostoslavsky R, Vann J, Park SK, Hartlerode A, Stegmuller J, Hafner A, Loerch P, Wright SM, Mills KD, Bonni A, Yankner BA, Scully R, Prolla TA, Alt FW, Sinclair DA (2008) SIRT1 redistribution on chromatin promotes genomic stability but alters gene expression during aging. Cell 135:907–918

O'Hagan HM, Mohammad HP, Baylin SB (2008) Double strand breaks can initiate gene silencing and SIRT1-dependent onset of DNA methylation in an exogenous promoter CpG island. PLoS Genet 4:e1000155

Pawelec G, Barnett Y, Forsey R, Frasca D, Globerson A, McLeod J, Caruso C, Franceschi C, Fülöp T, Gupta S, Mariani E, Mocchegiani E, Solana R (2002) T cells and aging, January 2002 update. Front Biosci 7:d1056–d1183

Pham TM, Winblad B, Granholm AC, Mohammed AH (2002) Environmental influences on brain neurotrophins in rats. Pharmacol Biochem Behav 73:167–175

Poon HF, Calabrese V, Calvani M, Butterfield DA (2006) Proteomics analyses of specific protein oxidation and protein expression in aged rat brain and its modulation by L-acetylcarnitine: insights into the mechanisms of action of this proposed therapeutic agent for CNS disorders associated with oxidative stress. Antioxid Redox Signal 8:381–394

Puerto M, Guayerbas N, Alvarez P, De la Fuente M (2005) Modulation of neuropeptide Y and norepinephrine on several leucocyte functions in adult, old and very old mice. J Neuroimmunol 165(1–2):33–40

Rattan SI (2008) Increased molecular damage and heterogeneity as the basis of aging. Biol Chem 389:267–272

Rattan SI (2010) Targeting the age-related occurrence, removal, and accumulation of molecular damage by hormesis. Ann N Y Acad Sci 1197:28–32

Roy V, Belzung C, Delarue C, Chapillon P (2001) Environmental enrichment in BALB/c mice: effects in classical tests of anxiety and exposure to a predatory odor. Physiol Behav 74:313–320

Sairanen M, Lucas G, Ernfors P, Castren M (2005) Brain-derived neurotrophic factor and antidepressant drugs have different but coordinated effects on neuronal turnover, proliferation and survival in the adult dentate gyrus. J Neurosci 25:1089–1094

Sastre J, Pallardo FV, Vina J (2003) The role of mitochondrial oxidative stress in aging. Free Radic Biol Med 35:1–8

Schenker C, Meier D, Wichmann W, Boesiger P, Valavanis A (1993) Age distribution and iron dependency of the T2 relaxation time in the globus pallidus and putamen. Neuroradiology 35:119–124

Schipper HM (2004) Brain iron deposition and the free radical-mitochondrial theory of aging. Aging Res Rev 3:265–301

Segovia G, Yagüe AG, García-Verdugo JM, Mora F (2006) Environmental enrichment promotes neurogenesis and changes the extracellular concentrations of glutamate and GABA in the hippocampus of aged rats. Brain Res Bull 70:8–14

Segovia G, Arco AD, Mora F (2009) Environmental enrichment, prefrontal cortex, stress, and aging of the brain. J Neural Transm 116:1007–1016

Sigueira IR, Fochesatto C, Lucena da Silva Torres I, Dalmaz C, Netto CA (2005) Aging affects oxidative state in hippocampus, hypothalamus and adrenal glands of Wistar rats. Life Sci 78:271–278

Singh R, Kanwar SS, Sood PK, Nehru B (2011) Beneficial effects of folic acid on enhancement of memory and antioxidant status in aged rat brain. Cell Mol Neurobiol 31:83–91

Small SA, Nava AS, Perera GM, Delapaz R, Stern Y (2000) Evaluating the function of hippocampal subregions with high-resolution MRI in Alzheimer's disease and aging. Microsc Res Tech 51:101–108

Stichel CC, Luebbert H (2007) Inflammatory processes in the aging mouse brain: participation of dendritic cells and T-cells. Neurobiol Aging 28:1507–1521

Sun LY, Bartke A (2007) Adult neurogenesis in the hippocampus of long-lived mice during aging. J Gerontol A Biol Sci Med Sci 62:117–125

Tien RD, Felsberg GJ, Ferris NJ, Osumi AK (1993) The dementias: correlation of clinical features, pathophysiology, and neuroradiology. AJR Am J Roentgenol 161:245–255

Toescu EC, Verkhratsky A (2003) Neuronal aging from an intraneuronal perspective: roles of endoplasmic reticulum and mitochondria. Cell Calcium 34:311–323

van Praag H, Kempermann G, Gage FH (2000) Neural consequences of environmental enrichment. Nat Rev Neurosci 1:191–198

Viña J, Sastre J, Pallardo F, Borras C (2003) Mitochondrial theory of aging: importance to explain why females live longer than males. Antioxid Redox Signal 5:549–556

von Bernhardi R (2007) Glial cell dysregulation: a new perspective on Alzheimer disease. Neurotox Res 12:215–232

von Gunten A, Ebbing K, Imhof A, Giannakopoulos P, Kövari E (2010) Brain aging in the oldest-old. Curr Gerontol Geriatr Res pii: 358531

Yankner BA, Lu T, Loerch P (2008) The aging brain. Annu Rev Pathol 3:41–66

Wayne SL, Rhyne RL, Garry PJ, Goodwin JS (1990) Cell-mediated immunity as a predictor of morbidity and mortality in subjects over 60. J Gerontol 45:M45–48

Zambrana Z, Marco EM, Arranz L, De Castro NM, Viveros MP, De la Fuente M (2007) Influence of aging and enriched environment on motor activity and emotional responses in mice. Ann N Y Acad Sci 1100:543–552

Zhu Y, Carvey PM, Ling Z (2006) Age-related change in glutathione and glutathione related enzymes in rat brain. Brain Res 1090:35–44

Chapter 7
Consequences of Altered Mortalin Expression in Control of Cell Proliferation and Brain Function

Renu Wadhwa and Sunil C. Kaul

Abstract Mortalin, a member of Hsp70 family, was first cloned as a mortality factor in mouse fibroblasts in 1993. It was subsequently determined as a key player of mitochondrial biogenesis, ATP production, stress responses, chaperoning, intracellular trafficking and continued proliferation of cancer cells. Besides its role in cancer, mortalin is also an important protein for the brain that utilizes high energy and depends heavily on mitochondrial functions. In a proteomic screening, mortalin was detected as a downregulated protein in Parkinson's disease and oxidized in Alzheimer's disease depicting that the "functional lack of mortalin" is related to these diseases. Knockdown of mortalin homologue in worms (*C. elegans*) caused abnormalities in mitochondria, premature senescence and progeria like phenotype. These studies have demonstrated that mortalin-mediated mitochondrial functions are not only the key factors in maintaining the continued proliferation of cancer cells but also the normal neuronal physiology. Lack of a functional mortalin leads to cancer cell death and neurodegenerative phenotype.

Keywords Mortalin • Cell proliferation • Stress • Cancer • Neurodegenerative disease

7.1 Introduction

Somatic cells have evolved mechanisms to put restrains on their proliferation. In the scenario of life-essential oxidation reactions accumulating to genetic and epigenetic errors, senescence (or cellular aging) could provide a fail-safe mechanism preventing cells from turning into cancers. In corollary, what characterizes the large majority of tumors is their ability to overcome the aging block and acquisition of

R. Wadhwa (✉) · S. C. Kaul
National Institute of Advanced Industrial Science & Technology (AIST),
Central 4, 1-1-1 Higashi, Tsukuba, Ibaraki 305-8562, Japan
e-mail: renu-wadhwa@aist.go.jp

M. K. Thakur, S. I. S. Rattan (eds.), *Brain Aging and Therapeutic Interventions*,
DOI 10.1007/978-94-007-5237-5_7,

unlimited potential to divide. In the last 2–3 decades, it has been established that the tumor suppressor pathways (Rb and/or p53, and their regulators, such as p16INK4a, p21WAF1 and ARF) regulate cellular senescence (Campisi 2005). A large number of studies support that stress is an essential regulatory component of aging and hence the stress chaperones have been assigned therapeutic value in aging and cancer treatment (Soti and Csermely 2002). Overall, cells derived from aged animals and those that have become senescent in the culture dish share the common features of a dysfunctional chaperone system (Nardai et al. 2002), baseline depression of stress and anti-oxidative protein levels (Kregel et al. 1995), weaker activation of inducible chaperones (Liu et al. 1989) and poorer binding of heat shock factor (HSF) to the heat shock element (Choi et al. 1990).

At our end, efforts to identify proteins involved in cellular mortal and immortal phenotypes, using normal and conditional mortal cells generated by fusion of mouse mortal and immortal mouse fibroblasts, led to the identification of a protein associated with cellular mortal phenotype and named it as 'mortalin'(Wadhwa et al. 1993a). The protein was isolated from mouse embryonic fibroblasts and antibodies were generated for (1) subcellular localization and (2) cloning of its cDNA from an expression library. These studies revealed that mortalin protein has pancytoplasmic distribution in normal fibroblasts (Wadhwa et al. 1993a) and is concentrated around the nucleus in immortal and transformed cells (Wadhwa et al. 1993b). cDNA cloning and homology search placed it in heat shock protein 70 (Hsp70) family (Wadhwa et al. 1993a) and assigned to chromosomes 18 and X in mouse, and chromosome 5q31.1 in human by fluorescence in situ hybridization (Kaul et al. 1995). Unlike other members of the Hsp70 family, mortalin is a heat un-inducible protein, but responds to glucose deprivation, oxidative injury, low-level radiation and some cytotoxins (Kaul et al. 2007). cDNAs from normal and immortal mouse cells showing pancytoplasmic and perinuclear mortalin staining were isolated by immunoscreening. Sequence analysis of these cDNAs revealed that the two forms of mouse mortalin, the pancytoplasmic (mot-1) and perinuclear (mot-2) differ by only two nucleotides in the carboxy-terminus of their open reading frame, resulting in two amino acid changes, V618M and R624G, in the protein. Mice breeding experiments showed that mot-1 and mot-2 segregated in F1 and F2 progenies, suggesting that these two proteins are encoded by two separate alleles in mouse (Kaul et al. 2000a; Wadhwa et al. 1996). Functional studies involving the expression of the cytoplasmic form by transfection of mot-1 cDNA (isolated from CD1-ICR mouse embryonic fibroblasts) to immortal NIH 3T3 cells induced cellular senescence. However, the perinuclear form expressed by mot-2 cDNA (isolated from NIH 3T3 cells) did not yield an equivalent effect. The data suggested that the senescence-inductive function is exclusive to cytoplasmic mortalin or mot-1 (Wadhwa et al. 1993c). In contrast to the identification of two mortalin cDNAs from mouse cells, human normal and transformed cells were seen to have identical cDNA sequence and yet exhibit differential protein distribution. Interestingly when senescence was induced in human transformed cells, mortalin distribution shifted from the perinuclear to the pancytoplasmic type (Wadhwa et al. 1995, 2000; Widodo et al. 2007). These findings have suggested that there are, at least, two kinds of mechanism for the differential distribution of mortalin in normal and transformed cells. The first one exists in mouse cells and is based on the different protein structures as discussed below, and the second one that exists in human cells and may involve differential mortalin-interacting cellular factors in normal and cancer cells that remains to be clearly characterized.

7.2 Mouse Mot-1 and Mot-2: Structures and Contrasting Activities in Cell Proliferation Control

Similar to its close relatives in Hsp70 family of proteins, mortalin consists of two inter-connected principal domains: the N-terminal ATPase and C-terminal regions. The structure of mortalin's N-terminus was deduced based on the X-ray data of bovine heat shock cognate protein (Hsc70) (Deocaris et al. 2006). Its N-terminal 44 kDa structure contains four sub-domains, I-IIA and I-IIB, that folds as a deep catalytic pocket stabilized by metal-binding (Sriram et al. 1997). Allosteric changes within the ATPase domain are communicated to the peptide-binding domain (PBD) through the chaperone's highly evolutionary conserved interdomain linker/interface (Jiang et al. 2005). This 18 kDa PBD is composed of two sets of four-stranded anti-parallel beta-sheets that form a twisted sandwich. When compared to the ATPase domain, there is a wider sequence variation in the PBD with other Hsp70s. This variation is believed to underlie the diversification of Hsp70 interacting clients (Rudiger et al. 2000). Flanking the PBD is a 10 kDa long C-terminal helix made-up of five helical domains (A–E). This interesting structure, called the "substrate lid", does not contact the peptide substrate directly and has the ability to flip-flop. This lid also functions as a molecular "latch" that locks-in substrates during an ADP-bound state (Zhu et al. 1996).

Given the opposing functions of mortalin: mot-1 being associated with limited lifespan and senescence (Wadhwa et al. 1993c), while mot-2 with lifespan extension, immortalization, malignant transformation, and late-stages of cancers (Kaul et al. 1998, 2003), it is remarkable that such subtle differences in two amino acids (V618M and R624G, for mot-1 and mot-2, respectively) result in these contrasting phenotypes. To appreciate how these changes could alter mortalin functions, the structure of the C-terminus peptide-binding domain (PBD) was understood in the context of its bacterial homologue, *E. coli* Hsp70 chaperone, DnaK. It appeared that apart from the flexible lid structure that 'flip-flops' above the substrate cleft, electrostatic "latches" between the lid and the cleft are critical for its chaperoning function. One "latch" consisting of Asp477, Arg513, Glu586 and His590 is common with other Hsp70s (Mayer et al. 2000), while an additional "latch" that we identified on the opposite end, consisting of Arg574, Arg578 and Glu628, appeared to be mortalin-specific. A replacement of Gly624 (in mot-2), located at the C-terminus of α-helix C, by Arg (in mot-1) is likely to extend the α-helix C. In contrast, Gly, a strong helix breaker, shortens the L3 (C–D) loop. The latter should perturb the structure of the "mortalin-specific latch", presumably pulling apart the electrostatic attractions that could result in the loss of chaperone action of the molecule. Additionally, the altered secondary structure of mot-1 and mot-2 proteins was also evident from their different mobility on SDS-PAGE (Kaul et al. 2000b). This electrophoretic behavior reflected the subtle changes in the flexibility of the proteins and was consistent with different chaperone and biological activities of the two proteins (Kaul et al. 1998, 2003; Wadhwa et al. 1993c).

7.3 Mortalin Functions as a Mitochondrial Import Machine and a Housekeeping Chaperone

Mortalin was independently cloned as the peptide binding protein, PBP74 (Domanico et al. 1993); mitochondrial heat shock protein, mtHsp70 (Bhattacharyya et al. 1995); and glucose-regulated protein, Grp75 (Webster et al. 1994), implying multifunctionality of this protein. Furthermore, independent studies have demonstrated the multiple sub-cellular localizations of mortalin that range from the mitochondria, ER, plasma membrane, vesicles and cytosol (Bhattacharyya et al. 1995; Ran et al. 2000; Domanico et al. 1993; Shin et al. 2003; Soltys and Gupta 2000; Pilzer and Fishelson 2005). Since majority of it is in mitochondria, this chaperone is widely regarded a major mitochondrial chaperone and import motor.

Majority of the mitochondrial proteins are encoded by the nuclear genome. The mitochondrial precursor proteins are rapidly transported across the mitochondrial membranes with the help from specific transport machines of which mortalin constitutes an important component to ensure that the proteins destined for the mitochondria are properly recognized, delivered and sorted to their proper compartments (Rehling et al. 2004). During the import of mitochondrial-targeted proteins, the proteins pass through the membranes via the 'Translocase of the Outer Membrane' (TOM). After crossing the outer membrane, precursor proteins segregate to two structurally distinct 'Translocases of the Inner Membrane' (TIM), TIM23 and TIM22. Transport of bulky proteins requires unfolding during shuttling and refolding to native conformers to regain function. Mortalin plays a key role in these processes. The fact that no cell can survive without mortalin (deletion mutations in Ssc1 were lethal) underscores the importance of mortalin to life (Craig et al. 1987). Due to the ROS-bathed cellular environment, mitochondrial proteins are extremely sensitive to oxidative damage and are required to undergo proteolytic degradation. Unlike in the cytosol that allows poly-ubiquitination of proteolytic substrates for targeting to the 26S proteasome, there is no evidence for existence of a similar system in the mitochondria. Instead, misfolded polypeptides are frequently found associated with mitochondrial chaperones (mortalin and Hsp60), matrix-localized PIM1 and membrane-bound proteases such as, m-AAA and i-AAA that facilitate degradation of misfolded polypeptides (Leonhard et al. 1999; Soti and Csermely 2002). Consistent with the major involvement of ROS-related mutational events in cancers, a study reported that the majority of mutations in the human colorectal cancer cell lines were somatically acquired mtDNA mutations. However, the detected mutations were not associated with major perturbations of mitochondrial functions, such as oxygen consumption and respiratory chain enzymatic activities (Polyak et al. 1998). Based on these, it was proposed that the chaperone buffering within the mitochondria might help in continued proliferation of cancer cells. Indeed, it has been shown that there are several differences between the mitochondria of transformed versus normal cells with regards to: (a) substrate preference for oxidation reactions, (b) degree of acceptor control ratios, (c) rates of electron and anion transport, (d) control of calcium holding and efflux, (e) mtDNA status, and (f) rates of mitochondrial biogenesis (Modica-Napolitano and Singh 2002; Wallace 2005). In this scenario, the mitochondrial mortalin has been shown to regulate mitochondrial biogenesis and ROS-induced stress.

7.4 Mortalin Functions Beyond the Mitochondrial Boundary

Several groups have reported that mortalin is also found in extra-mitochondrial sites. Confocal laser microscopy of the native protein with protein-specific antibodies in a variety of cell lines revealed its presence in the endoplasmic reticulum, cytoplasmic vesicles and cytosol (Domanico et al. 1993; Ran et al. 2000; Singh et al. 1997; Soltys and Gupta 2000; Wadhwa et al. 1995). Binding of mortalin to residents of different organelles may assist in its relocation to multiple subcellular sites. Far-western screening identified glucose regulated ER chaperone (Grp94) as one of its binding partners (Takano et al. 2001). It was also found to bind to membrane-associated proteins such as fibroblasts growth factor-1 (FGF-1)(Mizukoshi et al. 1999), IL receptor type-1 (Sacht et al. 1999) and the peroxisomal protein mevalonate pyrophosphate decarboxylase (MPD) (Wadhwa et al. 2003b). Interestingly, its interaction with FGF-1 was coupled to its cell-cycle dependent tyrosine phosphorylation (Mizukoshi et al. 2001) and was shown to regulate intracellular trafficking of FGF-1. Mortalin-IL receptor type-1 complex was shown to regulate the internalization of IL receptor type-1, critical in signaling pathway of the pro-inflammatory cytokine IL-1 (Sacht et al. 1999). More recently, serine/threonine kinase Akt, a key mediator of cell survival and cell growth, was shown to be a binding partner of mortalin (Vandermoere et al. 2007). By such interactions, mortalin has been shown to adopt essential roles in signal transduction, cell communication and neoplastic development.

7.5 Mortalin Inactivates p53 Functions in Cancer Cells

Expression profiling of mortalin in normal aging and large variety of cancer cell lines revealed bi-phasic expression pattern consisting of downregulation of mortalin during cellular senescence and an initial upregulation during immortalization followed by an elevation coinciding with the acquisition of an invasive phenotype (Wadhwa et al. 2006). Consistently, by analyzing the proteomics in tissue arrays, it was identified as a prognostic marker for colorectal cancers (Dundas et al. 2004). Global profiling of the cell surface proteome of cancer cells revealed the remarkable abundance of several chaperone proteins, including Grp78, mortalin, Hsp70, Hsp60, Hsp54, Hsp27 and protein disulfide isomerase (Shin et al. 2003). Immunohistochemistry of mortalin in serial grades of astrocyte tumors such as low-grade astrocytoma, anaplastic astrocytoma and glioblastoma revealed a correlation of its expression level with tumor aggressiveness (Takano et al. 1997). Indeed, forced upregulation of mortalin in breast cancers was shown to result into malignant and metastatic transformation of the tumor cells (Wadhwa et al. 2006). By a high-resolution proteomic approach, mortalin was found to be enriched in hepatocellular carcinoma (HCC) when compared to the adjacent non-tumor tissues. Clinico-pathological analysis further illustrated high tumor expression of mortalin associates with early recurrence of HCC in patients subjected to curative treatments (Yi et al. 2008). A second independent study in which 100 pairs of hepatic cancer tissues were examined by immunohistochemistry, revealed that mortalin was overexpressed in 61 % of the tumor tissues. It correlated with the tumor aggressiveness; there was a marked increase in mortalin level from early (stage I and stage II) to late (stage III and stage IV) stages. The clinico-pathological parameter analysis indicated that mortalin upregulation was significantly associated with HCC recurrence ($p=0.005$) and microsatellite formation ($p=0.028$), a consistent feature of intra-hepatic metastasis (Lu et al. 2011a, b). While there are a number of ways by which mortalin could potentially contribute to the continued proliferation of tumor cells, its impact in the activity of tumor suppressor protein p53 has been largely established. Mortalin and p53 interaction was first detected in human cancer cells by co-immunolocalization and co-immunoprecipitation of the two proteins; normal cells lacked this interaction (Kaul et al. 1998; Wadhwa et al. 1998, 2000, 2002). It was then shown that mortalin and p53 interact in the cytoplasm resulting in the nuclear exclusion and transcriptional inactivation of the latter (Wadhwa et al. 1998; Walker et al. 2006). Based on the studies using deletion mutants of mortalin (mot-2) and p53, their binding regions were assigned to an amino-terminus region of mortalin and the carboxy-terminus region of p53, the cytoplasmic sequestration domain (Kaul et al. 2001; Wadhwa et al. 2002). Indeed, small p53 peptides that bind to mortalin were able to act as binding antagonists resulting in translocation and reactivation of wild type p53 (Kaul et al. 2005). In addition to an inactivation of p53 function (Kaul et al. 2005), mortalin was shown to abrogate the control of p53 on centrosomal duplication, a hallmark of cancers (Ma et al. 2006; Kanai et al. 2007). Mortalin was shown to preferentially associate with duplicated centrosomes and its overexpression overrode the p53-dependent suppression of centrosome duplication (Ma et al. 2006). We undertook a study on the investigation of mortalin-p53 interaction in seven liver cancer cell lines (MHCC97H, MHCC97L, H2P, H2M, PLC/PRF/5, HepG2, Hep3B) and found that unlike most cancer cells, HepG2 hepatoma lacked mortalin-p53 interaction and hence further examined the regulation of mortalin-p53 interaction and their significance in these cancer cells. We found that mortalin-p53 interaction is a stress dependent event, also accompanied by phosphorylation of p53 (Lu et al. 2011b). HepG2 that lacked mortain-p53 interaction did not show ser/thr phosphorylation. HepG2 cells when subjected to stress by treatment with low doses of cisplatin, hydrogen peroxide and doxorubicin showed mortalin-p53 interaction. Based on these findings, a model on stress-regulation of mortalin-p53 interaction was proposed. In normal, immortalized and non-malignant cancer cells that are unstressed and have low p53, mortalin and p53 do not interact. In these cells, p53 freely translocates from cytoplasm to nucleus. Mortalin knockdown does not cause apoptosis in this category of cells. Mortalin-p53 interaction can be induced by exposure to the genotoxic stress that also results in p53 phosphorylation. In this category of cells, apoptotic ability of p53 is compromised by its binding to mortalin. Knockdown of mortalin in this category hence induces reactivation of p53-mediated apoptosis. Malignant cancer cells are physiologically stressed and accumulate p53 (mutant) that is highly phosphorylated and has mortalin-p53 interaction. According to this model, mortalin-p53 interaction is selective for stressed cancer cells (normal cells lack this interaction) and hence could serve as a safe target for cancer therapeutics (Lu et al. 2011b).

Mortalin-p53 interaction that causes inactivation of p53 function was also targeted by a small molecule (MKT-077, a cationic rhodacyanine dye) (Wadhwa et al. 2000; Deocaris et al. 2007; Lu et al. 2011a) and peptide (p53 312-352, carboxy-terminal amino acid resides 312-352 of p53), previously shown to bind to mortalin and reactivate wild-type p53 leading to growth arrest (Kaul et al. 2005; Wadhwa et al. 2000) and a phyto-extract (Widodo et al. 2007; Grover et al. 2012). All these reagents indeed caused growth arrest or apoptosis of cancer cells and qualified as potential anti-cancer reagents. Targeting mortalin with antisense, ribozyme or siRNA specific for mortalin also induced tumor cell-specific growth arrest and apoptosis (Wadhwa et al. 2003a, 2004; Yoo et al. 2010; Lu et al. 2011a, b), suggesting that the development of various modalities for targeting mortalin is therapeutically important for cancer treatment.

7.6 Mortalin Functions in Normal and Aging Brain

The brain is the most complex organ, consisting of billions of neurons connected by axons, synapses and signal pulses (action potential) that sense and communicate signals from one part of the body to the other.It exerts centralized control over the body by regulating muscular and hormonal activities and has very high caloric requirement as compared to rest of the body. Such continuous metabolic demand that supports the generation of action potentials in neuronal cells relies on the mitochondria. Though mitochondrial biogenesis is critical to brain physiology, this phenomenon remains largely a neglected theme in neurobiology. Initial immunohistochemical studies of mortalin in normal and tumor human brain sections revealed that mortalin expression was normally confined to neurons. Normal astrocytes showed undetectable expression of mortalin. This may reflect on the higher energy demand of the neurons. Large amounts of ATP are required by neurons for neurotransmission and maintenance of Na^+, K^+ and Ca^{2+} ionic gradients across its cell membrane (Erecinska and Silver 1994). Furthermore, mitochondria are continuously being trafficked to regions of nerve cells that have particularly high metabolic demands, such as the synapses, nodes of Ranvier and myelination/demyelination interface (Chang and Reynolds 2006). Such mitochondrial delivery to the synapses has been shown to be critical for learning and memory functions (Tong 2007). Mitochondria are also central to intracellular Ca^{2+} homeostasis, steroid synthesis, generation of free radical species and initiation of cell death, aging, metabolic and degenerative diseases including brain pathologies and cancer (Kann and Kovacs 2007; Wallace 2005). Calcium is a highly versatile intracellular messenger that drives membrane excitability, exocytosis of neurotrasmitters, vesicular trafficking, neurogenesis, metabolism, crosstalk between signaling pathways and apoptosis/necrosis. Through its reversible binding that results in specific conformational changes to proteins, Ca^{2+} regulates kinases, phosphatases, proteases, transcription factors and ion channels. Mortalin plays essential role in mitochondrial biogenesis and maintains mitochondrial protein integrity. Recent studies have connected this mitochondrial chaperone both to neurogenesis and neurodegeneration processes. One of the functions of mitochondria is to maintain intracellular calcium concentration through the interplay of its Na^+/Ca^{2+} exchanger and Ca^{2+}-uniporter, with the sarco-endoplasmic reticulum Ca^{2+}-ATPase and the plasma membrane Ca^{2+}-ATPase (Mattson 2007).

The adult brain retains at least two active germinal zones: the sub-granular zone of dentate gyrus that generates hippocampal interneurons and the forebrain subventricular zone that generates interneurons that migrate into the olfactory bulb (Temple and Qian 1995). The abundance of mortalin in neurons and its involvement in the processes of stress-resistance, bioenergetics and cell proliferation proposed it as a candidate player in the phenomenon of neurogenesis. Proteomic analysis of in vitro cultures of adult dorsal root ganglion (DRG) neurons by Willis et al. (2005) identified several cytoskeletal (β-actin, vimentin, etc.), chaperones (mortalin, Hsp60, Grp78/BiP, etc.), anti-oxidant (superoxide dismutase 1, peroxiredoxins 1 and 6) and metabolic (phosphoglyceratekinase 1, alpha enolase, etc.) proteins being synthesized abundantly in the axons. The level of mortalin protein was found to decrease in senescent human fibroblasts and in aged worms (Kimura et al. 2007). Overexpression leads to the lifespan extension in both systems, suggesting that the decline in mortalin level and thus its function(s) are closely related to the fixed proliferation potential of normal cells in vitro and longevity in vivo (Kaul et al. 2000c). In corollary, deletion mutations of SSC1, the yeast orthologue of mtHsp70, were lethal (Craig et al. 1989) and knockdown of mortalin with ribozyme or antisense inevitably led to cellular growth arrest (Wadhwa et al. 2003a, 2004). Worms treated with siRNA against Hsp-6 (hsp70F), a nematode orthologue of mortalin, caused a reduction in the level of ATP-2, Hsp60 and CLK-1, leading to abnormal mitochondrial morphology, lower ATP production and accelerated aging or progeria-like phenotypes (Kimura et al. 2007).

Massa et al. (1995) identified Grp75 from rat brain after exposure to metabolic stress. Subsequent cDNA cloning of this protein revealed its identity to mortalin. It was shown to be enriched in neurons of the basal forebrain, reticular and subthalamic nuclei, globus pallidus and amygdala. Furthermore, the expression of mortalin was upregulated following focal brain ischemia in a distinctive fashion. With low level of injury, induction of mortalin was restricted to the area of injury; however, with extensive injury, mortalin was upregulated in regions even outside the ischemic foci (Massa et al. 1995). To elucidate the functions of this molecular biomarker of brain ischemia, Zheng et al. (2000) overexpressed mortalin in CHL cells in glucose-free medium in order to simulate metabolic energy stress and demonstrated that with the increased levels of intracellular mortalin lead to greater resistance to glucose-deprivation. Furthermore, mortalin overexpression also resulted in decreased ROS production while maintaining cell viability during glucose deprivation in PC12 cells (Liu et al. 2005).

7.7 Mortalin in Neurodegenerative Diseases

Aging is associated with functional decline at molecular, cellular and organism level. Age-related brain pathologies are most frequently characterized by decreased protein degradation and accumulation of damaged proteins that result from decline in molecular repair. Unrepaired oxidized proteins initiate an exponential spread of molecular damage resulting in loss of their structural and catalytic functions of the proteome. While stress chaperones act as buffers assisting in refolding of denatured proteins and help in the degradation of the unrepaired proteins, they themselves are also vulnerable molecular targets of oxidative reactions and damaging free radicals generated in mitochondria. Two major neurodegenerative brain disorders, Alzheimer's (AD) and Parkinson's (PD) diseases, have recently been shown to be associated with functional inefficiencies of the mitochondrial chaperones.

Amyloid beta (Aβ) is known to poison the mitochondria in AD. Sub-lethal doses of Aβ peptide were shown to block mitochondrial import of mortalin and TOM20 that could contribute to the Alzheimer's pathology. In human AD brains, amyloid precursor protein (APP) also forms stable complexes with TOM40 and clogs the import complex (Devi et al. 2006). Using a proteomic approach combined with an immunological method for detecting protein carbonylation, Choi et al. (2004) reported AD-associated oxidative damage to mortalin, specifically in the hippocampus. They also showed that the hippocampus, but not the cortex in young (6-month old) ApoE KO mice had ~2-fold greater amount of total oxidized proteins compared to age matched wild type mice. Another study reported that the different mortalin isoforms that were differentially phosphorylated in the hippocampi of human APOE4 targeted replacement (TR) mice compared with the APOE3 (control) TR mice. The predominant mortalin isoforms were differentially expressed in the hippocampi of patients with AD (Osorio et al. 2007). Using a shotgun proteomics approach, Jin et al. (2006) found that the levels of mortalin significantly decreased in substantia nigra pars compacta in PD patients and in MES cells exposed to the mitochondrial Complex I inhibitor rotenone. In addition, nine candidate mortalin binding partners, including acyl-CoA dehydrogenase family member 9, phosphate carrier protein, thymidine kinase 2 and Hsp60 were identified as potential mediators of PD (Jin et al. 2006). Studies on the rotenone-induced cellular PD model revealed that mortalin is a target for oxidative damage (Jin et al. 2006). In an independent study, in vitro exposure of PC12 cells to reactive dopamine quinone that led to selective dopaminergic terminal degeneration also resulted in a rapid loss of several mitochondrial proteins including mortalin (Van Laar et al. 2008). Pathologic decline in mortalin level correlated with different stages of PD and Lewy body deposition in human brain (Shi et al. 2008). Furthermore, because of its abundance and "promiscuity" for client proteins, mortalin is highly susceptible to covalent modifications. Phosphorylation, oxidation and ubiquitination are among its documented post-translational changes. Examples of mortalin's cellular functions that are modulated by phosphorylation include its impact on centrosomal dynamics (Kuwabara et al. 2006) and FGF-1 activity (Mizukoshi et al. 1999, 2001). Altered phosphorylation patterns of mortalin were also found in AD that are suggestive of its altered function in disease pathology.

AD and PD pathologies are often mimicked in cellular chemical models that induce ROS generation. Besides, other environmental toxicants that target mitochondria are also known to alter mortalin functions. Mercuric chloride, a transition metal known to induce acute renal failure, associated with tubular impairment, induced mitochondrial deformities and altered both mortalin and Hsp60 expression in rat kidney (Goering et al. 2000; Stacchiotti et al. 2006). The toxicant tetrafluoroethylcysteine (TFEC), a by-product during the manufacturing of TeflonTM, is known to metabolize to an unstable difluorothioacetylfluoride (DFTAL) intermediate (Cooper et al. 2002) that covalently modifies some lysine residues of mortalin (Bruschi et al. 1993, 1998; Cooper et al. 2001). These covalent modifications may establish mortalin as a unique example of a "sick" chaperone. Sick chaperones accentuate the molecular damage in an exponential manner and contribute to disease pathology (Macario and Conway de Macario 2007). However, regardless of the primary mechanism, sick chaperones could greatly contribute to the progression of neurodegeneration by participating in a vicious cycle that could result in the accumulation of metabolic errors. Lack of mortalin in worms was shown to result into progeria like phenotype in which worms showed decreased motility and mitochondrial abnormalities (Kimura et al. 2007). Most recently, in Aβ peptide model of AD, mortalin overexpression was shown to protect SH-SY5Y cells against Aβ-induced neurotoxicity. Whereas mortalin-specific siRNA sensitized SH-SY5Y cells to Aβ-toxicity, mortalin overexpression inhibited the Aβ-induced depolarization of mitochondrial membrane potential and reversed the Aβ-induced reduction in cytochrome c oxidase activity and ATP generation. Aβ-induced ROS and lipid peroxidation were suppressed in mortalin overexpressing cells (Qu et al. 2011). In vivo study in which the overexpression of mortalin was achieved in rat brain reduced the infarct area resulted from middle cerebral artery occlusion and resulted in improved neurological outcome significantly as measured by neurological score, mitochondrial function, and levels of oxidative stress (Xu et al. 2009). Burbulla et al. (2010) identified novel PD-related mortalin mutations by genomic screening of PD patients. Functional characterization of these mutations, their impact on mitochondrial homeostasis and influence on adjacent signaling pathways, revealed that whereas increased level of wild type mortalin has a positive effect on essential mitochondrial functions, the mutant mortalins lacked the cytoprotective effect. Mortalin silencing severely reduced mitochondrial membrane potential and increased production of ROS. Complementation of mortalin knockdown with wild type, but not the mutant, mortalin resulted in a complete rescue of these defects. Furthermore, skin fibroblasts from a carrier of the mortalin variant showed an altered mitochondrial morphology, suggesting its structural role in mitochondria (Burbulla et al. 2010). Yang et al. (2011) also reported that the knockdown of mortalin in HeLa and HEK293T cells results in a collapse of mitochondrial membrane potential, abnormal accumulation of ROS and alterations in mitochondrial morphology under H_2O_2-induced stress conditions. Furthermore, mortalin was shown to interact with Parkin, E3-ubiquitin ligase gene that is involved in mitochondrial dynamics and mitophagy and is commonly mutated in autosomal recessive PD. It was suggested that in addition to the reduced expression level of mortalin observed in the affected brain regions of PD patients, it shows an altered interaction with a variety of PD-related mitochondrial proteins where it regulates the native folding and mitochondrial import under stressed conditions.

Taken together, it has become increasingly clear that multi-functionality of mortalin ranges from chaperoning, intracellular trafficking, mitochondrial import and ROS-management, regulation of apoptosis and stress response. In addition, its interaction with specific proteins such as p53 and Parkin mediate its role in cancers and PD, respectively. Mortalin-based therapeutic strategies hold potential not only for the treatment of cancer but also for the neurodegenerative disorders.

References

Bhattacharyya T, Karnezis AN, Murphy SP, Hoang T, Freeman BC, Phillips B, Morimoto RI (1995) Cloning and subcellular localization of human mitochondrial hsp70. J Biol Chem 270:1705–1710

Bruschi SA, West KA, Crabb JW, Gupta RS, Stevens JL (1993) Mitochondrial HSP60 (P1 protein) and a HSP70-like protein (mortalin) are major targets for modification during S-(1,1,2,2-tetrafluoroethyl)-L-cysteine-induced nephrotoxicity. J Biol Chem 268:23157–23161

Bruschi SA, Lindsay JG, Crabb JW (1998) Mitochondrial stress protein recognition of inactivated dehydrogenases during mammalian cell death. Proc Natl Acad Sci U S A 95:13413–13418

Burbulla LF, Schelling C, Kato H, Rapaport D, Woitalla D, Schiesling C, Schulte C, Sharma M, Illig T, Bauer P, Jung S, Nordheim A, Schöls L, Riess O, Krüger R (2010) Dissecting the role of the mitochondrial chaperone mortalin in Parkinson's disease: functional impact of disease-related variants on mitochondrial homeostasis. Hum Mol Genet 19:4437–4452

Campisi J (2005) Aging, tumor suppression and cancer: high wire-act! Mech Aging Dev 126:51–58

Chang DT, Reynolds IJ (2006) Mitochondrial trafficking and morphology in healthy and injured neurons. Prog Neurobiol 80:241–268

Choi HS, Lin Z, Li BS, Liu AY (1990) Age-dependent decrease in the heat-inducible DNA sequence-specific binding activity in human diploid fibroblasts. J Biol Chem 265:18005–18011

Choi J, Forster MJ, McDonald SR, Weintraub ST, Carroll CA, Gracy RW (2004) Proteomic identification of specific oxidized proteins in ApoE-knockout mice: relevance to Alzheimer's disease. Free Radic Biol Med 36:1155–1162

Cooper AJ, Wang J, Gartner CA, Bruschi SA (2001) Co-purification of mitochondrial HSP70 and mature protein disulfide isomerase with a functional rat kidney high-M(r) cysteine S-conjugate beta-lyase. Biochem Pharmacol 62:1345–1353

Cooper AJ, Bruschi SA, Anders MW (2002) Toxic, halogenated cysteine S-conjugates and targeting of mitochondrial enzymes of energy metabolism. Biochem Pharmacol 64:553–564

Craig EA, Kramer J, Kosic-Smithers J (1987) SSC1, a member of the 70-kDa heat shock protein multigene family of Saccharomyces cerevisiae, is essential for growth. Proc Natl Acad Sci U S A 84:4156–4160

Craig EA, Kramer J, Shilling J, Werner-Washburne M, Holmes S, Kosic-Smithers J Nicolet CM (1989) SSC1, an essential member of the yeast HSP70 multigene family, encodes a mitochondrial protein. Mol Cell Biol 9:3000–3008

Deocaris CC, Kaul SC, Wadhwa R (2006) On the brotherhood of the mitochondrial chaperones mortalin and heat shock protein 60. Cell Stress Chaperones 11:116–128

Deocaris CC, Widodo N, Shrestha BG, Kaur K, Ohtaka M, Yamasaki K, Kaul SC, Wadhwa R (2007) Mortalin sensitizes human cancer cells to MKT-077-induced senescence—revisiting a drug that had failed clinical trials. Cancer Lett 252:259–269

Devi L, Prabhu BM, Galati DF, Avadhani NG, Anandatheerthavarada HK (2006) Accumulation of amyloid precursor protein in the mitochondrial import channels of human Alzheimer's disease brain is associated with mitochondrial dysfunction. J Neurosci 26:9057–9068

Domanico SZ, DeNagel DC, Dahlseid JN, Green JM, Pierce SK (1993) Cloning of the gene encoding peptide-binding protein 74 shows that it is a new member of the heat shock protein 70 family. Mol Cell Biol 13:3598–3610

Dundas SR, Lawrie LC, Rooney PH, Murray GI (2004) Mortalin is over-expressed by colorectal adenocarcinomas and correlates with poor survival. J Pathol 205:74–81

Erecinska M, Silver IA (1994) Ions and energy in mammalian brain. Prog Neurobiol 43:37–71

Goering PL, Fisher BR, Noren BT, Papaconstantinou A, Rojko JL, Marler RJ (2000) Mercury induces regional and cell-specific stress protein expression in rat kidney. Toxicol Sci 53:447–457

Grover A, Priyandoko D, Gao R, Shandilya A, Widodo N, Bisaria VS, Kaul SC, Wadhwa R, Sundar D (2012) Withanone binds to mortalin and abrogates mortalin-p53 complex: Computational and experimental evidence. Int J Biochem Cell Biol (in press)

Jiang J, Prasad K, Lafer EM, Sousa R (2005) Structural basis of interdomain communication in the Hsc70 chaperone. Mol Cell 20:513–524

Jin J, Hulette C, Wang Y, Zhang T, Pan C, Wadhwa R, Zhang J (2006) Proteomic identification of a stress protein, mortalin/mthsp70/GRP75: relevance to Parkinson disease. Mol Cell Proteomics 5:1193–1204

Kanai M, Ma Z, Izumi H, Kim SH, Mattison CP, Winey M, Fukasawa K (2007) Physical and functional interaction between mortalin and Mps1 kinase. Genes Cells 12:797–810

Kann O, Kovacs R (2007) Mitochondria and neuronal activity. Am J Physiol Cell Physiol 292:C641–657

Kaul SC, Wadhwa R, Matsuda Y, Hensler PJ, Pereira-Smtih OM, Komatsu Y, Mitsui Y (1995) Mouse and human chromosomal assignments of mortalin, a novel member of the murine hsp70 family of proteins. FEBS Lett 361:269–272

Kaul SC, Duncan EL, Englezou A, Reddel RR, Mitsui Y, Wadhwa R (1998) Malignant transformation of NIH3T3 cells by overexpression of mot-2 protein. Oncogene 17:907–911

Kaul SC, Duncan E, Sugihara T, Reddel RR, Mitsui Y, Wadhwa R (2000a) Structurally and functionally distinct mouse hsp70 family members Mot-1 and Mot-2 proteins are encoded by two alleles. DNA Res 7:229–231

Kaul SC, Takano S, Reddel RR, Mitsui Y, Wadhwa R (2000b) Transcriptional inactivation of p53 by deletions and single amino acid changes in mouse mot-1 protein. Biochem Biophys Res Commun 279:602–606

Kaul SC, Reddel RR, Sugihara T, Mitsui Y, Wadhwa R (2000c) Inactivation of p53 and life span extension of human diploid fibroblasts by mot-2. FEBS Lett 474:159–164

Kaul SC, Reddel RR, Mitsui Y, Wadhwa R (2001) An N-terminal region of mot-2 binds to p53 in vitro. Neoplasia 3:110–114

Kaul SC, Yaguchi T, Taira K, Reddel RR, Wadhwa R (2003) Overexpressed mortalin (mot-2)/mthsp70/GRP75 and hTERT cooperate to extend the in vitro lifespan of human fibroblasts. Exp Cell Res 286:96–101

Kaul SC, Aida S, Yaguchi T, Kaur K, Wadhwa R (2005) Activation of wild type p53 function by its mortalin-binding, cytoplasmically localizing carboxyl terminus peptides. J Biol Chem 280:39373–39379

Kaul SC, Deocaris CC, Wadhwa R (2007) Three faces of mortalin: a housekeeper, guardian and killer. Exp Gerontol 42:263–274

Kimura K, Tanaka N, Nakamura N, Takano S, Ohkuma S (2007) Knockdown of mitochondrial heat shock protein 70 promotes progeria-like phenotypes in caenorhabditis elegans. J Biol Chem 282:5910–5918

Kregel KC, Moseley PL, Skidmore R, Gutierrez JA, Guerriero V Jr (1995) HSP70 accumulation in tissues of heat-stressed rats is blunted with advancing age. J Appl Physiol 79:1673–1678

Kuwabara H, Yoneda M, Hayasaki H, Nakamura T, Mori H (2006) Glucose regulated proteins 78 and 75 bind to the receptor for hyaluronan mediated motility in interphase microtubules. Biochem Biophys Res Commun 339:971–976

Leonhard K, Stiegler A, Neupert W, Langer T (1999) Chaperone-like activity of the AAA domain of the yeast Yme1 AAA protease. Nature 398:348–351

Liu AY, Lin Z, Choi HS, Sorhage F, Li B (1989) Attenuated induction of heat shock gene expression in aging diploid fibroblasts. J Biol Chem 264:12037–12045

Liu Y, Liu W, Song XD, Zuo J (2005) Effect of GRP75/mthsp70/PBP74/mortalin overexpression on intracellular ATP level, mitochondrial membrane potential and ROS accumulation following glucose deprivation in PC12 cells. Mol Cell Biochem 268:45–51

Lu WJ, Lee NP, Kaul SC, Poon RTP, Wadhwa R, Luk JM (2011a) Induction of mutant p53-dependent apoptosis in human hepatocellular carcinoma by targeting stress protein mortalin. Intl J Cancer 129:1806–1814

Lu WJ, Lee NP, Kaul SC, Lan F, Poon RT, Wadhwa R, Luk JM (2011b) Mortalin–p53 interaction in cancer cells is stress dependent and constitutes a selective target for cancer therapy. Cell Death Different 18:1046–1056

Ma Z, Izumi H, Kanai M, Kabuyama Y, Ahn NG, Fukasawa K (2006) Mortalin controls centrosome duplication via modulating centrosomal localization of p53. Oncogene 25:5377–5390

Macario AJ, Conway de Macario E (2007) Chaperonopathies and chaperonotherapy. FEBS Lett 581:3681–3688

Massa SM, Longo FM, Zuo J, Wang S, Chen J, Sharp FR (1995) Cloning of rat grp75, an hsp70-family member, and its expression in normal and ischemic brain. J Neurosci Res 40:807–819

Mattson MP (2007) Calcium and neurodegeneration. Aging Cell 6:337–350

Mayer MP, Rudiger S, Bukau B (2000) Molecular basis for interactions of the DnaK chaperone with substrates. Biol Chem 381:877–885

Mizukoshi E, Suzuki M, Loupatov A, Uruno T, Hayashi H, Misono T, Kaul SC, Wadhwa R, Imamura T (1999) Fibroblast growth factor-1 interacts with the glucose-regulated protein GRP75/mortalin. Biochem J 343:461–466

Mizukoshi E, Suzuki M, Misono T, Loupatov A, Munekata E, Kaul SC, Wadhwa R, Imamura T (2001) Cell-cycle dependent tyrosine phosphorylation on mortalin regulates its interaction with fibroblast growth factor-1. Biochem Biophys Res Commun 280:1203–1209

Modica-Napolitano JS, Singh K (2002) Mitochondria as targets for detection and treatment of cancer. Expert Rev Mol Med 2002:1–19

Nardai G, Csermely P, Soti C (2002) Chaperone function and chaperone overload in the aged. A preliminary analysis. Exp Gerontol 37:1257–1262

Osorio C, Sullivan PM, He DN, Mace BE, Ervin JF, Strittmatter WJ, Alzate O (2007) Mortalin is regulated by APOE in hippocampus of AD patients and by human APOE in TR mice. Neurobiol Aging 28:1853–1862

Pilzer D, Fishelson Z (2005) Mortalin/GRP75 promotes release of membrane vesicles from immune attacked cells and protection from complement-mediated lysis. Int Immunol 17:1239–1248

Polyak K, Li Y, Zhu H et al (1998) Somatic mutations of the mitochondrial genome in human colorectal tumours. Nat Genet 20: 291–293

Qu M, Zhou Z, Xu S, Chen C, Yu Z, Wang D (2011) Mortalin overexpression attenuates beta-amyloid-induced neurotoxicity in SH-SY5Y cells. Brain Res 1368:336–345

Ran Q, Wadhwa R, Kawai R, Kaul SC, Sifers RN, Bick RJ, Smith JR, Pereira-Smith OM (2000) Extramitochondrial localization of mortalin/mthsp70/PBP74/GRP75. Biochem Biophys Res Commun 275:174–179

Rehling P, Brandner K, Pfanner N (2004) Mitochondrial import and the twin-pore translocase. Nat Rev Mol Cell Biol 5:519–530

Rudiger S, Mayer MP, Schneider-Mergener J, Bukau B (2000) Modulation of substrate specificity of the DnaK chaperone by alteration of a hydrophobic arch. J Mol Biol 304:245–251

Sacht G, Brigelius-Flohe R, Kiess M, Sztajer H, Flohe L (1999) ATP-sensitive association of mortalin with the IL-1 receptor type I. Biofactors 9:49–60

Shi M, Jin J, Wang Y, Beyer RP, Kitsou E, Albin RL, Gearing M, Pan C, Zhang J (2008) Mortalin: a protein associated with progression of parkinson disease? J Neuropathol Exp Neurol 67:117–124

Shin BK, Wang H, Yim AM, Le Naour F, Brichory F, Jang JH, Zhao R, Puravs E, Tra J, Michael CW, Misek DE, Hanash SM (2003) Global profiling of the cell surface proteome of cancer cells uncovers an abundance of proteins with chaperone function. J Biol Chem 278:7607–7616

Singh B, Soltys BJ, Wu ZC, Patel HV, Freeman KB, Gupta RS (1997) Cloning and some novel characteristics of mitochondrial Hsp70 from Chinese hamster cells. Exp Cell Res 234:205–216

Soltys BJ, Gupta RS (2000) Mitochondrial proteins at unexpected cellular locations: export of proteins from mitochondria from an evolutionary perspective. Int Rev Cytol 194:133–196

Soti C, Csermely P (2002) Chaperones and aging: role in neurodegeneration and in other civilizational diseases. Neurochem Int 41:383–389

Sriram M, Osipiuk J, Freeman B, Morimoto R, Joachimiak A (1997) Human Hsp70 molecular chaperone binds two calcium ions within the ATPase domain. Structure 5:403–414

Stacchiotti A, Borsani E, Ricci F, Lavazza A, Rezzani R, Bianchi R, Rodella LF (2006) Bimoclomol ameliorates mercuric chloride nephrotoxicity through recruitment of stress proteins. Toxicol Lett 166:168–177

Takano S, Wadhwa R, Yoshii Y, Nose T, Kaul SC, Mitsui Y (1997) Elevated levels of mortalin expression in human brain tumors. Exp Cell Res 237:38–45

Takano S, Wadhwa R, Mitsui Y, Kaul SC (2001) Identification and characterization of molecular interactions between glucose-regulated proteins (GRPs) mortalin/GRP75/peptide-binding protein 74 (PBP74) and GRP94. Biochem J 357:393–398

Temple S, Qian X (1995) βFGF, neurotrophins, and the control or cortical neurogenesis. Neuron 15: 249–252

Tong JJ (2007) Mitochondrial delivery is essential for synaptic potentiation. Biol Bull 212:169–175

Van Laar VS, Dukes AA, Cascio M, Hastings TG (2008) Proteomic analysis of rat brain mitochondria following exposure to dopamine quinone: implications for Parkinson disease. Neurobiol Dis 29:477–489

Vandermoere F, El Yazidi-Belkoura I, Demont Y, Slomianny C, Antol J, Lemoine J, Hondermarck H (2007) Proteomic exploration reveals that actin is a signaling target of the kinase akt. Mol Cell Proteomics 6:114–124

Wadhwa R, Kaul SC, Ikawa Y, Sugimoto Y (1993a) Identification of a novel member of mouse hsp70 family. Its association with cellular mortal phenotype. J Biol Chem 268:6615–6621

Wadhwa R, Kaul SC, Mitsui Y, Sugimoto Y (1993b) Differential subcellular distribution of mortalin in mortal and immortal mouse and human fibroblasts. Exp Cell Res 207:442–448

Wadhwa R, Kaul SC, Sugimoto Y, Mitsui Y (1993c) Induction of cellular senescence by transfection of cytosolic mortalin cDNA in NIH 3T3 cells. J Biol Chem 268:22239–22242

Wadhwa R, Pereira-Smith OM, Reddel RR, Sugimoto Y, Mitsui Y, Kaul SC (1995) Correlation between complementation group for immortality and the cellular distribution of mortalin. Exp Cell Res 216:101–106

Wadhwa R, Akiyama S, Sugihara T, Reddel RR, Mitsui Y, Kaul SC (1996) Genetic differences between the pancytosolic and perinuclear forms of murine mortalin. Exp Cell Res 226:381–386

Wadhwa R, Takano S, Robert M, Yoshida A, Nomura H, Reddel RR, Mitsui Y, Kaul SC (1998) Inactivation of tumor suppressor p53 by mot-2, a hsp70 family member. J Biol Chem 273:29586–29591

Wadhwa R, Sugihara T, Yoshida A, Nomura, H, Reddel RR, Simpson R, Maruta H, Kaul SC (2000) Selective toxicity of MKT-077 to cancer cells is mediated by its binding to the hsp70 family protein mot-2 and reactivation of p53 function. Cancer Res 60:6818–6821

Wadhwa R, Yaguchi T, Hasan MK, Mitsui Y, Reddel RR, Kaul SC (2002) Hsp70 family member, mot-2/mthsp70/GRP75, binds to the cytoplasmic sequestration domain of the p53 protein. Exp Cell Res 274:246–253

Wadhwa R, Ando H, Kawasaki H, Taira K, Kaul SC (2003a) Targeting mortalin using conventional and RNA-helicase-coupled hammerhead ribozymes. EMBO Rep 4:595–601

Wadhwa R, Yaguchi T, Taira K, Kaul SC (2003b). Mortalin-MPD (mevalonate pyrophosphate decarboxylase) interactions and their role in control of cellular proliferaction. Biochem Biophys Res Commun 302:735–742

Wadhwa R, Takano S, Taira K, Kaul SC (2004) Reduction in mortalin level by its antisense expression causes senescence-like growth arrest in human immortalized cells. J Gene Med 6:439–444

Wadhwa R, Takano S, Kaur K, Deocaris C, Pereira-Smith OM, Reddel RR, Kaul SC (2006) Upregulation of mortalin/mthsp70/Grp75 contributes to human carcinogenesis. Int J Cancer 118:2973–2980

Walker C, Bottger S, Low B (2006) Mortalin-based cytoplasmic sequestration of p53 in a nonmammalian cancer model. Am J Pathol 168:1526–1530

Wallace DC (2005) A mitochondrial paradigm of metabolic and degenerative diseases, aging, and cancer: a dawn for evolutionary medicine. Annu Rev Genet 39:359–407

Webster TJ, Naylor DJ, Hartman DJ, Hoj PB, Hoogenraad NJ (1994) cDNA cloning and efficient mitochondrial import of pre-mtHSP70 from rat liver. DNA Cell Biol 13:1213–1220

Widodo N, Kaur K, Shrestha BG, Takagi Y, Ishii T, Wadhwa R, Kaul SC. (2007) Selective killing of cancer cells by leaf extract of Ashwagandha: identification of a tumor-inhibitory factor and the first molecular insights to its effect. Clin Cancer Res 13:2298–2306

Willis D, Li KW, Zheng JQ, Chang JH, Smit A, Kelly T, Merianda TT, Sylvester J, van Minnen J, Twiss JL (2005) Differential transport and local translation of cytoskeletal, injury-response, and neurodegeneration protein mRNAs in axons. J Neurosci 25:778–791

Xu L, Voloboueva LA, Ouyang Y, Emery JF, Gillard RG (2009) Overexpression of mitochondrial Hsp70/Hsp75 in rat brain protects mitochondria, reduces oxidative stress, and protects from focal ischemia. J Cerebral Blood Flow Metabol 29:365–374

Yang H, Zhou X, Liu X, Yang L, Chen Q, Zhao D, Zuo J, Liu W (2011) Mitochondrial dysfunction induced by knockdown of mortalin is rescued by Parkin. Biochem Biophys Res Commun 410:114–120

Yi X, Luk JM, Lee NP, Peng J, Leng X, Guan XY, Lau GK, Beretta L, Fan ST (2008) Association of mortalin (HSPA9) with liver cancer metastasis and prediction for early tumor recurrence. Mol Cell Proteomics 7:315–325

Yoo JY, Ryu J, Yaguchi T, Kaul SC, Wadhwa R, Yun C-O (2010) Enhanced tumor killing by a mortalin targeting modified adeno-oncolytic virus. J Gene Medicine 12:586–595

Zheng DH, Zuo J, Yang ZJ, Xia BL, Zhang XN (2000) Grp75 protects cells from injuries caused by glucose deprivation. Yi Chuan Xue Bao 27:666–671

Zhu X, Zhao X, Burkholder WF, Gragerov A, Ogata CM, Gottesman ME, Hendrickson WA (1996) Structural analysis of substrate binding by the molecular chaperone DnaK. Science 272:1606–1614

Chapter 8
Age-Induced Alterations in Biological Clock: Therapeutic Effects of Melatonin

Anita Jagota

Abstract The suprachiasmatic nucleus (SCN) in hypothalamus contains a light-entrained circadian clock, the master pacemaker that orchestrates mammalian circadian rhythms in physiology and behavior. SCN consists of core circadian machinery genes that regulate melatonin synthesis in pineal from precursor neurotransmitter serotonin. The circadian melatonin signal functions as hands of the clock to inform all cells in the organism and in consequence the organism as a whole, about the passage of time and also regulate SCN through a feedback loop. Aging is associated with changes in several basic parameters of circadian rhythms leading to sleep disturbances. The endogenous melatonin levels decline gradually with age. The melatonin has been identified as an antiaging drug due to its multitasking role as rhythm synchronizer, an immunoregulator, an antioxidant- a potent free radical scavenger with beneficial effects on sleep as well as age related diseases. This review aims to summarize the current knowledge on the changes of the circadian system in advanced age and the therapeutic effects of antioxidant melatonin on such changes.

Keywords Antioxidant • Melatonin • Aging • Circadian rhythms • Suprachiasmatic nucleus

8.1 Circadian Time Keeping System: Biological Clock

Extensive physiological and behavioral studies have indicated that the circadian pacemaker, the endogenous clock is characterized by a cycle with a period of approximately 24 h duration. Such clocks have been localized to discrete sites in central nervous system (CNS) and, in mammals, to the bilaterally paired suprachiasmatic nucleus (SCN) in hypothalamus (Jagota et al. 2000; Reiter et al. 2010;

A. Jagota (✉)
Neurobiology and Molecular Chronobiology laboratory, Department of Animal Sciences, School of Life Sciences, University of Hyderabad, Hyderabad 500046, India
e-mail: ajsl@uohyd.ernet.in; anita_jagota@yahoo.com

M. K. Thakur, S. I. S. Rattan (eds.), *Brain Aging and Therapeutic Interventions*,
DOI 10.1007/978-94-007-5237-5_8,

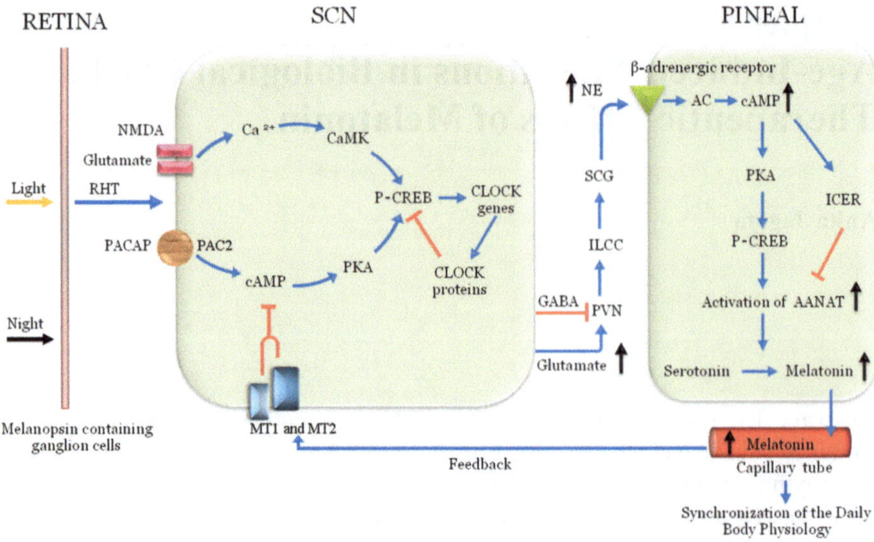

Fig. 8.1 Mammalian circadian timing system: melanopsin-containing ganglion cells in retina relay photic information via RHT to SCN by releasing glutamate and PACAP which act on CaMK and PKA via NMDA and PAC2 receptors respectively to increase P-CREB thus entraining and regulating clock gene expression clock proteins in SCN. The time information from SCN through GABA reaches PVN and then to SCG via ILCC. Then during night the time information travels from SCG by NE to β-adrenergic receptors at pineal, stimulating AC resulting in increased cAMP which activate PKA and hence increased P-CREB activating AANAT resulting in melatonin synthesis. The cAMP also triggers the expression of a negative transcription factor, ICER. Both blood and CSF melatonin acts on SCN via MT1 and MT2 receptors for resetting the circadian pacemaker. *RHT* retinohypothalamic tract, *PACAP* pituitary adenylate cyclase activating polypeptide, *cAMP* cyclic adenosine monophosphate, *CREB* cAMP response element-binding, *P-CREB* phosphorylated CREB, *CaMK* calmodulin kinase, *PKA* protein kinase A, *GABA* gamma-amino butyric acid, *PVN* periventricular nucleus, *SCG* superior cervical ganglion, *ILCC* intermediolateral cell column, *NE* norepinephrin, *AC* adenylate cyclase, *AANAT* arylalkylamine N-acetyltransferase, *ICER* inducible cAMP early repressor

Welsh et al. 2010). These clocks are periodically synchronized to the geophysical time. Photoperiod is the most dominant environmental zeitgeber (time giver) for the phase entrainment of the circadian oscillator. The photic information reaches SCN via the retinohypothalamic tract (RHT). The electrical information is converted into chemical information that alters the phase of clock gene expression in a subset of SCN neurons which then regulates both synthesis and release of melatonin (hormonal message for darkness) from pineal. The time information from SCN passes to the pineal via a multisynaptic pathway for the synthesis of melatonin from serotonin (5-hydroxy tryptamine; 5-HT) (Fig. 8.1). This pathway is actually activated during night without light stimuli. In pinealocytes, tryptophan is converted into serotonin via 5-hydroxytryptophan. Then N-acetylation of serotonin by arylalkylamine N-acetyltransferase (AANAT) followed by methylation of the 5-hydroxy moiety by hydroxyindole-O-methyl-transferase (HIOMT) results in melatonin synthesis. Melatonin helps to regulate other hormones and maintains the body's circadian rhythm through its receptors. The rhythm of melatonin production is endogenous such that melatonin levels are high at night and low during the day (Reiter et al. 2010; Yonei et al. 2010).

Melanopsin-containing ganglion cells in retina relay light information to the SCN via the retinohypothalamic tract (RHT) by releasing glutamate and pituitary adenylate cyclase activating polypeptide (PACAP) which causes entrainment of clock gene expression in the SCN. Information from SCN neurons passes to the periventricular nucleus (PVN) of the hypothalamus where they release gamma-amino butyric acid (GABA). The PVN gives message of darkness to pineal via intermediolateral cell column (ILCC) and superior cervical ganglion (SCG). The sympathetic nerve fibres from the SCG release norepinephrine (NE) which acts on both α1- and β-adrenergic receptors present on the pinealocytes. The β-adrenergic receptors stimulate adenylate cyclase (AC) and α1 adrenergic receptors potentiate the β- induced cAMP production. Increased levels of cAMP lead to the activation of cAMP-dependent protein kinase A (PKA). The PKA phosphorylates a group of transcription factors such as cAMP response element-binding (CREB). Phosphorylated-CREB (P-CREB) binds to the cAMP-responsive elements (CREs) present on the cAMP response genes such as AANAT and stimulates its transcription leading to 100–150 folds increase in Nat mRNA levels and translation with 70 folds nocturnal increase in protein levels and also maintains the enzyme in its active form. Activation of AANAT results in a 10-fold increase in melatonin synthesis and secretion, approximately 5–6 h after the onset of night. The cAMP also triggers the expression of a negative transcription factor, an inducible cAMP early repressor (ICER) which competes with P-CREB for the CREs in the AANAT promoter. AANAT gene expression is suppressed when there is a decrease in P-CREB together with an increase in ICER. Increased ICER levels inhibit transcription of CRE-induced genes late in the night. The mechanism involved in photoperiodic control of pineal metabolism involves two important links: photoperiodic regulation of AANAT gene expression and HIOMT activity occurs at the transcriptional level (Simonneaux and Ribelayga 2003). The mRNA levels of HIOMT exhibit circadian variation with a peak at mid-light phase in *in vivo* as well as *in vitro* conditions. The SCN controls melatonin rhythm in the pineal by using inhibitory signal, GABA during day time and stimulatory signal, glutamate at night time. The decrease in melatonin synthesis at the end of the night depends on post-translational mechanisms triggered by termination of NE release from SCG terminals (Perreau-Lenz et al. 2005). Melatonin is transported into the blood and cerebrospinal fluid (CSF) of the third ventricle.

Melatonin receptors inhibit neuronal activity and phase shift circadian firing rhythms in the SCN (Dubocovich et al. 2003). Melatonin receptors are G protein-coupled receptors with two types of G-proteins (Gi (inhibitory- activates K^+ channels, inhibits adenylate cyclase) and Go (inhibits Ca^{2+} channels)). G proteins activate AC which in turn activates second messenger molecules for regulation of various physiological functions. In mammals, three types of melatonin receptor have been identified: MT1 (or Mel1A or MTNR1A), MT2 (or Mel1B or MTNR1B) and MT3 (or Mel1C or MTNR1C) (Sugden et al. 2004).

Both blood and CSF melatonin acts on SCN via MT1 and MT2 receptors for resetting the circadian pacemaker and regulating circadian processes such as sleep (Reiter et al. 2010; Yonei et al. 2010). Melatonin when it binds to its receptors, there is an influx of Ca^{2+} which then activates calmodulin by binding to it. This Ca^{2+} calmodulin complex binds to Calmodulin kinase II (CaMKII) and activates it. CaMKII also gets autophosphorylated and phosphorylates intracellular targets such as tryptophan hydroxylase. SCN is rich in CaMKII and it is known to be involved in transmission of photic information and phase resetting of the circadian clock upon light exposure. Phosphorylation of CaMKII is rhythmic both under free-running and entrained conditions with peak levels during the subjective day (Agostino et al. 2004).

The basic function or nature of an oscillatory system is to return the system when it moves away from its regular manner. This is achieved by involvement of positive and negative feedback loops. Several putative clock genes, *clock, per1, per2, per3, bmal1, cry1* and *cry2* are expressed abundantly in the SCN (Takahashi et al. 2008; Dibner et al. 2010; Welsh et al. 2010). The positive regulators include *clock, bmal1* and *rorα*, whereas the negative elements comprise of *per, cry* and *rev-erbα*. All genes are expressed rhythmically except *clock* that is constitutively expressed. When CLOCK and BMAL1 reach critical concentrations, they dimerise. The CLOCK/BMAL1 hetrodimers then act at E-box elements to promote transcription of Period (*per1, per2, per3*) and Cryptochrome (*cry1, cry2*) genes, leading to increased PER and CRY levels. PER and CRY in the cytoplasm are phosphorylated in the presence of caesin kinase 1 ε and δ, heterodimerize and then enter the nucleus and inhibit transcription of their own genes by interacting with CLOCK/BMAL1 heterodimer complex. The clock proteins are regulated dynamically in both spatial (nuclear and cytoplasmic) and temporal (production and degradation) dimensions. Delays could be associated with transcription, translation, dimerization, nuclear entry of PER/CRY heterodimers. The main oscillatory clock proteins shuttling between nucleus and cytoplasm are degraded by ubiquitination and the proteasome pathway. Further, ubiquitin ligase complexes β-TrCP1 and FBXL3 are responsible for decline in cytoplasmic PER and CRY levels (Yagita et al. 2002). In addition to this core loop, negative feedback loop, with REV-ERBα acting on ROR elements to inhibit *bmal1* transcription, also contributes to clock precision and robustness. Core clock output involves in addition to the central loop involving CLOCK/BMAL1, another indirect pathway, consisting of antagonistic regulation of PAR proteins and E4 BP4 (Mitsui et al. 2001). Thus daily cycling of clock gene mRNA, clock protein and other clock controlled genes and their protein products is characteristic of circadian systems (Welsh et al. 2010).

Interestingly, sirtuin 1 (SirT1) has been linked recently to the circadian rhythm machinery through direct deacetylation activity as well as through the NAD^+ salvage pathway (Jung-Hynes et al. 2010). In addition, the post-translational modifications of clock proteins are important for ensuring the maintenance of circadian rhythms, as they can modulate the activity and turnover of major clock components (Bellet and Sassone-Corsi 2010).

8.2 Age-Induced Circadian Rhythm Disruptions

Disruption of circadian rhythms is both the cause and the consequence of many diseases. Aging is the progressive deterioration in the behavioral, biochemical, physiological, morphological and anatomical aspects of an organism (Jagota 2005; Kirkwood 2005). Aging and circadian rhythms were linked initially by studies on circadian rhythms of release of hormones such as cortisol, thyroid stimulating hormone (TSH), melatonin, prolactin, growth hormone (GH) and sleep pattern of young and healthy elderly men. These alterations in the rhythmicity of these hormones can be related to modification in the kinetics of the activation of signaling pathways in the SCN; a reduction in the amplitude of photic information from the retina to the clock as well as age-related changes within the clock mechanism of the SCN itself. Early onset of activity, i.e., phase advance has been also reported in hamsters and mice with aging. Some workers have reported altered locomotor and wheel running activity, feeding, drinking, and core body temperature (CBT) in old rats and decreased melatonin synthesis and its outflow (Mishima et al. 2001). Thus, the circadian clock properties and functioning are altered with aging with the desynchronization of rhythms and the efficacy of input and output pathways to and from the SCN. The diurnal rhythm of $\alpha 1$ adrenergic receptor expression, characteristic of young rats, disappears by middle age (Smith et al. 2005). Aging results in neuronal deterioration, reduction of dendritic surface, decrease in protein levels as well as changes in the glucose rhythms. These changes lead to the aperiodic pattern of firing in the SCN neurons. Circadian disruptions associated with aging lead to poor health consequences and hastened senescence in elderly people. The decline in physiological function with aging may be associated with malfunctioning of various autonomic systems in the body. Aging is linked with the decreased robustness in the functioning of the circadian system in humans with reduced sensitivity of the SCN to retinal stimulations, loss of temporal coordination among bodily systems, leading to deficits in homeostasis and sub-optimal functioning of the physiology. Such alterations accelerate the aging process and contribute to senescence with neuronal degeneration of SCN leading to organic deterioration of the circadian oscillator and is characterized by loss of precision, decreased synchronization, a shorter period of the endogenous oscillator, reduced exposure to synchronizing stimuli such as light, or altered responsiveness to zeitgeber (Benloucifa et al. 2006; Gibson et al. 2009). Various studies on human aging show a decrease in pacemaker output and that the symptomatic expression of this abnormality is circadian rhythm sleep disorders (CRSD) (Fig. 8.2; Table 8.1) responsible for decrease in daytime alertness with a decline in actual sleep time, leading to system wide changes affecting physiology, e.g., digestion, mood and fatigue (Jagota 2005; Gibson et al. 2009). Temporal isolation experiments revealed that there is a negative relationship between the period of clock and age of the individual. Interestingly about 80 % of subjects in the 50–80 year age group have been found to show spontaneous internal desynchronization of rhythms that may affect sleep patterns and other aspects of aging (Wu et al. 2007). The phase advance in various rhythms with aging in older people such as sleep

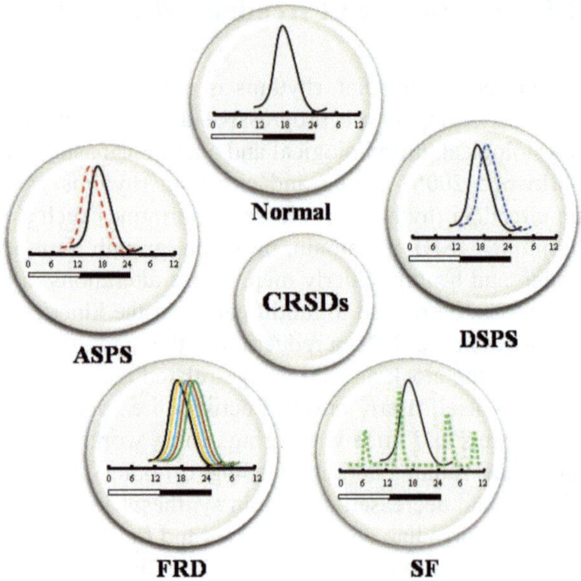

Fig. 8.2 Circadian rhythm sleep disorders (CRSDs): *ASPS* advanced sleep phase syndrome, *DSPS* delayed sleep phase syndrome, *FRD* free running disorder, *SF* sleep fragmentation

Table 8.1 Age induced circadian rhythm disorders

Disease
Circadian rhythm sleep disorders (CRSD)
Advanced sleep phase syndrome (ASPS)
Delayed sleep phase syndrome (DSPS)
Non 24 h sleep wake disorder: free running disorder (FRD)
Sleep fragmentation (SF): irregular sleep wake pattern
Periodic leg movements in sleep (PLMS)
Sleep disordered breathing (SDB)
REM sleep behavior disorder (RBD)
Restless leg syndrome (RLS)
Narcolepsy
Alzheimer's disease: sundowning
Insomnia
Chronic obstructive pulmonary disease (COPD)
Dementia: mild cognitive impairment (MCI)
Depression: affective disorders
Mood disorders
Unipolar affective disorder
Bipolar affective disorder
Seasonal affective disorder
Major depressive disorder (MDD)
Cardiovascular disorders
Cancer
Congenital blindness
Metabolic syndrome

wake, body temperature and hormone rhythms have been reported. Sleep disturbance is also a frequent symptom in patients with age associated neurodegenerative diseases such as Parkinson's disease (PD), Alzheimer's disease (AD) and Dementia (Harper et al. 2005; Whitehead et al. 2008). Many AD patients also suffer from severe circadian system related behavioral disturbances such as daytime agitation and night restlessness that they are linked to mental decline. Cellular senescence has been reported to impair circadian expression of clock genes due to decrease in ability of cells to transmit circadian signals to their clocks. The impairment is associated with decreased responsiveness of CREB-dependent signaling (Kunieda et al. 2006). Altered sleep/activity patterns can affect the function of the central and peripheral oscillators leading to alterations in metabolism. Altered sleep patterns can lead to arrhythmic exposure to light and thus constant resetting of the central oscillator which in turn may alter normal feeding patterns and desynchronize peripheral oscillators in metabolic tissues, such as liver and pancreas (Bellet and Sassone-Corsi 2010). Aging has also been linked with onset of menopause accompanied with changes in biological rhythms. The biological rhythms appear compromised by the middle age. We have also previously reported age induced alterations in daily rhythms of 5-HT levels in brain as well as SCN starting at middle age (Jagota and Kalyani 2008, 2010).

8.3 Age-Induced SCN Dysfunction at Neurotransmitter Level

It has been reported that aging causes a diminished function with decrease in the concentration of various neurotransmitters in the brain leading to various behavioural changes. The SCN contains one of the densest serotoninergic terminal plexus of the brain (Jagota 2006). Serotonin is an important neurotransmitter associated not only with circadian function but also with various physiological functions such as growth, neuroprotection, neurogenesis, behavior abnormalities such as aggression, insomnia, depression, suicidal or criminal behavior, loss of sex drive, despair and/or misery in elderly and modifications of the fine wiring of brain connections. In addition, serotonin metabolism plays an important role in regulation of food intake, reproduction, immunity, neurological function and anti-stress responses (Chen et al. 2007; Jagota and Reddy 2007; Yao et al. 2011).

The age related decline in brain serotonin levels has been reported in rats and monkeys (Kakiuchi et al. 2001) as well as human (Van Dyck et al. 2000). The age related alterations in serotonin have been related by some workers with psychiatric disorders such as depression, psychosis as well as neurodegenerative disorders such as PD and AD (Rehman and Masson 2001). We have previously reported progressive decline with age in mean 5-HT levels in brain as well as SCN and reduced amplitude of daily rhythmicity with disintegration at middle age. Such changes in loss of daily serotonin rhythmicity in brain and SCN in aging rats were linked earlier to age related circadian and sleep disorders (Jagota and Kalyani 2008, 2010).

As age induced decrease in serotonin levels has been linked to decrease in melatonin levels which in turn influence serotonin levels through feedback mechanisms, leading to disturbed physiological function and senescence. Decreased serotonin levels have been also related to the decreased transport of precursor amino acid i.e. tryptophan across the blood-brain-barrier; diminished activity of the anabolic enzymes and/or enhanced activity of catabolic enzymes which could be responsible for lower serotonin levels in the aging brain (Hussain and Mitra 2000). Many workers have reported the age related change in the morphology of serotonergic neurons in rat brain stem nuclei, frontal cortex, striatum, hypothalamus and in various brain regions, decline in melatonin and norepinephrine levels and MT1 melatonin receptor in SCN (Wu et al. 2007). The age induced decreased serotonin levels could also be responsible for age related increased MAO-B levels and neurodegeneration (Toussaint et al. 2000). A similar change in neurotransmitter serotonin receptors 5-HT7 and loss of sensitivity to the circadian effects of 8-OH-DPAT (Serotonin agonist) and decreased density of α-adrenergic receptors in SCN of aging hamsters have been reported. The functional activity of the SCN is also altered with a loss of day/night differences in vasoactive polypeptide mRNA levels of aged rats (Aujard et al. 2001).

The amplitude of release of neurotransmitters and neuropeptides declines and the rhythms of release become more erratic. Aging alters the rhythmic expression of vasoactive intestinal peptide (VIP) in the SCN though Arginine vasopressin (AVP) rhythm persists. Aging and AD have been reported to show degeneration of SCN with decrease in vasopressin levels as well as its mRNA level with decreased melatonin levels (Doi et al. 2011).

8.4 Aging and Clock Gene Expression

The age related desynchronization and deterioration occurs at the level of individual cells and is related with decreased expression of several genes involved in the molecular machinery of the circadian clock. Both *clock* and *bmal1* show reduced expression with aging. The involvement of *bmal1* in the aging has been demonstrated by some workers through experiments such as that *bmal1* null mutant mice show early signs of aging. It is an important protein required for normal tissue homeostasis in mice (Kondratov et al. 2006). Interestingly, reductions in *bmal1* expression are not yet linked with changes in *per1, per2* and *cry1* amplitude in the aged SCN, thus indicating the involvement of downstream targets of *bmal1* responsible for circadian disruption with advanced age (Asai et al. 2001). Mice mutant for *per1* and *per2* showed early onset of aging with faster decline of fertility and loss of soft tissue (Lee 2005). Clock gene expression of peripheral tissues such as liver and heart has also been reported to decrease with aging. Some experiments have been reported to show no change in *per1* and *per2* in constant darkness and *per1*-driven luciferase with aging (Hofman and Swaab 2006). The existence of a complex interconnection between aging and individual components of the circadian clock machinery has been highlighted by some workers (Antoch et al. 2008). Recently, SirT1 has been identified as regulator of aging, inflammation and metabolism (Bellet and Sassone-Corsi 2010). In addition, many studies provide strong evidence that the circadian clock and circadian rhythmicity regulate aging and cancer through circadian clock gene expression and their products as well as epigenetic modifications (Yu and Weaver 2011).

8.5 Age-Induced Disruptions in Melatonin Production

The circadian organization of body is mediated through the rhythmic release of various hormones, especially melatonin, and the secretion pattern change during aging so does the temporal organization of physiological and behavioral function. Interestingly age has been associated with a gradual waning of the nocturnal melatonin rhythm in all species including humans examined to date. Since melatonin secretion decreases with aging, some workers called this condition as "pinealpause". Decreased melatonin leads to disturbances in the circadian pacemaker, which causes internal temporal desynchronization inducing a variety of chronopathologies and leads to generalized deterioration of health (Fig. 8.3). We have found reduced melatonin levels with aging in both SCN and pineal in aging rats with loss of rhythmicity in middle age. Reduced melatonin concentration during aging, especially nocturnal levels, has been extensively reported in the pineal gland, plasma, CSF and urine as 6-hydroxymelatonin. The variations in the nocturnal serum melatonin peak at the age of 60 with decline by 70 year of age onward has been reported by many workers with change in timing of melatonin rhythm. Interestingly, older subjects enter sleep and awake earlier relative to their nightly melatonin secretory episode which indicates that aging is also associated with a change in the internal phase relationship between the sleep-wake cycle and the output of the circadian pacemaker. The decreased melatonin levels with age have been related to increased calcification in pineal gland in human leading to disturbed circadian rhythmicity in the sleep-wake cycle. However, no relationship between plasma melatonin or the metabolite 6-hydroxymelatonin in urine has been reported by some workers (Pandi-Perumal et al. 2005; Cardinali et al. 2008; Hill et al. 2011).

The peripheral melatonin levels have been reported to have auto-regulatory effects on receptor expression in the SCN, i.e. decreasing circulating melatonin levels by pinealectomy increases melatonin receptor expression in the SCN, whereas a single melatonin injection results in decreased melatonin receptor expression in the SCN. The melatonin levels decrease in the course of aging and even more dramatically in AD. Interestingly, autoregulatory feedback loop has been reported to be disturbed during aging and AD due to degeneration of the SCN neurons (Wu et al. 2007).

There is decline in melatonin and its precursor serotonin with aging. Melatonin deficiency especially in relation to serotonin may be responsible for the promotion of aging in the organism. Disturbed circadian melatonin rhythms have profound ef-

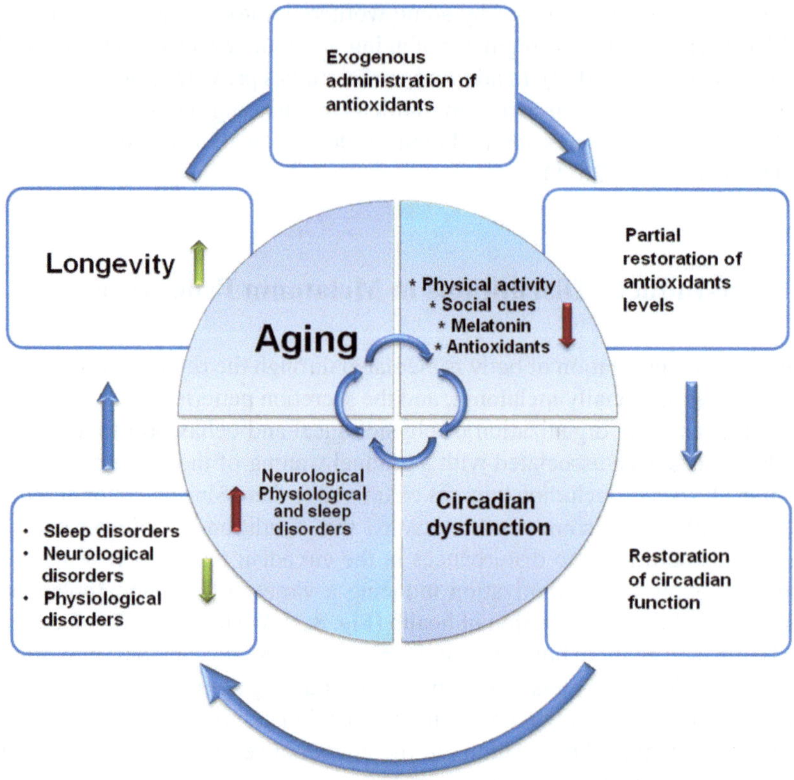

Fig. 8.3 Therapeutic effects of antioxidant melatonin. The diagrammatic representation of senescence induced decline in health and physiological functions responsible for circadian dysfunction leading to aging and effects of melatonin in restoring such functions leading to longevity

fects on the health and well-being of the elderly subjects (Poeggeler 2005; Wu et al. 2007). Healthy elderly subjects showed earlier clock time for melatonin circadian rhythms, which could be responsible for advanced wake time, cortisol, body and temperature peaks (Smith et al. 2005). Circadian disruptions have been related to decrease in MT1 receptor in aged subjects and late stage clinical AD patients. Similarly, alterations in circadian rhythms as well as production of the pineal hormone melatonin have been linked to aging and cancer risk (Wu et al. 2007).

8.6 Aging, Circadian Rhythms and Oxidative Stress

Age associated increase in oxidative stress or damage and inflammation are assumed to be a central phenomenon of aging (Fig. 8.3). Their attenuation is an aim for both healthy aging and life extension. Though, how clocks influence aging is not yet understood, there appears a relation between oxidative processes and reductive protection, detoxification, recharging and restoration (Rollo 2009).

Aging is linked with selective cell death in the brain. This could be associated with oxidative stress due to increased free radical generation and accumulation of reactive oxygen species (ROS) and nitrogen species (RNS) leading to onset of many age related neurodegenerative diseases. The gradual reduction with aging in melatonin, which functions as an autocoid, paracoid, hormone, antioxidant and a tissue factor could be responsible for accumulation of oxidatively modified molecules leading to mitochondria related disorders. Impaired mitochondrial dysfunction is regarded as the driving force for aging process with enhanced production of ROS. This could be responsible for possible accumulation of mitochondrial DNA mutations in postmitotic cells which are considered to be contributory factors to age related degeneration.

Melatonin has been reported to exist in higher plants (edible plants) and is inadvertently obtained from daily meals. Melatonin administration leads to sleep promoting effect in addition to lowering deep body temperatures not only in those with rhythm disorders but also in healthy individuals from children to elderly people, shortens the time required to fall asleep; improves sleep. In addition, melatonin functions as an antioxidant and acts in bone metabolism. It has been reported to inhibit age related visceral adiposity. Melatonin inhibits lipid peroxidation and blocks the production of isoprostanes. It is involved in free radical (OH., O_2., and NO.) scavenging (Poeggeler 2005). In addition, the endogenous melatonin also stimulates the antioxidant enzymes such as glutathione peroxidase (GPx), superoxide dismutase (SOD) and catalase (CAT) as well as modulates the daily rhythm patterns of glutathione levels in rat liver and brain (Baydas et al. 2002). Hence melatonin has its own antioxidant effect and also intensifies the activity of endogenous antioxidant enzymes, which together exert a powerful antioxidant effect. Considering that melatonin is secreted during the night time and passes through the blood brain barrier, it may play a preventive role against oxidation disorders of cerebral nerve cells during nocturnal sleep (Yonei et al. 2010). Recently, melatonin has been reported to regulate synthesis of 7α-hydroxypregnenolone which plays a central role in the circadian rhythms of activity (Tsutsui et al. 2009).

As melatonin has marked beneficial actions at cellular level particularly in mitochondria, various modes of action have been identified at different levels, from anti-excitatory/anti-excitotoxic and anti-inflammatory effects to regulation of anti- and pro-oxidative enzymes and direct radical detoxification (Hardeland et al. 2012). The relationship between radical formation to circadian function has many aspects such as age associated decline in the amplitude of circadian oscillations and dysphasing due to progressive shortening of spontaneous circadian period resulting in phase advance as well as the steady decline in nocturnal rhythmic secretion of melatonin levels. The survival signal pathways have been reported to be activated by melatonin. One such pathway is the Bcl-2 pathway, which stabilizes mitochondrial function by anti-apoptotic Bcl-2 family modulators. Since melatonin can readily reach the mitochondria due to its high lipophilicity, upon entry into the cell, it could become concentrated at a superficial position in lipid layers near the polar heads of phospholipids, a key place to function as a free radical scavenger (Rebrin et al. 2005).

The oxidative stress, DNA damage, mitochondrial dysfunction and altered cellular and subcellular activities of various organ systems are accompanied with mammalian aging (Judge et al. 2005). Decreased endogenous melatonin levels in aging may contribute to free radical-mediated brain aging (Reiter et al. 2010). The deteriorated free radical scavenging system due to oxidative/nitrosative stress in aged individuals plays a role in altered circadian rhythms pattern (Hardeland et al. 2011, 2012). The altered circadian behavior of endogenous antioxidants and lipid peroxidation levels in blood of wistar rats has been reported during aging process (Nachiyar et al. 2011). The decreased antioxidant levels in aged individuals result in accumulation of ROS leading to lipid peroxidation of membranes by damaging polyunsaturated fatty acids present in the membrane phospholipids (Sohal 2002; Yoon et al. 2002). Thus free radicals generated during aging are detoxified by stimulating the intracellular antioxidants glutathione, SOD, CAT and GPx through administration of antioxidants such as lipoate (Arivazhagan et al. 2000) or melatonin (Mauriz et al. 2007; Baeza et al. 2010).

8.7 Effect of Exogenous Melatonin Administration on Age-Induced Circadian Disruption

Melatonin is a multitasking molecule. It is an endogenous synchronizer and has widespread integrative and regenerative effects with numerous functions as a free radical scavenger, potent antioxidant and an antiaging drug. Melatonin not only functions as a hormone and a circadian mediator for time information but also eliminates free radicals. Melatonin is used for the treatment of various diseases and disorders such as cancer, immune disorders, cardiovascular diseases, depression, seasonal affective disorder (SAD), CRSDs and sexual dysfunction. Melatonin has been found to act as a differentiating agent in some cancer cells and to lower their invasive and metastatic status.

Interestingly, melatonin as well as its metabolites (cyclic 3-hydroxymelatonin, AFMK and AMK) are highly effective in scavenging for variety of toxic radicals such as ONOO– (Peroxynitrite), O_2.– (Superoxide anion), H_2O_2 (Hydrogen peroxide), $1O_2$ (Singlet oxygen), NO. (Nitric oxide), LOO. (Lipid peroxyl) and HClO (Hypochlorous acid), thus protecting cells from oxidative damage. Oxygen (O_2) is the precursor for generating various free radicals in mitochondrial electron transport chain (ETC). Melatonin is found to be successful in reducing cellular damage and death by detoxifying the free radical generated in ETC from O_2. Melatonin therapy has been shown to improve sleep disturbances in the elderly, indicating that a complex interaction of decreased pacemaker output as well as responsiveness of effector systems to pacemaker outputs play a major role in aging (Miller et al. 2005; Davidson et al. 2008).

Interestingly, melatonin has been reported to have actions which are non-genomic i.e. do not require a receptor or formation of a complex with another molecule. This receptor- independent action i.e. radical scavenging has been related to presence of melatonin in vicinity of a ROS when it is generated. As mitochondria are site of free radical production, it would be advantageous if concentrations of melatonin were high within the mitochondria. Martin et al. (2000) have reported higher concentrations of melatonin in mitochondria compared to other portions of cell or blood. Melatonin highly resists mitochondrial oxidative damage and cellular apoptosis, portends its use in clinical medicine to treat septic shock, neurodegeneration, ischemia, ionizing radiation, toxin, heavy metal exposure, etc. Interestingly, a number of studies have compared melatonin with classic antioxidants such as glutathione, mannitol, vitamin C, vitamin E and reported that melatonin is a better antioxidant (Reiter et al. 2010).

In addition, melatonin has been reported to inhibit free radical formation in microglia exposed to amyloid β1-42 by preventing the phosphorylation of the p47 Nox subunit via the P13/Akt pathway, thus giving support to the hypothesis that melatonin has a protective effect at the level of radical generation (Srinivasan et al. 2011).

The exogenous administration of melatonin helps in resetting the circadian clock as the endogenous melatonin declines with age for several reasons (Revell et al. 2006; Jagota and Kalyani 2008, 2010). External administration of melatonin is associated with treatment of cancer, age related and circadian rhythm disorders due to its potent antioxidant activity (Reiter et al. 2010). Various reports proved that melatonin acts as an antiaging agent (Touitou 2001; Tajes et al. 2009; Reiter et al. 2010; Hardeland et al. 2012). We have recently reported effect of exogenous melatonin administration on age induced alterations in serotonin rhythms in SCN. Our studies indicated an age related decrease in the mean serotonin levels and daily 5-HT rhythmicity in SCN. Melatonin administration restored differentially altered serotonin levels and amplitude of rhythmicity in variable age groups. Interestingly, we found age related loss of sensitivity of melatonin in restoration of 5-HT levels and its rhythmicity and that the restoration was relatively better in middle age groups (Jagota and Kalyani 2010).

The use of melatonin has received extraordinary attention as a novel pharmacological approach to treat circadian rhythm disturbances in aging and age related disorders such as PD, AD and dementia (Table 8.2). Melatonin has been shown to be effective in treatment of seasonal affective disorder and is being considered for bipolar and other disorders where circadian disturbances are involved. Studies have found that the use of melatonin can help entrain the circadian clock to environmental cycles and have beneficial effects for the treatment of certain forms of insomnia (Turek and Gillette 2004; Wade et al. 2007). In another study, researchers concluded that melatonin is effective in treating delayed sleep phase syndrome (Buscemi et al. 2006).

Melatonin has been reported to increase survival and inhibit oxidative and amyloid pathology in a transgenic mouse model of AD. In AD patients, melatonin has been suggested to improve circadian rhythmicity, decreased agitated behavior, confusion and sundowning in uncontrolled studies (Maurizi 2001; Zisapel 2001)

Table 8.2 Therapeutic effects of melatonin administration on age induced circadian disorders

Disease	Reference
Alzheimer's disease (AD): decreased "sundowning," improved sleep, slowing of the disease	Maurizi 2001
Advanced sleep phase syndrome (ASPS)	Zisapel 2001
Sleep disturbances in PD: improvement in total night time sleep	Dowling et al. 2005
Sleep problems in chronic obstructive pulmonary disease (COPD): improvement in sleep	Nunes et al. 2008
Rapid eye movement (REM) sleep behavior disorder and narcolepsy	Billiard 2009
Delayed sleep phase syndrome (DSPS): synchronization of sleep-wake rhythm	van Geijlswijk et al. 2010
Restless leg syndrome (RLS): significant improvement of leg discomfort	Whittom et al. 2010
Mild cognitive impairment (MCI) in AD: improves sleep quality and cognitive performance	Cardinali et al. 2011

(Table 8.2). Recently, ramelteron, a potent agonist for the melatonin receptors has been reported in its efficacy towards management of chronic insomnia, sleep latency, total sleep time, etc. (Spadoni et al. 2011).

Melatonin administration has been demonstrated to improve blood levels of neutral fat, free fatty acids, total cholesterol and to reduce TNF-α by 50 % in experimental rat model of diabetes. Pinealectomy resulted in increased insulin resistance and induced hyperinsulinemia accelerating disease progression in type 2 diabetes. Thus, melatonin improves insulin resistance (Nishida et al. 2003). Long term administration of melatonin to middle aged and old humans and experimental animal models of hypercholesterolemia as well as diabetes reduces blood and liver cholesterol and LDL-cholesterol levels. In addition, treatment of peri- and postmenopausal women with melatonin increased HDL-cholesterol. Hence, melatonin favourably affects lipid metabolism also. Melatonin plays very important role in bone metabolism. It accelerates the proliferative differentiation of osteoblasts and increased collagen production and prevents osteoporosis and accelerates fracture healing. Melatonin administration has been related with prevention of brain damage during fetal and neonatal period (Yonei et al. 2010).

Circadian rhythms also affect the time dependent therapeutic efficacy and toxicity of drugs by influencing both the pharmacokinetics and pharmacodynamics. As melatonin has been associated with chronotherapy, understanding and characterizing the complexities of circadian rhythmicity will help in timely administration of chemotherapy agents in various age induced disorders (Jung-Hynes et al. 2010).

8.8 Summary and Conclusion

Senescence decreases the ability of cells to transmit circadian signals with decline in endogenous melatonin. The circadian dysfunction with aging is linked to human pathophysiology both as a contributing factor as well as consequence. Information collected here displays a window on therapeutic effects of melatonin with the potential as rhythm synchronizer, an anti inflammatory, an antioxidant, a potent free radical scavenger and an antiaging drug with beneficial effects on sleep as well as age related diseases (Fig. 8.3). The sirtuins have emerged as potential therapeutic targets for treatment of human pathologies involving circadian dysfunction such as neurodegenerative, cardiovascular, metabolic diseases and cancer. As circadian rhythms also affect the time dependent therapeutic efficacy and toxicity of drugs, understanding and characterizing the circadian rhythmicity in gene expression in various tissues will play an important role in both optimizing the timing of drug administration and in the development of new therapeutics targeting the molecular clock. With the huge increase in the development of antibody and antisense oligonucleotide based therapeutics, characterizing the circadian rhythmicity in mRNA and protein expression will become more prominent in the future. Thus, there is need for more basic and clinical research and lifestyle that can increase melatonin with age.

Acknowledgements AJ is thankful to Prof MK Thakur and Prof Suresh IS Rattan for giving this opportunity. This work is supported by UGC (Ref: F. No.: 32-613/2006(SR), DST (Do No.: SR/SO/AS-47/2004), DST-Nano (Ref: 8.18), ICMR (Ref. No. BMS/NTF/14/2006-2007) and DBT (Ref No. BT/PR 3974/MED/30/813/2012) grants to AJ.

References

Agostino PV, Ferreyra GA, Murad AD, Watanabe Y, Golombek DA (2004) Diurnal, circadian and photic regulation of calcium/calmodulin-dependent kinase II and neuronal nitric oxide synthase in the hamster suprachiasmatic nuclei. Neurochem Int 44:617–625

Antoch MP, Gorbacheva VY, Vykhovanets O, Toshkov IA, Kondratov RV, Kondratova AA (2008) Disruption of the circadian clock due to the *Clock* mutation has discrete effects on aging and carcinogenesis. Cell Cycle 7:1197–1204

Arivazhagan P, Thilakavathy T, Panneerselvam C (2000) Antioxidant lipoate and tissue antioxidants in aged rats. J Nutr Biochem 11:122–127

Asai M, Yoshinobu Y, Kaneko S, Mori A, Nikaido T, Moriya T, Akiyama M, Shibata S (2001) Circadian profile of *per* Gene mRNA expression in the Suprachiasmatic Nucleus, Paraventricular Nucleus, and Pineal Body of aged rats. J Neurosci Res 66:1133–1139

Aujard F, Dkhissi-Benyahya O, Fournier I, claustrat B, Schilling A, Cooper HM, Perret M (2001) Artificially accelerated aging by shortened photoperiod alters early gene expression (*fos*) in the suprachiasmatic nucleus and sulfatoxymelatonin excretion in a small primate, microcebus murinus. Neuroscience 105:403–412

Baeza I, Fdez-Tresguerres J, Ariznavarreta C, De la Fuente M (2010) Effects of growth hormone, melatonin, oestrogens and phytoestrogens on the oxidized glutathione (GSSG)/reduced glutathione (GSH) ratio and lipid peroxidation in aged ovariectomized rats. Biogerontology 11:687–701

Baydas G, Gursu MF, Yilmaz S, Canpolat S, Yasar A, Cikim G, Canatan H (2002) Daily rhythm of glutathione peroxidase activity, lipid peroxidation and glutathione levels in tissues of pinealectomized rats. Neurosci Lett 323:195–198

Bellet MM, Sassone-Corsi PP (2010) Mammalian circadian clock and metabolism—the epigenetic link. Cell Sci 23:3837–3848

Benloucifa S, Greena K, L'Hermite-Balériaux M, Weintraub S, Wolfed LF, Zee PC (2006) Responsiveness of the aging circadian clock to light. Neurobiol Aging 27:1870–1879
Billiard M (2009) REM sleep behavior disorder and narcolepsy. CNS Neurol Disord Drug Targets 8:264–270
Buscemi N, Vandermeer B, Hooton N, Pandya R, Tjosvold L, Hartling L, Vohra S, Klassen TP, Baker G (2006) Efficacy and safety of exogenous melatonin for secondary sleep disorders and sleep disorders accompanying sleep restriction: meta-analysis. BMJ 332:385–393
Cardinali DP, Esquifino AI, Srinivasan V, Seithikurippu R, Pandi-Perumal (2008) Melatonin and the immune system in aging. Neuroimmunomodulation 15:272–278
Cardinali DP, Pagano ES, Scacchi Bernasconi PA, Reynoso R, Scacchi P (2011) Disrupted chronobiology of sleep and cytoprotection in obesity: possible therapeutic value of melatonin. Neuro Endocrinol Lett 32:588–606
Chen SJ, Kao CL, Chang YL, Yen CJ, Shui JW, Chien CS, Chen IL, Tsai TH, Ku HH, Chiou SH (2007) Antidepressant administration modulates neural stem cell survival and serotoninergic differentiation through bcl-2. Curr Neurovasc Res 4:19–29
Davidson AJ, Yamazaki S, Arble DM, Menaker M, Block GD (2008) Resetting of central and peripheral circadian oscillators in aged rats. Neurobiol Aging 29:471–477
Dibner C, Schibler U, Albrecht U (2010) The mammalian circadian timing system: organization and coordination of central and peripheral clocks. Annu Rev Physiol 72:517–549
Doi M, Ishida A, Miyake A, Sato M, Komatsu R, Yamazaki F, Kimura I, Tsuchiya S, Kori H, Seo K, Yamaguchi Y, Matsuo M, Fustin JM, Tanaka R, Santo Y, Yamada H, Takahashi Y, Araki M, Nakao K, Aizawa S, Kobayashi M, Obrietan K, Tsujimoto G, Okamura H (2011) Circadian regulation of intracellular G-protein signalling mediates intercellular synchrony and rhythmicity in the suprachiasmatic nucleus. Nat Commun 2:327–336
Dowling GA, Mastick J, Colling E, Carter JH, Singer CM, Aminoff MJ (2005) Melatonin for sleep disturbances in Parkinson's disease. Sleep Med 6:459–466
Dubocovich ML, Rivera-Bermudez MA, Gerdin MJ, Masana MI (2003) Molecular pharmacology, regulation and function of mammalian melatonin receptors. Front Biosci 1:1093–1098
Gibson MV, Fritz J, Kachur V (2009) Practical strategies for management of hypertension in the elderly. Geriatrics 64:10–19
Hardeland R, Cardinali DP, Srinivasan V, Spence DW, Brown GM, Pandi-Perumal SR (2011) Melatonin—a pleiotropic, orchestrating regulator molecule. Prog Neurobiol 93:350–384
Hardeland R, Madrid JA, Tan DX, Reiter RJ (2012) Melatonin, the circadian multioscillator system and health: the need for detailed analyses of peripheral melatonin signaling. J Pineal Res 52:139–166
Harper DG, Volicer L, Stopa EG, Mckee AC, Nitta M, Satlin A (2005) Disturbance of endogenous circadian rhythm in aging and Alzheimer disease. Am J Geriatr Psychiatry 13:359–368
Hill V, Dunn L, Dunning K, Page SJ (2011) A pilot study of rhythm and timing training as a supplement to occupational therapy in stroke rehabilitation. Top Stroke Rehabil 18:728–737
Hofman MA, Swaab DF (2006) Living by the clock: the circadian pacemaker in older people. Aging Res Rev 5:33–51
Hussain AM, Mitra AK (2000) Effect of aging on tryptophan hydroxylase in rat brain: implications on serotonin level. Drug Metab Dispos 28:1038–1042
Jagota A (2005) Aging and Sleep Disorders. I J Gerontol 19:415–424
Jagota A (2006) Suprachiasmatic nucleus: the center for circadian timing system in mammals. Proc Indian Natl Sci Acad B71:275–288
Jagota A, Kalyani D (2008) Daily serotonin rhythms in rat brain during postnatal development and aging. Biogerontology 9:229–234
Jagota A, Kalyani D (2010) Effect of melatonin on age induced changes in daily serotonin rhythms in suprachiasmatic nucleus of male wistar rat. Biogerontology 11:299–308
Jagota A, Reddy MY (2007) The effect of curcumin on ethanol induced changes in suprachiasmatic nucleus (SCN) and pineal. Cell Mol Neurobiol 27:997–1006
Jagota A, de la Iglesia HO, Schwartz WJ (2000) Morning and evening circadian oscillations in the suprachiasmatic nucleus in vitro. Nat Neurosci 3:372–376

Judge S, Jang YM, Smith A, Hagen T, Leeuwenburgh C (2005) Age-associated increases in oxidative stress and antioxidant enzyme activities in cardiac interfibrillar mitochondria: implications for the mitochondrial theory of aging. FASEB J 19:419–421

Jung-Hynes B, Reiter RJ, Ahmad N (2010) Sirtuins, melatonin and circadian rhythms: building a bridge between aging and cancer. J Pineal Res. 48:9–19

Kakiuchi T, Ohba H, Nishiyama S, Sato K, Harada N, Nakanishi S, Tsukada H (2001) Age-related changes in muscarinic cholinergic receptors in the living brain: a PET study using N-[11C] methyl-4-piperidyl benzilate combined with cerebral blood flow measurement in conscious monkeys. Brain Res 916:22–31

Kirkwood TB (2005) Time of our lives. What controls the length of life? EMBO Rep Spec:S4–8

Kondratov RV, Kondratova AA, Gorbacheva VY, Vykhovanets OV, Antoch MP (2006) Early aging and age-related pathologies in mice deficient in BMAL1, the core componentof the circadian clock. Genes Dev 20:1868–1873

Kunieda T, Minamino T, Katsuno T, Tateno K, Nishi J, Miyauchi H, Orimo M, Okada S, Komuro I (2006) Cellular senescence impairs circadian expression of clock genes *in vitro* and *in vivo*. Circ Res 98:532–539

Lee CC (2005) The circadian clock and tumor suppression by mammalian period genes. Methods Enzymol 393:852–861

Martin J, Marler M, Shochat TAncoli-Israe S (2000) Circadian rhythms of agitation in institutionalized patients with Alzheimer's Disease. Chronobiol Internat. 17:405–418

Mauriz JL, Molpeceres V, Garcıa-Mediavilla MV, Gonzalez P, Barrio JP, Gonzalez-Gallego J (2007) Melatonin prevents oxidative stress and changes in antioxidant enzyme expression and activity in the liver of aging rats. J Pineal Res 42:222–230

Maurizi CP (2001) Alzheimer's disease: roles for mitochondrial damage, the hydroxyl radical, and cerebrospinal fluid deficiency of melatonin. Med Hypotheses 57:156–160

Miller JP, Mcauley JD, Pang KCH (2005) Spontaneous *fos* expression in the Suprachiasmatic nucleus of young and old mice. Neurobiol Aging 26:1107–1115

Mishima K, Okawa M, Shimizu T, Hishikawa Y (2001) Diminished melatonin secretion in the elderly caused by insufficient environmental illumination. J Clin Endocrinol Metab 8:129–134

Mitsui S, Yamaguchi S, Matsuo T, Ishida Y, Okamura H (2001) Antagonistic role of E4BP4 and PAR proteins in the circadian oscillatory mechanism. Genes Dev 15:995–1006

Nachiyar RK, Subramanian KP, Manivasagam TT (2011) Influence of aging on the circadian patterns of thiobarbituric acid reactive substances and antioxidants in Wistar rats. Biol Rhythm Res 42:147–154

Nishida S, Sato R, Murai I, Nakagawa S (2003) Effect of pinealectomy on plasma levels of insulin and leptin and on hepatic lipids in type 2 diabetic rats. J Pineal Res 35:251–256

Nunes DM, Mota RM, Machado MO, Pereira ED, Bruin VM, Bruin PF (2008) Effect of melatonin administration on subjective sleep quality in chronic obstructive pulmonary disease. Braz J Med Biol Res 41:926–931

Pandi-Perumal SR, Zisapel N, Srinivasan V, Cardanali DP (2005) Melatonin and sleep in aging population. Exp Gerontol 40:911–925

Perreau-Lenz S, Kalsbeek A, Van Der Vliet J, P'evet P, Buijs RM (2005) In vivo evidence for a controlled offset of melatonin synthesis at dawn by the suprachiasmatic nucleus in the rat. Neuroscience 130:797–803

Poeggeler B (2005) Melatonin, aging, and age-related diseases: perspectives for prevention, intervention, and therapy. Endocrine 27:201–212

Rebrin I, Zicker S, Wedekind KJ, Paetau-Robinson I, Packer L, Sohal RS (2005) Effect of antioxidant-enriched diets on glutathione redox status in tissue homogenates and mitochondria of the senescence-accelerated mouse. Free Radic Biol Med 39:549–557

Rehman H, Masson E (2001) Neuroendocrinology of aging. Age Aging 30:279–287

Reiter RJ, Tan DX, Fuentes-Broto L (2010) Melatonin: a multitasking molecule. Prog Brain Res 181:127–151

Revell VL, Burgess HJ, Gazda CJ, Smith MR, Fogg L, Eastman CI (2006) Advancing human circadian rhythms with afternoon melatonin and morning intermittent bright light. J Clin Endocrinol Metab 91:54–59
Rollo CD (2009) Dopamine and aging: intersecting facets. Neurochem Res 34:601–629
Simonneaux V, Ribelayga C (2003) Generation of the melatonin endocrine message in mammals: a review of the complex regulation of melatonin synthesis by norepinephrine, peptides, and other pineal transmitters. Pharmacol Rev 55:325–395
Smith CP, Walton A, Loveland AD, Umberger GH, Kryscio RJ, Gash DM (2005). Memories that last in old age: motor skill learning and memory presentation. Neurobiol Aging 26:883–890
Sohal RS (2002) Role of oxidative stress and protein oxidation in the aging process. Free Radic Biol Med 33:37–44
Spadoni G, Bedini A, Rivara S, Mor M (2011) Melatonin receptor agonists: new options for insomnia and depression treatment. CNS Neurosci Ther 17:733–741
Srinivasan V, Pandi-Perumal SR, Brezezinski A, Bhatnagar KP, Cardinali DP (2011) Melatonin, immune function and cancer. Recent Pat Endocr Metab Immune Drug Discov 5:109–123
Sugden D, Davidson K, Hough KA, Teh MT (2004) Melatonin, melatonin receptors and melanophores: a moving story. Pigment Cell Res 17:454–460
Tajes M, Gutierrez-Cuesta J, Ortuño-Sahagun D, Camins A, Pallàs M (2009) Anti-aging properties of melatonin in an in vitro murine senescence model: involvement of the sirtuin 1 pathway. J Pineal Res 47:228–237
Takahashi JS, Hong HK, Ko CH, Mcdearmon EL (2008) The genetics of mammalian circadian order and disorder: implications for physiology and disease. Nat Rev Genet 9:764–775
Touitou Y (2001) Human aging and melatonin. Clinical relevance. Exp Gerontol 36:1083–1100
Toussaint O, Dumont P, Dierick JF, Pascal T, Frippiat C, Chainiaux F, Sluse F, Eliaers F, Remacle J (2000) Stress-induced premature senescence. Essence of life, evolution, stress, and aging. Ann N Y Acad Sci 908:85–98
Tsutsui K, Inoue K, Miyabara H, Suzuki S, Ogura Y, Tobari Y, Haraguchi S (2009) Discovery of a novel avian neurosteroid, 7alpha-hydroxypregnenolone, and its role in the regulation of the diurnal rhythm of locomotor activity in Japanese quail. Gen Comp Endocrinol 163:117–122
Turek FW, Gillette MU (2004) Melatonin, sleep, and circadian rhythms: rationale for development of specific melatonin agonists. Sleep Med 5:523–532
Van Dyck CH, Malison RT, Seibyl JP, Laruelle M, Klumpp H, Zoghbi SS, Baldwin RM, Innis RB (2000) Age-related decline in central serotonin transporter availability with [(123)I]beta-CIT SPECT. Neurobiol Aging 21:497–501
van Geijlswijk IM, Korzilius HP, Smits MG (2010) The use of exogenous melatonin in delayed sleep phase disorder: a meta-analysis. Sleep 33:1605–1671
Wade AG, Ford I, Crawford G, Mcmahon AD, Nir T, Laudon M, Zisapel N (2007) Efficacy of prolonged release melatonin in insomnia patients aged 55–80 years: quality of sleep and next-day alertness outcomes. Curr Med Res Opin 23:2597–2605
Welsh DK, Takahashi JS, Kay SA (2010) Suprachiasmatic nucleus: cell autonomy and network properties. Annu Rev Physiol 72:551–577
Whitehead DL, Davies AD, Playfer JR, Turnbull CJ (2008) Circadian rest-activity rhythm is altered in Parkinson's disease patients with hallucinations. Mov Disord 23:1137–1145
Whittom S, Dumont M, Petit D, Desautels A, Adam B, Lavigne G, Montplaisir J (2010) Effects of melatonin and bright light administration on motor and sensory symptoms of RLS. Sleep Med 11:351–355
Wu YH, Zhou JN, Van Heerikhuize J, Jockers R, Swaab DF (2007) Decreased MT1 melatonin receptor expression in the suprachiasmatic nucleus in aging and Alzheimer's disease. Neurobiol Aging 28:1239–1347
Yagita K, Tamanini F, Yasuda M, Hoeijmakers JH, Van Der Horst GT, Okamura H (2002) Nucleocytoplasmic shuttling and mCRY-dependent inhibition of ubiquitylation of the mPER2 clock protein. EMBO J 21:1301–1314
Yao K, Fang J, Yin YL, Feng ZM, Tang ZR, Wu G (2011) Tryptophan metabolism in animals: important roles in nutrition and health. Front Biosci 3:286–297

Yonei Y, Hattori A, Tsutsui K, Okawa M, Ishizuka B (2010) Effects of melatonin: basic studies and clinical applications. Anti Aging Med 7:85–91

Yoon SO, Yun CH, Chung AS (2002) Dose effect of oxidative stress on signal transduction in aging. Mech Aging 123:1597–1604

Yu EA, Weaver DR (2011) Disrupting the circadian clock: gene-specific effects on aging, cancer, and other phenotypes. Aging 3:479–493

Zisapel N (2001) Circadian rhythm sleep disorders: pathophysiology and potential approaches to management. CNS Drugs 15:311–328

Yoneto Y, Hattori A, [illegible] Ohtsuka M, Ishibashi [illegible] (2010) Effects of melatonin: basic studies and clinical applications. Anti Aging Med 7:85 [illegible]
[illegible] Mar CH, Cortner A (2003) Dose effect of oxidative stress on signal transduction in aging. Mech Ageing Dev [illegible]
Yu [illegible] (2011) Uncoupling the circadian clock: gene-specific [illegible] and other phenotypes. Ageing [illegible] 479–493
Zisapel N (2001) Circadian rhythm sleep disorders: pathophysiology and potential approaches to management. CNS Drugs [illegible]

Chapter 9
Neurolipofuscin in Aging and Aluminum-Induced Aging: Possible Therapeutic Interventions

Mahdi Hasan, Sandeep Tripathi and Abbas A. Mahdi

Abstract Neurolipofuscin is considered a reliable biomarker of aging. Accumulating evidence indicates that it is not simply an inert, harmless, wear and tear pigment but it distorts the protein building machinery of the cell and interferes with the important autophagic process. Numerous forms of cellular stresses activate macroautophagy. Increased autophagic vacuoles (AVs) are associated with not only aging and ceroid disorders but also Alzheimer's disease. Mitochondria may have means for specifically targeting macroautophagy degradation which would be particularly important for the healthy long axons and distal terminals. The decomposition of mitochondrial material is not only an important source of lipofuscin, but is at the same time a key to the understanding of mechanism of aging. Lipofuscin may become indigestible because the proteins are 'fixed' via aldehyde bridges between amino groups. The increasing proportion of defective mitochondria and an ever decreasing supply of functional lysosomes are postulated to hasten the senescence and/or demise of the postmitotic cells. Oxidatively damaged mitochondria may contain some already peroxidized undegradable macromolecules. Brain aluminum content is known to increase with age Aluminum toxicity might be one of the underlying causes of Alzhemier's disease. Accumulation of this element in aged neurons has been demonstrated along with increment of lipofuscin. Both aluminum and iron bind to transferrin receptor before crossing the blood-brain barrier via transferrin mediated endocystosis. High level of iron, concomitant with increased aluminum content, has been detected in the aged rat brain. Accumulating evidence indicates that chronic aluminum administration accelerates aging process. A number of antioxidants have been reported to decrease lipofuscin content of neurons. Centrophenoxine facilitates elimination of lipofuscin. Also, citiolone retards lipofus-

M. Hasan (✉)
Department of Anatomy, CSM Medical University, Lucknow 226003, India
e-mail: drmahdihasan36@gmail.com

Sandeep Tripathi · Abbas A. Mahdi
Department of Biochemistry, CSM Medical University, Lucknow 226003, India

Sandeep Tripathi
Department of Biotechnology (IAST), NIMS University, Jaipur 303121, India

M. K. Thakur, S. I. S. Rattan (eds.), *Brain Aging and Therapeutic Interventions,*
DOI 10.1007/978-94-007-5237-5_9,

cinogenesis. Recently, some Ayurvedic herbal remedies, such as Maharishi Amrit Kalash, have been found to reduce lipid peroxidation and lipofuscin deposition. Administration of extract of *Bacopa monnieri*, which possesses strong antioxidant activity, has also successfully reduced lipofuscin content of neurons subjected to aluminum-induced lipofuscinogenesis. We thus conclude that accumulation of lipofuscin, mitochondrial dysfunctioning and increased reactive oxygen species may be significant indicator of aging—perhaps even central to our understanding of the complex phenomenon of aging.

Keywords Neurolipofuscin • Aluminum accelerated-aging • Oxidative-stress • Antioxidants

9.1 Introduction

The age-dependent accumulation of lipofuscin in brain cells is one of the most consistent features of aging (Glees and Hasan 1976; Hasan et al. 2009). Accumulation of lipofuscin may be the result of an imbalance between formation and removal mechanisms. Lipofuscin is often considered a hallmark of aging, showing an accumulation rate that inversely correlates with longevity (Terman and Brunk 2004). Aside from large lipid content, lipofuscin is known to contain sugars and metals, mercury, aluminum, iron, copper and zinc (Takutake 1997). In the aging human brain, deposits of lipofuscin are not uniformly distributed but are concentrated in specific regions of functional interest. Robust evidence suggests that lipofuscin is not benign but can distort and displace the endoplasmic reticulum, the protein building machinery of the cell. By interfering with the important autophagic process by which most worn out cellular components are degraded, it may prevent renewal of cells and advance the accumulation of damaged cellular constituents due to binding of transition metals, such as iron and copper. Lipofuscin also seems to sensitize lysosomes and cells to oxidative stress. Of importance in pathogenesis of age-related macular degeneration, lipofuscin deposition interferes with the phagocytic activity of retinal pigment epithelial cells and also sensitizes their lysosomes to blue light (Terman and Brunk 2004). Additionally, it can impair the functioning of seemingly unrelated cellular systems, including the ubiquitin/proteasome pathway. The inhibition of proteasomal system is one of the major aspects of the cytotoxic effects of lipofuscin, which inhibits the proteasome by binding to surface motif (Hohn et al. 2011). This membrane-bound cellular waste can neither be degraded nor ejected from the cell.

9.2 Perturbed Proteolytic Degradation

The protease inhibitor, leupeptin, has been shown to cause an accumulation of lysosomally associated intracytoplasmic dense bodies resembling lipofuscin when administered intraventricularly to the brains of young rats (Ivy et al. 1989). These findings support the idea that lipofuscin formation during normal aging involves perturbed proteolytic degradation.

9.3 Autophagic Vacuoles (AVs)

The term 'autophagy' is used specifically for the lysosomal degradation by a cell of its own components. One form, macroautophagy, in which AVs accumulate cytosolic components including proteins, lipids and nucleic acids for degradation, provides the only means by which a cell can degrade its own large organelles such as mitochondria (Sulzer et al. 2008). Macroautophagy occurs by the formation of autophagosomes, double-membrane vesicles that sequester organelles, proteins or portions of the cytoplasm, which they fuse with lysosomes. As a result of this process, the sequestered contents are degraded by lysosomal enzymes and recycled as source of energy. Autophagy may occur either as a general phenomenon, for instance, when cells lack nutrients and mobilize their energy reserves, or it can specifically target distinct cellular structures such as damaged mitochondria ("mitophagy") (Green et al. 2011). Numerous forms of cellular stresses activate macroautophagy, and increased AVs are associated not only with aging and ceroid disorders but also in Alzheimer's disease (Salminen et al. 2011). Macroautophagy consists of steps highly conserved from yeast to mammals, including (1) a triggering via inhibition of mTOR (mammalian target of rapamycin) or regulation of insulin receptor substrate-2 or extracellular signal-regulated kinases (ERKs) that activate the Vps34/beclin complex to promote the formation and elongation of the membrane forming the AV, (2) sequestration of cytoplasmic content for degradation, and (3) acidification and fusion of the AV with the lysosome for proteolytic degradation of its content by lysosomal hydrolases.

9.4 Sequestration of Cytoplasmic Content

Although macroautophagy was long considered a purely non-specific bulk degradation pathway, recent results suggest specific recognition of some cargo. Preferential targeting of proteins to AVs may occur by a form of polyubiquitination in which ubiquitin subunits are linked via their K63 residues, in contrast to polyubiquitination at the K48 site which confers delivery of a substrate to the proteasome (Tan et al. 2008). Mitochondria may have means for specifically targeting macroautophagic degradation, which would be particularly important for the health of long axons and distal terminals. 'Mitophagy' of damaged and dysfunctional mitochondria can undergo degradation by an ERK2- dependent signaling pathway independent from mTOR (Zhu et al. 2007). There may be multiple substrate recognition/targeting mechanisms that target additional damaged organelles and pigment components to AVs, serving both for degradation and to sequester reactive catecholamine and lipids away from the cyotosol.

9.5 Lipofuscin (LF) Ontogeny

Contrary to the lysosomal hypothesis of lipofuscin formation supported by Sekhon et al. (1969), Glees and Hasan (1976) stressed that "The decomposition of mitochondrial material is not only an important source of lipofuscin, but is at the same time a key to the understanding of one mechanism of aging." Their conclusion is now well supported by Gray and Woulfe (2005) in the following words. In neurons, LF is generally thought to result from incomplete digestion of mitochondrial products. When mitochondria are exposed to UV, a non-degradable substance can be pelleted that has properties of LF pigment. A mitochondrial constituent, lipoic acid, is associated with neuronal LF in Alzheimer's disease (Moreira et al. 2007). Lipofuscin's principal lipid components are suggested to stem from reactions of a highly reactive lipid derivative, 4-hydroxy-2-nonenal, and malonaldehyde as well as an accumulation of dolichols (Ng Ying Kin et al. 1983). 4-Hydroxy-2-nonenal reacts with lysine, histidine and cystine residues to form so-called Michael adducts, Schiff-base cross-links, and fluorescent fluorophores, and has been reported to block proteasome activity (Okada et al. 1999). Peroxide and iron-mediated oxidation may play important roles; cell cultures exposed to low oxygen or iron produce LF, whereas iron chelators and antioxidants block the pigment synthesis (Brunk and Terman 2002a). In contrast to the short lifetime of typical AVs, pigmented AVs accumulate over a lifetime (Sulzer et al. 2008).

9.6 Lipofuscin is Indigestible

Lipofuscin may become indigestible because the proteins are 'fixed' via aldehyde bridges between amino groups, a form of cross-link that is not a good substrate for lysosomal hydrolases (Gray and Woulfe 2005). A trimethyl lysine modification in subunit C is proposed to contribute to the resistance of ceroid pigment to degradation in Batten disease (Katz et al. 1995). It has been suggested that with advancing age there may be some slow 'slippage' as the rate of free radical damage increases, which could block AV/lysosome fusion, while protease activity decreases (Harman 1989), leading to a buildup of indigestible material.

9.7 Evidence for Lysosomal Dysfunction in Aging

There is much evidence for disrupted lysosomal function over aging (Massey et al. 2006), which may further contribute to pigment accumulation. As mentioned, Batten's disease is caused by mutations of lysosomal proteases, e.g. CLN8 (cathepsin D) (Tyynela et al. 2000). The CLN2 mutation of a lysosomal serine protease appears to specifically inhibit lysosomal degradation of subunit C and possibly an analogous subunit of the secretory vesicle ATPase (Tanner et al. 1997). In addition to mutations of lysosomal enzymes, pharmacologic inhibition of lysosomal proteases with leupeptin produces AVs (Nunomura and Miyagishi 1993).

9.8 Inhibition of Lysosomal Fusion

The number of AVs increases when their fusion with lysosomes is disrupted, e.g., when microtubules are disrupted by colchicine. This may occur if organelle traffic through the axon is overcrowded, resulting in steady hindrance or problems in organelle transport. Sulzer et al. (2008) observed many instances in video microscopy of labeled AVs that appear to be stuck in axons, sometimes bouncing off each other as they attempt retrograde transport. Given the cross-talk between degradation pathways, so that inhibition of one pathway stimulates another, it may not be surprising that proteasome inhibition also induces LF (Terman and Sandberg 2002), perhaps via enhancing AV formation. The fusion of endosomes or AVs with lysosomes could be blocked by alkalinization within these organelles, as the acidic pH and the ATP-driven vacuolar proton pump is required for the fusion of endocytic structures with the central vacuole (Peters et al. 2001).

9.9 The Free Radical Model of Lipofuscin Accumulation

The recent free-radical theory of aging, as set out by Harman in 1956, casts oxygen radicals produced by interaction of the respiratory enzymes involved in the direct utilization of molecular oxygen. Harman's paper cites the work of Fenton, whose eponymous chemistry is based on the reactive properties of ferrous iron in the generation of the highly reactive hydroxyl radical (Fig. 9.1). Much subsequent work has localized this iron to mitochondria, residing in the cytoplasm or within autophagolysosomes, wherein damaged mitochondria are disassembled for recycling (Terman and Brunk 1998). Regulation of mitochondrial division (fission) is poorly understood. However, it is likely to be impaired by oxidative damage to mitochondrial DNA and proteins. Mitochondria are the main source of reactive oxygen species formation, as well as the main target for free radical attack. Although mitochondrial fission is not absolutely dependent on mtDNA replication (as is the case for cell division which requires nuclear DNA replication); the amount of normal DNA per mitochondrion apparently must not be too low. Consistent with this, mtDNA-depleted cells usually contain substantially enlarged mitochondria. Therefore, age dependent accumulation of mutations in mtDNA, perhaps especially in the control region for replication, may also diminish mitochondrial fission which latter could govern the appearance of abnormal, large mitochondria (Fig. 9.2). The cascade of events initiated by the hydroxyl radical is thought to culminate with the formation of aldehydes such as malondialdehyde (a quantifiable product of lipid peroxidation

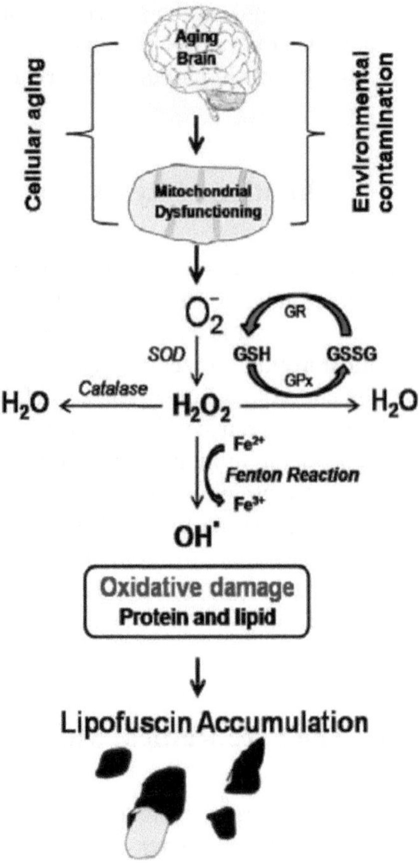

Fig. 9.1 Mitochondrial dysfunctioning and production of reactive oxygen species during aging which could promote increased accumulation of lipofuscin granules in the aging brain

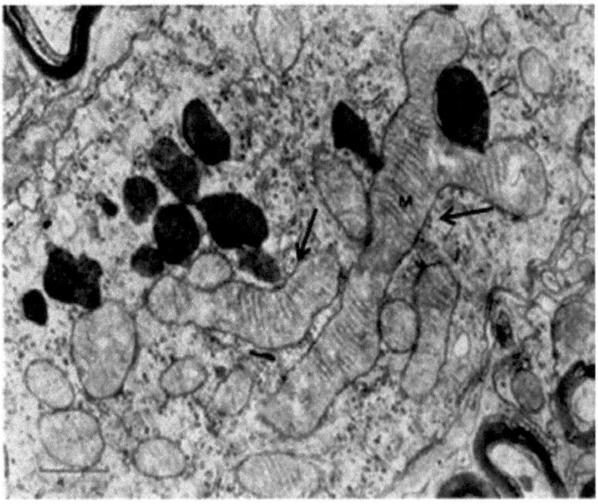

Fig. 9.2 Electron micrograph of perikaryon of a monkey lateral geniculate neuron showing long mitochondria in right half of a figure. The magnification indicator line on the left represents 1 μm (This figure is reproduced from Glees and Hasan 1976, with the permission of the authors)

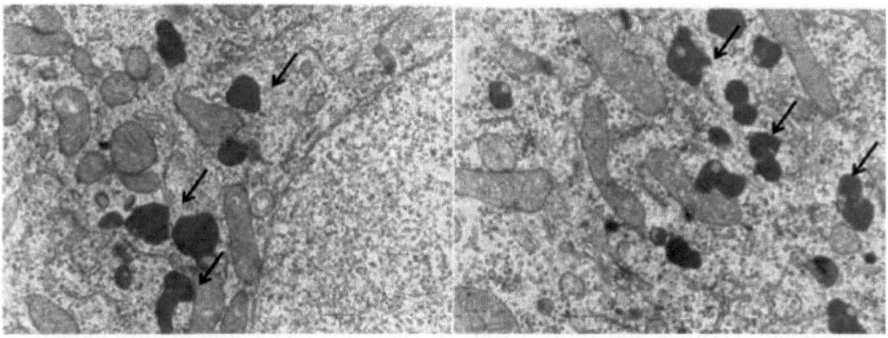

Fig. 9.3 On the left hand side, electron micrograph shows part of a nucleus on the right and lipofuscin granules of variegated forms, mostly electron disks mingled with the mitochondrial profiles from lateral geniculate body of a monkey. Magnification 40,000×. On the right hand side part of a perikaryon of a monkey hippocampal neuron is depicted with a number of electron dense lipofuscin granules. Three of them possess electron lucid vacuoles. Magnification 40,000×. (This figure is reproduced from Glees and Hasan 1976 with the permission of the authors)

and a suitable proxy for reactive oxygen status within mitochondria). It is probably the aldehyde bridges linking amino groups that make the proteinaceous component of lipofuscin so refractory to lysosomal degradation. The mitochondrial-lysosomal axis theory of aging (Brunk and Terman 2002b) posits that the futile task of attacking lipofuscin acts as a sink for lysosomal enzymes, impeding the degradation of damaged mitochondria. The increasing proportion of defective mitochondria and an ever-decreasing supply of functional lysosomes are postulated to hasten the senescence and/or demise of the postmitotic cell. Lipofuscin granules are detectable in a small percentage of neurons in the brains of young children but become progressively and markedly more abundant between the 2nd and 9th decade of life. This age associated increase in the sheer amount of lipofuscin in brain cells is attended by alterations in its biochemical composition. The topographic pattern of distribution of lipofuscin accumulation in the human brain is not uniform but displays a particular predilection for certain areas. Lipofuscin is present in virtually every type of neuron but is most abundant in the largest neurons. It is prominent in areas of the brain and spinal cord involved in initiating, monitoring, and controlling movement, including the inferior olivary nucleus, the dentate nucleus of the cerebellum, the globus pallidus, and the motor neurons in the anterior horn of the spinal cord and brainstem. The latter directly innervate muscles and provide the signals necessary for voluntary movement of the face, eyes, limbs and trunk. Lipofuscin abundance increases with age in the cerebral cortex. Conversely, neurons in certain brain areas appear to be resistant to age-associated lipofuscin accumulation, including neurons in certain regions of the hypothalamus involved in fluid balance and cardiovascular control.

Using electron microscopy, lipofuscin granules appear as osmiophilic, preferentially, perinuclear and irregularly shaped profiles of variable electron density (Fig. 9.3). Another important property of lipofuscin is its broad fluorescence. Because of the difficulties inherent in the analysis of lipofuscin fluorophores, their nature and composition has not yet been fully defined. Nevertheless, test tube experiments suggest that reactions between carbonyl (mainly aldehyde, resulting from lipid peroxidation reaction) and amino compounds produce Schiff bases that display autoflourescent properties. Mitochondria are the main site of ROS formation and also the main target of their attack (Harman 1956). Autophagocytosis of mitochondria seems be a major contributor to lipofuscin formation. Oxidatively damaged mitochondria may contain some already peroxidized, undegradable macromolecules. Moreover, such effete mitochondria are not only ferruginous (being rich in heme proteins) but also may generate larger amounts of superoxide than do functional mitochondria (Brunk and Terman 2002a). Their involvement in lipofuscinogenesis is supported by fact that a least one mitochondrial protein—ATP synthase subunit C (SCMAS) is a predominant component of lipofuscin.

9.10 Aluminum-Induced Lipofuscin

Humans are exposed to Aluminum (Al) from various environmental sources and interventions, e.g., ingestion of antacids and dialysis. Aluminum compounds enter our bodies through mouth, nose and skin. This metal can also be encountered in cookware, some foods, dust and other sources, including drinking water (Nayak 2002). Aluminum sulphate is commonly used in water purification plants. Humans consume on an average 7,600 μg/day of Al from drinking water and food (Yoon and McNiven 2001). Evidences from clinical and animal model studies demonstrate that brain aluminum content increases with age (Struys-Ponsar et al. 1993). It may be either due to increased exposure with age or decreased ability to remove Al from the body (Markesberry et al. 1984). Al is a potent neurotoxic element, which has been suggested to play an important role in the degeneration of nerve cells of experimental animals as well as human brain. It has been implicated in several human neurodegenerative disorders, including Alzheimer's disease (AD). Also, Al exposure is reported to be associated with memory loss, tremor, jerky movements and generalized convulsions (Zatta et al. 2003). Furthermore, a decline in visual memory has been reported in hemodialyzed patients who exhibited higher serum Al (Vander et al. 1991). Some researcher noted the striking similarity of dementia dialytica to Alzheimer's dementia, so naturally they posited that Al toxicity might be the underlying cause of AD.

The possible mechanism of Al induced neurotoxicity has been related to cell damage via free radical production. Increased lipid peroxidation (LPO) is one of the major consequences of oxidative stress (Oteiza et al. 1993). Lipofuscin, a morphological biomarker of lipid peroxidation, represents an end-product of oxidative degradation of lipids by free radical mechanism. This so-called age-pigment, contains derivatives of lipid peroxidation e.g., malondialdehyde (Jung et al. 2007) as well as metal ions, e.g., Cu, Fe, Zn and Al (Tokutake 1997). Excessive accumulation of

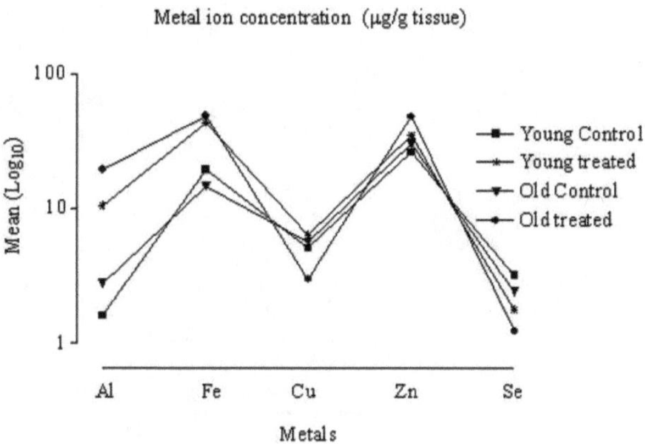

Fig. 9.4 The concentration of different metals (Al, Fe, Cu, Zn and Se) in frontal cortex is expressed as mean in six rats of each group (young control, young Al treated, aged control and aged Al treated). The significant ($p<0.05$) comparison using one-way ANOVA followed by Student Newman-Keuls post hoc test between young controls (■), young Al treated (*), aged control (▼) and aged control (●)

some metal ions (e.g., Fe, Cu, Zn, Mg and Mn) and competition between Al and these essential elements can, however, result in chronic or acute toxicity.

Studies on age associated and Al mediated toxic effects are very important as there are several reports that, on one hand the efficiency of the blood-brain barrier (BBB) may decline with advancing age (Mooradian 1988), and on the other hand, cognitive decline may account for functional and morphological changes in the central nervous system (CNS) (Tripathi et al. 2011). In one of our previous studies, we found that Al was able to alter the energy pathways and was responsible for cognitive decline in young rats (Tripathi et al. 2008) and these changes may correlate with the finding of Mahdi et al. (2008).

Although toxic effects of Al are well established, but its mechanism of action is poorly understood. Following oral administration, retention of Al is reported in the brain, bone, kidney, muscle and heart (Nayak 2002). Tripathi et al. (2009) observed accumulation of this metal in neurons showing ultrastructural changes. Interestingly, Levesque et al. (2000) also reported similar electron microscopic findings in Al treated rat brain. Al, while in circulation, is reported to cause reduction of erythrocyte formation and diminution of their iron content (Nasiadek and Chmielnicka 2000). It has been reported that Fe and Al bind to transferrin receptor before crossing the blood-brain barrier via transferrin-mediated endocytosis and thus enter into the brain, where they are retained for a prolonged period (Mooradian 1988). Tripathi et al. (2009) detected high Al content in the rat brain along with significantly increased levels of iron and zinc in the frontal cortex (Fig. 9.4). It is notable that the Al accumulation in treated aged group was far greater than that of young rats. Moreover, it has also been observed reduced concentration of Se in both the aged and young Al treated rats, but these changes were insignificant when we compared them with the young and aged control rats. Furthermore, our results showed that there was reduced concentration of Cu in Al treated aged rats. It may be recalled that Cu and Se are the cofactors of antioxidative enzymes SOD and GSHPx, respectively. Therefore, any reduction in Cu and Se content may lead to reduction of antioxidative capacity of brain following Al administration. Our findings of incre-

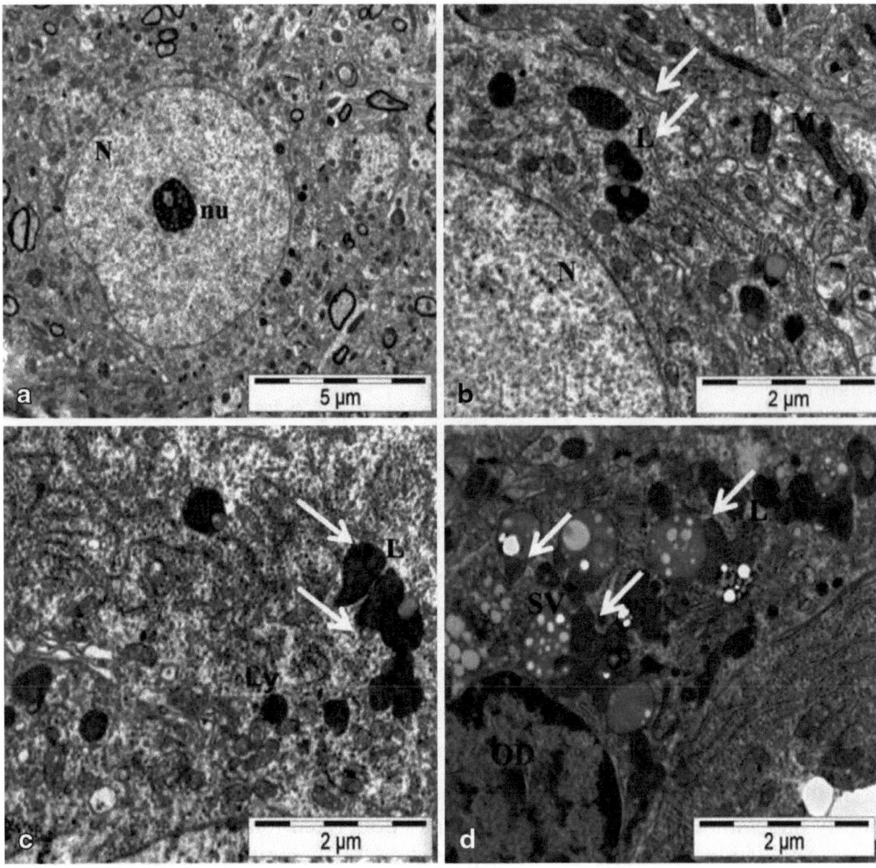

Fig. 9.5 **a** Electron micrograph (EM) of part of a neuron of frontal cortex of young rat (prominent nucleus (*N*) and nucleolus (*nu*). **b** Micrograph of the frontal cortex of Al intoxicated young rat. Its perikaryon shows a number of variegated lipofuscin (*L*) pigment granules in the vicinity of nucleus. **c** EM of aged rat showing cluster of three pleomorphic lipofuscin granules (*L*) mingled with a few lysosomes (*Ly*) and mitochondrial profiles. **d** EM showing a peripheral segment of perikaryon of a neuron with part of satellite oligodendrocyte (*OD*) from frontal cortex of Al intoxicated aged rat. A large number of pleomorphic irregular lipofuscin granules showing spongy form vacuolation (*SV*) are seen

ment of Al, Fe and Zn and decreased level of Cu and Se in the brain are in consistent with the observation of Zeeca et al. (2001). Taken together, they are in conformity with the hypothesis of Yokel (2006) that metal ion dysfunction in the brain is the hallmark of neurodegenerative changes. Furthermore, aged rats were more prone to Al-induced alterations in metal ion homeostasis, had elevated lipid peroxidation and increased lipofuscinogenesis. The number and size of granules remarkably increased in Al treated aged rats (Fig. 9.5). Increasing intraneuronal accumulation of lipofuscin is the most consistent cytological change, which has been correlated with Al neurotoxicity and aging. It may be noted here that spongiform and clustered lipofuscin granules were also found in the aged Al treated rats which had higher Al and Fe content quantitatively (Fig. 9.5d). Furthermore, changes observed in Al treated young rats resembled those of old control animals which indicate that Al is responsible for premature aging of animals. Lipofuscin in itself is a cytotoxic agent which may induce a variety of ultra structural changes, like cell vacuolization, mitochondrial swelling and demyelination in brain tissue (Deloncle et al. 2001). Hence an elevated Al content along with high neurolipofuscin levels may possibly play a role in the development of neurodegenerative disorders. Also, Deloncle et al. (2001) reported that after chronic administration of aluminum L-glutamate to rats, the aging process was accelerated. It is apparent that Al may play a role in the premature aging of animals.

9.11 Effects of Drugs on Neurolipofuscin

In recent years, significant attempts have been made to decelerate physiological aging by chemical intervention. These attempts have been in the form of studies, inter alia of tissue cultures, antioxidants, lipofuscin and cross-link inhibitors, hormones and compounds enhancing learning.

9.11.1 Antioxidants

As the rate of free radical reactions in cells are reduced by antioxidants, 2-mercaptoethylamine (2 MEA) and butylated hydroxytoluene (BHT) are capable of trapping free radical intermediates. Harman's (1989) observation that diets including these agents increase the mean lifespan of mice by 20–40 %, without affecting the maximum lifespan, is not surprising. Chronic Vitamin E deficiency, an antioxidant is known to produce accumulation of lipofuscin in neurons. Under certain conditions, it has also been shown that Vit. E will retard or temporarily inhibit pigment formation, although once formed its removal cannot be accelerated.

9.11.2 Lipofuscin inhibitors

Nandy and Bourne (1966) observed that meclofenoxate (centrophenoxine) decreased the amount of brain lipofuscin in aged guinea pigs; a marked elimination of the pigment was noticeable in animals under treatment for 12 weeks. Later electron microscopic investigations by Hasan et al. (1974) provided detail information regarding the drug induced diminution and dissolution of neuronal lipofuscin. Magnesium orotate (100 mg/kg) also inhibited lipofuscin and a functional improvement was observed in the affected animals (Varkonyi et al. 1970).

Deprenyl (selegiline) is an irreversible monoamine-oxidase B (MAO-B) inhibitor which has antioxidant and neuroprotective effects (Kitani et al. 2002). Kiray et al. (2006) examined the effects of chronic deprenyl administration at a dose of 1 mg/kg/day on spatial memory, oxidant stress markers and total neuron count of hippocampus CA1 region of aged male rats. Age-related deficits in learning and memory are associated with hippocampal structural and biochemical changes. In their study, they showed that the total number of neurons in the CA1 hippocampus region was significantly higher in deprenyl-treated rats. The correlation between spatial memory performance and total number of CA1 neurons was significant. Their results indicated that the effect of deprenyl on spatial memory may be related to the prevention of age-dependent neuronal loss. Although apoptosis may play a role in the normal aging process, both apoptosis and aging were affected by oxidant stress. As deprenyl has antioxidant and anti-apoptotic effects, it may decrease or delay the age-related neuronal death. Apoptosis is suggested to be considerable in normal aging and neurodegenerative disorders. Kiray et al. (2006) showed that deprenyl treatment significantly decreased lipid peroxidation in all brain regions investigated by them.

Some other pharmacological products, such as potassium orotate (25 mg/day) removed lipofuscin from neurons of nucleus reticularis gigantocellularis (Low et al. 1974). Also, nordihydroguaiaretic acid (NDGA), a natural antioxidant, observed to partially correct and/or prevent vitamin E deficiency symptoms in chicks restricted pigment accumulation in natural death mutant of *Neurospora Crassa* (Munkres and Rana 1978). A free radical scavenger, citiolone (N-homocysteine thiolactone) has also been observed to retard pigment accumulation and favour its removal (Aloj Totaro and Pisanti 1981). Patro et al. (1992) made a comparative study of the undermentioned four neuritropic agents for their lipofuscinolytic activity. Dimethylaminothanol, chlorpromazine, centrophenoxine and encephabol depleted the lipofuscin in Purkinje neuronal area by 21 %, 27 %, 42 % and 61 %, respectively, after 3 months of treatment.

9.12 Effect of Ayurvedic Herbal Remedies

Unfortunately, not much work has been done on the effects of Ayurvedic herbal remedies in this thrust area of research. Vohra et al. (2001) reported the effects of Maharishi Amrit Kalash (MAK), an Ayurvedic herbal mixture, on two biomarkers of aging, lipid peroxidation and lipofuscin, in aging guinea pig brain. Brain regions studied were cerebral cortex, hypothalamus, cerebellum and spinal cord. Treatment with MAK (500 mg/kg body weight/day for 2 months) reduced the lipid peroxide and lipofuscin pigment significantly in brain regions and also helped in restoring normal oxygen consumption in the older animals. They concluded that their results indicated antioxidant properties of MAK. Later, Vohra et al. (2002) investigated age-dependent alterations in a dark Purkinje neuronal population of guinea pigs (10 months and 32 months old) and rats 3 months, 6 months, 12 months,

15 months and 28 months. Dark neurons are considered a manifestation of neuronal injury and although they cover various grades of damage, their mode of formation is not yet clear. Their electron microscopic analysis revealed a significant increase ($P<0.05$) in the number of dark Purkinje neurons with age in both guinea pigs and rats. Treatment of guinea pigs with MAK (500 mg/kg body wt/day for 2 months) significantly inhibited ($P<0.05$) the activity of cathepsin-D and lipid peroxidation, and decreased the number of dark neurons. Their findings suggest that the number of dark neurons increases with age and MAK prevents the conversion of light to dark Purkinje neurons due to its inhibitory effects on cathepsin-D activity and antioxidant properties.

9.12.1 Administration of *Bacopa monnieri* extract

The whole plant (*B. monnieri*) was dried in shade and then powdered. The powder was extracted with distilled water. The aqueous extract was discarded and the residual plant material was extracted thrice with 90 % ethanol. The residue obtained after removing the solvent was dried in vacuo and macerated with acetone to give a free flowing powder. The Bacopa extract so prepared contained 40 % bacosides estimated as bacoside A by high pressure thin liquid chromatography (Deb et al. 2008). Tripathi et al. (2011) directly introduced a dose of *B. monnieri* extract, 40 mg/kg body weight with 100 mg $AlCl_3$/kg body wt into the rat pharynx via a feeding cannula to the experimental group for 90 days. Their results clearly demonstrated that *B monniera* inhibits anticholinergic enzyme AChE, almost to the same extent as donepezil, and this may be responsible for protection of synaptic morphology leading to enhancement in the behavioral performance (Singh and Dhawan 1997). An elevated AChE activity in cerebellum was observed following Al administration and this may be directly correlated with cholinergic sign and symptoms (Kaizer et al. 2008). It may be pointed out that loss of cholinergic neuronal activity is one of the cardinal features of dementia. Tripathi et al. (2011) found elevated lipid peroxide levels in Al treated rats. Earlier it has been reported that the increased lipid peroxidation and protein oxidation in Al neurotoxicity may be due to the accumulation of excess iron and it may further lead to an increase in Fe catalyzed Fenton reaction resulting in generation of more reactive oxygen species (ROS) (Tripathi et al. 2008). Tripathi et al. (2008) also detected elevated lipofuscin levels in Al treated rats. Increased lipifuscinogenesis is one of the well known biomarker of neuronal aging (Jung et al. 2007). Earlier Kumar et al. (2008) had also reported that increased Al and lipofuscin concentration could deleteriously affect the neurons, leading to depletion of antioxidants. However, Tripathi et al. (2008) reported that in *B. monnieri* treated rat cerebellum, there was significantly reduced level of lipid and protein peroxidation products and reduced lipofuscin content (Fig. 9.5b). They also detected levels of the enzymes involved in antioxidant defense, viz. SOD, CAT and GPx in Al treated rats. These findings are consistent with the earlier reports (Tripathi et al. 2011), which also documented a significant decrease in the activities of SOD and CAT in brain after Al insult. Additionally, they noted a significant reversal in above stated changes by the co-administration of *B. monnieri*. These biochemical modifications indicate that *B. monnieri* possesses strong antioxidative property and it also acts as an anti-aging agent.

Acknowledgements We are grateful to Indian National Science Academy, New Delhi for sanctioning Honorary Scientist Scheme, to one of us (MH) and to Indian Council of Medical Research, New Delhi. Authors will also thank to Era's Lucknow Medical College, Lucknow, India for providing facilities during research work.

References

Aloj Totaro E, Pisanti FA (1981) Quantitative evaluation of lipofuscin in relation to age and meclofenoxate treatment. Electron microscopic study of "*Torpedo M.*" neurons. Acta Neurol (Napoli) 3:453–459

Brunk UT, Terman A (2002a) Lipofuscin: mechanisms of age related accumulation and influence on cell function. Free Radic Biol Med 33:611–619

Brunk UT, Terman A (2002b) The mitochondrial-lysosomal axis theory of aging: accumulation of damaged mitochondria as a result of imperfect autophagocytosis. Eur J Biochem 269:1996–2002

Deb DD, Kapoor P, Dighe RP, Padmaja R et al (2008) In vitro safety evaluation and anticlastogenic effect of BacoMind on human lymphocytes. Biomed Environ Sci 1:7–23

Deloncle R, Huguet F, Fernandez B, Quellard N et al (2001) Ultrastructural study of rat hippocampus after chronic administration of aluminum l-glutamate: an acceleration of the aging process. Exp Gerontol 36:231–244

Glees P, Hasan M (1976) Lipofuscin in neuronal aging and diseases. Stuttgart Norm Pathol Anat (Stuttg) 32:1–68

Gray DA, Woulfe J (2005) Lipofuscin and aging: a matter of toxic waste. Sci Aging Knowledge Environ 5:re1

Green DR, Galluzzi L, Kroemer G (2011) Mitochondria and the autophagy-inflammation-cell death axis in organismal aging. Science 333:1109–1112

Harman D (1956) A theory based on free radical and radiation chemistry. J Gerontol 11:298–300

Harman D (1989) Lipofuscin and ceroid formation: the cellular recycling system. Adv Exp Med Biol 266:3–15

Hasan M, Glees P, El-Ghazzawi E (1974) Age-associated changes in the hypothalmus of the guinea pig: effect of dimethylaminoethyl p-chlorophenoxyacetate an electron microscopic and histochemical study. Exp Gerontol 9:153–159

Hasan M, Tripathi S, Mahdi AA, Mitra K et al (2009) Lipofuscin, lipid peroxidation and antioxidant status in discrete brain regions of the aged rat brain. Proc Indian Natl Sci Acad 75:1–9

Hohn S, Dallerac G, Faure A, Urbach YK et al (2011) Behavioral and in vivo electrophysiological evidence for presymptomatic alteration of prefrontostriatal processing in the transgenic rat model for huntington disease. J Neurosci 15:8986–8997

Ivy GO, Kanai S, Ohta M, Smith G et al (1989) Lipofuscin-like substances accumulate rapidly in brain, retina and internal organs with cysteine protease inhibition. Adv Exp Med Biol 266:31–45

Jung T, Bader N, Grune T (2007) Lipofuscin: formation, distribution, and metabolic consequences. Ann N Y Acad Sci 1119:97–111

Kaizer RR, Correa MC, Gris LR, da Rosa CS et al (2008) Bohrer D, Morsch VM, Schetinger MR. Effect of long-term exposure to aluminum on the acetylcholinesterase activity in the central nervous system and erythrocytes. Neurochem Res 33:2294–2301

Katz ML, Gao CL, Tompkins JA, Bronson RT et al (1995) Mitochondrial ATP synthase subunit c stored in hereditary ceroid-lipofuscinosis contains trimethyl-lysine. Biochem J 310:887–892

Kiray M, Bagriyanik HA, Pekcetin C, Ergur BU et al (2006) Deprenyl and the relationship between its effects on spatial memory, oxidant stress and hippocampal neurons in aged male rats. Physiol Res 55:205–212

Kitani K, Minami C, Isobe K, Maehara K (2002) Why (--) deprenyl prolongs survivals of experimental animals: increase of anti-oxidant enzymes in brain and other body tissues as well as mobilization of various humoral factors may lead to systemic anti-aging effects. Mech Aging Dev 123:1087–1100

Kumar P, Taha A, Sharma D, Kale RK et al (2008) Effect of dehydroepiandrosterone (DHEA) on monoamine oxidase activity, lipid peroxidation and lipofuscin accumulation in aging rat brain regions. Biogerontology 9:235-246

Levesque L, Mizzen CA, McLachlan DR, Fraser PE (2000) Ligand specifc effects on aluminum incorporation and toxicity in neurons and astrocytes. Brain Res 877:191–202

Low S, Lengsfeld AM, Wieland T (1974) Prevention by aging or by cytochalasin B of phalloidin stimulated formation of microfilaments in cell membrane preparations of rat liver. Histochemistry 38:253–258

Mahdi AA, Annarao S, Tripathi S, Nawab A et al. (2008) Correlation of age-related metabonomic changes in 1H NMR serum and urine profiles of rats with cognitive function. Open Magn Resonance 1:71–76

Markesberry WR, Ehmann WD, Alaudin M, Hoosain T (1984) Brain trace element concentrations in aging. Neurobiol Aging 5:19–28

Massey AC, Zhang C, Cuervo AM (2006) Chaperone-mediated autophagy in aging and disease. Curr Top Dev Biol 73:205–235

Mooradian AD (1988) Effect of aging on the blood brain-barrier. Neurobiol Aging 9:31–39

Moreira PI, Harris PL, Zhu X, Santos MS et al (2007) Lipoic acid and N-acetyl cysteine decrease mitochondrial-related oxidative stress in Alzheimer disease patient fibroblasts. J Alzheimers Dis 12:195–206

Munkres K, Rana RS (1978) Antioxidants prolong life span and inhibit the senescence-dependent accumulation of fluorescent pigment (lipofuscin) in clones, of Podospora anserina. Mech Aging Dev 7:407–415

Nandy K, Bourne GH (1966) Effect of centrophenoxine on the lipofuscin pigments in the neurones of senile guinea-pigs. Nature 210:313–314

Nasiadek M, Chmielnicka J (2000) Interaction of aluminum with exogenous and endogenous iron in the organism of rats. Ecotoxicol Environ Saf 45:284–290

Nayak P (2002) Aluminum: impacts and disease. Environ Res 89:111–115

Ng Ying Kin NM, Palo J, Haltia M and Wolfe LS (1983) High levels of brain dolichols in neuronal ceroid-lipofuscinosis and senescence. J Neurochem 40:1465–1473

Nunomura A, Miyagishi T (1993) Ultrastructural observations on neuronal lipofuscin (age pigment) and dense bodies induced by a proteinase inhibitor, leupeptin, in rat hippocampus. Acta Neuropathol 86:319–328

Okada K, Wangpoengtrakul C, Osawa T, Toyokuni S et al (1999) 4-Hydroxy-2-nonenal-mediated impairment of intracellular proteolysis during oxidative stress. Identification of proteasomes as target molecules. J Biol Chem 274:23787–23793

Oteiza PL, Keen CL, Han B, Golub MS (1993) Aluminium accumulation and neurotoxicity in swiss-webster mice after long-term dietary exposure to aluminium and citrate. Metabolism 42:1296–1300

Patro N, Sharma SP, Patro IK (1992) Lipofuscin accumulation in aging myocardium & its removal by meclophenoxate. Indian J Med Res 96:192–198

Peters C, Bayer MJ, Buhler S, Andersen JS et al (2001). Trans-complex formation by proteolipid channels in the terminal phase of membrane fusion. Nature 409:581–588

Salminen A, Kaarniranta K, Haapasalo A, Hiltunen M, Soininen H, Alafuzoff I (2011) Emerging role of p62/sequestosome-1 in the pathogenesis of Alzheimer's disease. Prog Neurobiol 96(1):87-95

Sekhon SS, Andrews JM, Maxwell DS (1969) Accumulation and development of lipofuscin pigment in the aging central nervous system of the mouse. J Cell Biol 43:123a

Singh HK, Dhawan BN (1997) Neuropsychopharmacological effects of the ayurvedic nootropic *Bacopa monniera* Linn. (Brahmi). Indian J Pharmacol 29:S359–365

Struys-Ponsar C, Florence A, Gauthier A, Crichton RR et al (1993) Degeneration changes induced in the rat brain by administration of aluminum citrate: a model for the study of cerebral aging involution. Behav Process 29:113–114

Sulzer D, Mosharov E, Talloczy Z, Zucca FA et al (2008) Neuronal pigmented autophagic vacuoles: lipofuscin, neuromelanin, and ceroid as macroautophagic responses during aging and disease. J Neurochem 106:24–36

Tan JM, Wong ES, Kirkpatrick DS, Pletnikova O et al (2008) Lysine 63-linked ubiquitination promotes the formation and autophagic clearance of protein inclusions associated with neurodegenerative diseases. Hum Mol Genet 17:431–439

Tanner A, Shen BH, Dice JF (1997) Turnover of F1F0-ATP synthase subunit 9 and other proteolipids in normal and Batten disease fibroblasts. Biochim Biophys Acta 1361:251–262

Terman A, Brunk UT (1998) Ceroid/lipofuscin formation in cultured human fibroblasts: the role of oxidative stress and lysosomal proteolysis. Mech Aging Dev104;277–291

Terman A, Brunk UT (2004) Lipofuscin. Int J Biochem Cell Biol 36:1400–1404

Terman A, Sandberg S (2002) Proteasome inhibition enhances lipofuscin formation. Ann N Y Acad Sci 973:309–312

Tokutake S (1997) Accumulation of aluminum and silicon in lipofuscin granules suggests retardation of blood-brain barrier function by aging. Ann N Y Acad Sci 826:510–512

Tripathi S, Somashekar BS, Mahdi AA, Gupta A et al (2008) Aluminum mediated metabolic changes in rat serum and urine: a proton magnetic resonance study. J Bio Mol Toxicol 22:119–127

Tripathi S, Mahdi AA, Nawab A, Chander R et al (2009) Influence of age on aluminium induced lipid peroxidation and neurolipofuscin in frontal cortex of rat brain: a behavioral, biochemical and ultrastructural study. Brain Res 1253:107–116

Tripathi S, Mahdi AA, Hasan M, Mitra K et al (2011) Protective potential of Bacopa monniera (Brahmi) extract on aluminum induced cerebellar toxicity and associated neuromuscular status in aged rats. Cell Mol Biol (Noisy-le-grand) 57:3–15

Tyynela J, Sohar I, Sleat DE, Gin RM et al (2000) A mutation in the ovine cathepsin D gene causes a congenital lysosomal storage disease with profound neurodegeneration. EMBO J 19:2786–2792

Vander VGB, Marani E, Tio S, De Wolff FA (1991) Aluminum neurotoxicity. Prog Histochem Cytochem 23:235–242

Varkonyi T, Zoltan OT, Foldi M (1970) Studies on the brain edema induced by triethyltinsulfate in rats. 8. The effect of theophylline on the fine structural alterations in experimental triethyltinsulfate-induced poisoning in rats. Arzneimittelforschung 20:1594–1595

Vohra BP, Sharma SP, Kansal VK, Gupta SK (2001) Effect of Maharishi Amrit Kalash an ayurvedic herbal mixture on lipid peroxidation and neuronal lipofuscin accumulation in aging guinea pig brain. Indian J Exp Biol 39:355–359

Yokel RA (2006) Blood-brain barrier flux of aluminum, manganese, iron and other metals suspected to contribute to metal-induced neurodegeneration. J Alzheimers Dis 10:223–53

Yoon Y, McNiven MA (2001) Mitochondrial division: new partners in membrane pinching. Curr Biol 11:R67–70

Zatta P, Lucchini R, Van RSJ, Taylor A et al (2003) The role of metals in neurodegenerative processes: aluminum, manganese, and zinc. Brain Res Bull 62:15–28

Zeeca L, Gallorini M, Schunemann V, Trautwein AX et al (2001) Iron, neuromelanin and ferritin content in the substancia nigra of normal subjects at different ages: consequence for iron storage and neurodegenerative processes. J Neurochem 76:1766–1733

Zhu JH, Horbinski C, Guo F, Watkins S et al (2007) Regulation of autophagy by extracellular signal-regulated protein kinases during 1-methyl-4-phenylpyridinium-induced cell death. Am J Pathol 170:75–86

Chapter 10
Dietary Restriction as a Potential Intervention to Retard Age-associated Impairment of Brain Functions

Gurcharan Kaur and Sukhwinder S. Lakhman

Abstract The search for interventions to improve or slow down the age-associated decline in cognitive abilities has interested human beings forever. Out of the various environmental factors that are known to facilitate healthy aging process, dietary restriction (DR) seems to be the most promising regimen as it is known to prolong the lifespan, attenuate aging and prevent and/or delay the onset of numerous age associated diseases in model systems. In our recent studies, we have provided a scientific evidence for cognition and motor coordination enhancing properties of late onset short term intermittent fasting DR (IF-DR) regimen in aging rats. The improvement in motor coordination and memory task by IF-DR in aging rat brain was further linked to reversal/decline in protein and DNA damage by reducing mitochondrial ROS generation. The promise of dietary interventions to enhance plasticity can open a new line of non-invasive treatments to improve age-related functional impairments. The life-style interventions such as dietary restriction could be used to improve mental health and quality of life during normal aging. Further, the implementation costs of these strategies are rather economical and affordable almost to everyone. Moreover, late onset short term DR has the ability to resist cognitive decline and neurodegeneration, and hence may be a potential intervention to partially reverse age-related impairment of brain functions.

Keywords Brain aging • Lifestyle Interventions • Physical activity • Dietary Supplements • Environmental enrichment • DR/CR • Phytochemicals as hormetins

---

G. Kaur (✉)
Department of Biotechnology, Guru Nanak Dev University, Amritsar, Punjab, India
e-mail: kgurcharan.neuro@yahoo.com

S. S. Lakhman
Department of Pharmaceutical, Social and Administrative Sciences,
DYC School of Pharmacy, Buffalo, USA

M. K. Thakur, S. I. S. Rattan (eds.), *Brain Aging and Therapeutic Interventions*,
DOI 10.1007/978-94-007-5237-5_10,

10.1 Introduction

Aging is an inevitable universal phenomenon involving a series of complex molecular mechanisms, which accompany decline in many physiological functions of the body and pose a major risk for many neurodegenerative diseases. With the rapidly growing population of elderly people and associated increase in incidence of dementia and cognitive decline, a major challenge facing mankind is how to ensure healthy brain aging. The research in biogerontology has provided us with insights into the possible interventional therapies against challenging age-related pathologies. This review focuses on the interventional regimens/therapies principally contributing to disease prevention and/or reversing the age related changes once they have occurred. Several studies suggest the critical link between aging and diseases like cancer, atherosclerosis, cardiovascular defects, cataract, diabetes, dementia, stroke, Alzheimer and neurodegeneration along with deceleration in cognitive functions accompanied by memory loss (Matsumoto et al. 2000; Farooqui and Farooqui 2009; Lee and Wei 2012).

Age-associated neuropathologies are mainly due to enhanced oxidative stress, neuronal degeneration and inflammation, glutamate excitotoxicity and many other factors (Hamilton et al. 2001). The key repair mechanisms depend on the level of antioxidants, tissue repair by neurite associated proteins, improved brain plasticity marker's expression, angiogenesis and role of growth factors. Mechanisms may seem vivid and unclear but the free radical theories or mitochondrial damage theories provide an insight to the targets that need to be taken care of. The therapeutic interventions currently being tested in animal models as well as being put to practice on human subjects are environmental enrichment, pharmacological interventions, physical activity/exercise, calorie/dietary restriction etc. It may be further suggested that the simultaneous focus of animal model studies on "biological" and "behavioral" mechanisms that contribute to the potential beneficial effects of lifestyle interventions may have greater clinical applications.

10.2 Lifestyle Interventions—Road to Healthy Brain Aging

An ideal solution for healthy aging and delaying the onset of age associated pathologies lies in the implementation of lifestyle interventions such as caloric/dietary restriction, pharmacological, environmental enrichment, physical activity, etc. In a recent study, Chakravarty et al. (2012) suggested that the life style habits of middle age determine disabilities and mortalities associated with later life. Several recent studies have confirmed the potential beneficial role of physical activity and environmental enrichment in improvement of life expectancy and healthy aging (reviewed by Volkers and Scherder 2011; Charansonney 2011; Scali et al. 2012). Individuals living in an enriched environment with physical and social activity, perform much better on cognitive tests compared to animals in impoverished environment. Sedentary and lonely people show decline in cognitive functioning as compared to physically and socially active people. Another well focused and established intervention is physical activity or exercise, which when appropriately undertaken is one of the most successful anti-aging interventions known to delay aging and improving general health status and fitness. The physically active aged individuals showed better cognitive performance and growth factor gene expression compared to their counterparts (Yaffe et al. 2001; Barnett 2012). Exercise has been reported to provide protection against many fatal diseases like atherosclerosis, diabetes, cancer, ischemic heart disease (Jolliffe et al. 2000; Piepoli et al. 2004). The physical exercise offered beneficial results and enhanced hippocampal neurogenesis, synaptic plasticity (Farmer et al. 2004), neurotransmission (Cotman and Berchtold 2002), and improved learning and memory by neurotrophic factors like brain-derived neurotrophic factor (BDNF), nerve growth factor (NGF) and fibroblast growth factor-2 (FGF-2) in the hippocampus of the brain, which are known to be involved in the brain plasticity functions and learning and memory activities.

Epidemiological studies also verify that exercise reduces the risk of stroke and stimulates brain recovery after injury in rats and humans. Similarly, voluntary wheel running has been found to increase angiogenesis in the motor cortex, cerebellum and hippocampus of the rat (Swain et al. 2003; Lopez-Lopez et al. 2004). In a recent study by O'Callaghan et al. (2009), it was suggested that there is a link between functional neuronal plasticity and improved expression of neurotrophin BDNF, thus indicating the ability of brain to respond positively to the physical exercise across lifespan. Another aspect of physical exercise also includes environmental enrichment, which is often related with intelligence. The animal studies prove that the animals maintained in enriched environment exhibit increased synaptic plasticity along with the resistance of neurons against injury. Environmental enrichment increases new cell numbers in aged animals (Kempermann et al. 2002) and has been reported to stimulate synaptic plasticity and synaptic strength.

Genetic manipulation may be another useful intervention and some possible candidates are like mutating genes involved in insulin pathways (Tatar et al. 2003; Liang et al. 2003), increasing expression of antioxidant genes (Mitsui et al. 2002), heat shock genes (Munoz 2003) or sirtuins (Tissenbaum and Guarantee 2001) which have been reported for increasing longevity. Shimokawa et al. (2008) reviewed the concept of conserved mechanisms that influence aging and the possible role of longevity genes or signals like FoxO transcription factors that contribute to DR. The identification of longevity genes evoked a new understanding of the possible role of genes or SNPs on the longevity or longevity influencing factors. The notion that longevity genes confer resistance to stress or attenuate accrual of tissue damage is important but identification of longevity signals that would stand against odds like ROS generation, macromolecular damage and mitochondrial function preservation is still a question of concern and needs to be addressed critically.

Besides, few potential pharmacological interventions have also been identified including antioxidants (Melov et al. 2000) and compounds that modulate protein deacetylase activity (Howitz et al. 2003; Wood et al. 2004). Despite the discrepancies with dosage and administration modes, few drugs have been successfully reported to extend lifespan in animal models, e.g. propargylamines (Kitani et al. 2002), though the only worry is applicability to humans with no side effects. Similarly, sirtuins have recently gained much attention due to their impact as physiological targets for treating age associated diseases (Lappalainen 2011). Sirtuins interact with metabolic pathways and have been proposed to act as potential targets of caloric restriction as well as pharmacological interventions. It is suggested that sirtuins may also provide a novel approach to exercise physiology. Quercetin, a natural polyphenolic flavonoid that induces sirtuins also has potential health benefits, which may be useful for disease prevention.

10.3 Dietary Restriction and Healthy Brain Aging

Aging is a complex, heterogeneous, and multifactorial phenomenon, which is the consequence of multiple interactions between genes and environment. The spectacular advances in functional genomics in the recent past have greatly accelerated the research on the effects of environmental factors as interventional strategies for healthy lifespan (Qiu et al. 2010; Fontana et al. 2010b; Katewa and Kapahi 2010). Life expectancy of the world population has increased dramatically during the last century and it is expected that the number of older adults will rise, while the number of youths will decline in the near future. This demographic shift has considerable public health and economic implications since aging is associated with the development of serious chronic diseases (reviewed by Omodei and Fontana 2009). In non-human and human primates, CR regimen without under nutrition is known to reduce abdominal obesity as well as protect against diabetes, hypertension and cardiovascular diseases.

The most reliable and effective anti aging intervention in almost all organisms studied so far to extend mean and maximum lifespan is dietary restriction. Besides being anti aging regimen, the ongoing studies also suggest it as potent anti cancer therapy (Suttie et al. 2005) as well as effective against many traumatic injuries (Kumar et al. 2009) or diseases like cardiovascular (Ripple et al. 2009) or immune functions deficits (Volk et al. 1994). It is well known that DR can retard the aging process in organisms ranging from yeast to non-human primates as well as delay the onset of many age-related diseases including neurodegenerative disorders. Knowledge gained from DR research in animal models may help to translate this information to design new therapeutic approaches for disease prevention strategies in humans. Signaling pathways induced by DR/CR are therefore potentially new therapeutic targets for neurodegenerative diseases. Many recent reviews have summarized the evidence on key biological mechanisms underlying the beneficial effects of DR/CR based on our current understanding, with particular emphasis on the recent impact of CR on neuroprotection, and on the emerging development of pharmacological agents that target signaling pathways induced by CR. DR seems to possibly work by establishing an adaptive conditioning response that maintains the survival mode in the organism, focusing on the energy conservation, which causes shift in metabolic status from growth to maintenance activities and hence promotes anti aging effects.

DR may be implemented either as a reduction of total nutrient intake without causing malnutrition or restriction of major dietary components (protein, lipid or carbohydrates). Another regimen which is based on the temporal variations of food intake (intermittent fasting) has recently gained much attention of gerontologists. Understanding the molecular mechanisms of how DR slows aging and age-associated diseases has gained pace in the last few years. Though there are queries about various aspects of DR regimen like duration, short or long term and onset or initiation age, young, middle or in aged animals, the beneficial effects still stand. DR regimen was capable to prevent an age-related decline in the expression of genes involved in fatty acid oxidation (Park et al. 2006; Zhu et al. 2007; Solomon et al. 2008), including decreased body temperature, decreased heart rate and blood pressure, and decreased glucose and insulin levels (Mattson 2003; Kaur et al. 2008).

Of all the other interventional strategies being explored, DR is the most robust nongenetic, non-pharmacological intervention known to increase active and healthy lifespan in a variety of species. Although the exact molecular mechanism(s) remains to be elucidated, the significant popularity of the regimen stems from the wide beneficial effects on the energy related molecules like cytochrome oxidase (Cerqueira et al. 2011) and creatine kinase (Shinmura et al. 2007) and stress chaperons, HSP-70, GRP-78 and Gadd153, brain plasticity related molecules and oxidative status of cell (Mattson et al. 2001, 2003; Kaur et al. 2008; Sharma et al. 2010). DR causes decrease in the ROS production and attenuates the accrual of age associated oxidative damage in brain, liver, heart and skeletal muscle (Gredilla et al. 2001; Sanz et al. 2005; Lopez-Lluch et al. 2006; Singh et al. 2011). Evidence further supports that DR can mitigate mitochondrial dysfunction by increasing antioxidant activities (Sharma et al. 2010; Goto et al. 2002; Radak et al. 2002; Araki and Goto 2004; Goyary and Sharma 2008), mitochondrial respiration and turnover (Nisoli et al. 2005; Hepple et al. 2006; Miwa et al. 2008) enhancing removal of damaged mitochondria. The beneficial effect of DR further extends on the reduction of mitochondrial free radical generation and proton leak and enhanced activity of complex IV in aged rats, suggesting the compensatory loop helping efficient enzyme activity and decrease in ROS generation (Gredilla et al. 2001; Ayala et al. 2007; Singh et al. 2011).

Emerging data from our lab has focused mainly on the potential beneficial effects of late onset intermittent fasting dietary restriction (IF-DR) regimen to improve age associated impairment of brain functions. IF-DR regimen initiated in late age for short term (12 weeks) was seen to compensate for age related increase in oxidative stress and induction of stress chaperone HSP-70. Age associated decline in the neuronal and synaptic plasticity related molecules like synapsin 1, synaptophysin, calcineurin and CamKinase were found to be effectively restored in rats on IF-DR regimen in the middle and late age (Kaur et al. 2008; Sharma et al. 2010; Singh et al. 2011). Results are summarized in Fig. 10.1. Further the beneficial effects of DR were found to be effective against reactive gliosis as indicated by decreased expres-

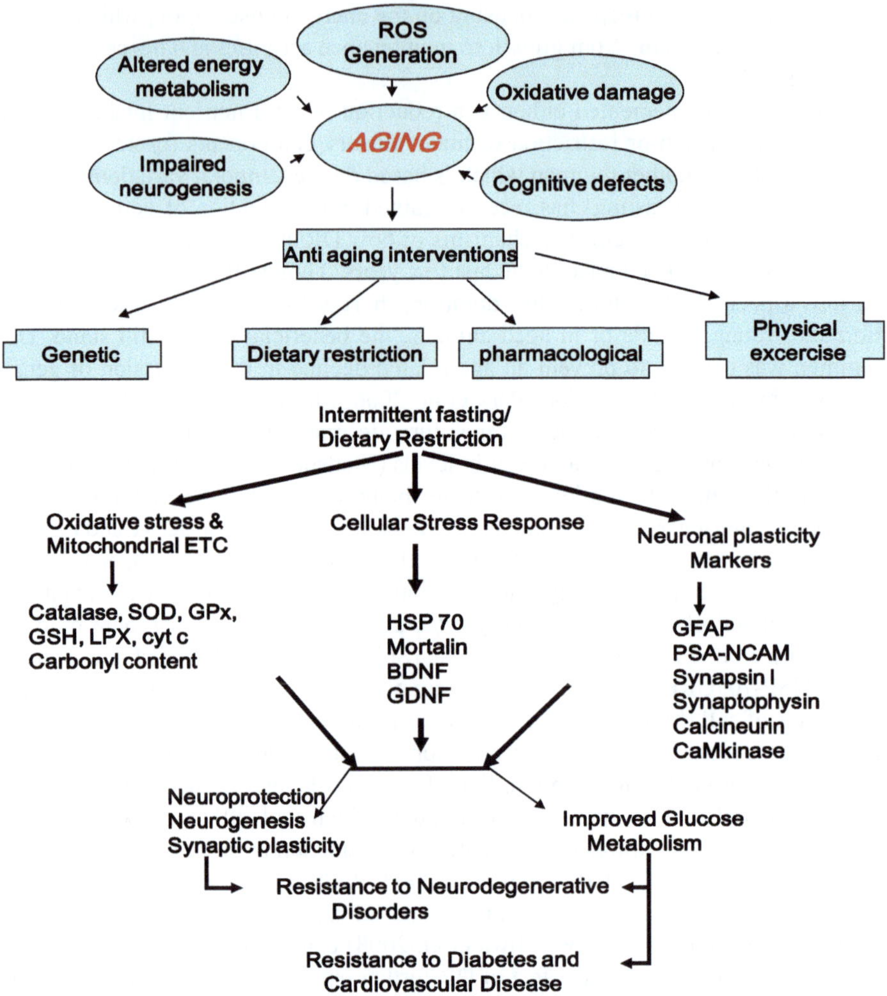

Fig. 10.1 Summary of the potential beneficial effects of intermittent fasting dietary restriction regimen. (Sharma et al. 2010; Singh et al. 2011)

sion of GFAP, an astrocytic marker along with upregulation of NCAM and PSA-NCAM, markers of neuronal plasticity (Kaur et al. 2008). Our studies on animal model of IF-DR regimen simultaneously focused on "biological" and "behavioral" mechanisms to establish the potential beneficial effects of this lifestyle intervention, which may have greater clinical applications and can be easily implemented in human subjects. Also based on the previous theories linking oxidative stress, mitochondrial dysfunction, behavioral performance and synaptic plasticity, we observed correlation of the DR regimen with various regulatory or stress response pathways with learning, memory and brain plasticity, all crucially important for healthy aging.

Another important pro-longevity factor reported for mediating lifespan extension by DR regimen is sirtuins, protein deacetylases or ADP ribosyltransferases (Lin et al. 2000). SIRT1 has been reported to be directly linked to the mammalian aging and can regulate physiological processes like stress response and energy metabolism, known to be affected by aging and moderated by DR (Tissenbaum and Guarantee 2001; Rogina and Helfand 2004; Guarantee 2006; Haigis and Guarantee 2006; Schwer and Verdin 2008). Recent literature reports sirtuins as key antiaging genes in different model organisms which is attributed to their NAD-dependence, thus linking to the metabolic activity of cells. Similarly, mammalian sirtuins have been associated with stress resistance and many of the metabolic pathways such as adipogenesis, gluconeogenesis, and insulin and glucose homeostasis are reported to play an important role as an antiapoptotic factor in the survival of neurons (Luo et al. 2001, Motta et al. 2004).

The experimental regimen DR particularly depends on the reduction of the calories per se and not upon the reduction of consumption of dietary components, so besides the success of IF-DR regimen, the applicability to humans stills remains the question of concern. Colman et al. (2009) carried out a 20-year longitudinal study in non-human primates and reported that CR improves health span in rhesus macaques. They divided adult rhesus monkeys into two groups which were given either control or CR diet (30 % reduction of total food). The important observations of this study are that the CR animals looked subjectively younger and showed a statistically significant decrease in the impairment of muscle function with age, glucose homeostasis and incidence of neoplasia and cardiovascular disease. Further, caloric restriction was also seen to reduce the age-associated brain atrophy in regions believed to regulate motor behavioral function.

Some recent studies have also examined the long-term effects of CR on human subjects. Fontana et al. (2010b) compared three groups including (a) 28 human volunteers who had consumed a CR diet for an average of 6.9 ± 5.5 years, (b) endurance runners who ran an average of 48 miles per week who had been training regularly for an average of 21 years and (c) sedentary controls (regular exercise < 1 h per week). Both interventions i.e. CR and endurance exercise resulted in significant reduction in body weight, BMI, total body fat, lower fasting level of insulin as well as higher insulin sensitivity as compared to controls. This study further reported that the individuals in the CR group also had lower levels of fasting glucose, high serum level of adiponectin and free fatty acids and lower serum levels of inflammatory mediators including IL-6, TNFR-I and TNFR-II.

Another landmark study has been reported by Lefevre et al. (2009) which suggested that CR might reduce the risk factors for cardiovascular disease and memory decline in humans. The Comprehensive Assessment of Long-Term Effects of Reducing Intake of Energy (CALERIE) research team is looking at effects of short-term (6 months) CR on risk factors for cardiovascular disease. The study included 36 individuals who were assigned randomly to one of three groups: (a) controls, (b) 25 % calorie restriction and (c) CR+EX (12.5 %CR+12.5 % increase in energy expenditure via structured aerobic exercises). The study reported that CR, with or without exercise, showed significant changes in several risk factors usually associated with cardiovascular health, including the ratio of total cholesterol to HDL cholesterol and systolic blood pressure. Another recent study examined the effect of CR on memory function (Witte et al. 2009). Fifty normal to overweight elderly subjects were divided into three groups: (a) consuming a 30 % CR diet, (b) one consuming an increased proportion of unsaturated fatty acids and (c) served as control. The CR diet led to a significant (20 %) increase in verbal memory score, as well as decrease in fasting plasma levels of insulin and C-reactive protein.

Mild DR mediated stress whether due to restriction of meal size or frequency is based on the hormetic effects of DR, which is known to increase the cellular stress resistance. The recent data from our lab suggests that late onset short term IF-DR regimen has the potential to retard age associated detrimental effects on brain functions, which involve decline in cognitive and motor performance as well as oxidative molecular damage to protein. DR may be used as a novel approach for therapeutic intervention in several diseases after information is made available by clinical trials on the effects of mild dietary stress on human health. To add strength and support to the hypothesis, the idea of DR mimetics has also been introduced, with which one can induce DR like state with resistance to the aging associated pathologies and improving late life health. To ascertain link between meal frequency and healthy aging, we need to conduct more well designed studies on human subjects using intermittent fasting paradigm e.g. skipping meals regimens especially dinner at least on alternate days and study the beneficial effects on health predictors.

References

Ayala V, Naudı A, Sanz A, Caro P, Portero-Otin M, Barja G, Pamplona R (2007) Dietary protein restriction decreases oxidative protein damage, peroxidizability index, and mitochondrial complex I content in rat liver. J Gerontol A Biol Sci Med Sci 62:352–360

Araki S, Goto S (2004) Dietary restriction in aged mice can partially restore impaired metabolism of apolipoprotein A-IV and C-III. Biogerontology 5:445–450

Barnett F (2012) The effect of excersice on affective and self efficacy responses in older and younger women. J Phys Act Health (Epub ahead of print).

Cerqueira FM, Laurindo FR, Kowaltowski AJ (2011) Mild mitochondrial uncoupling and calorie restriction increase fasting eons, akt and mitochondrial biogenesis. PLoS One 6:e18433

Chakravarty EF, Hubert HB, Krishnan E, Bruce BB, Lingala VB, Fries JF (2012) Lifestyle risk factors predict disability and death in healthy aging adults. Am J Med 125:190–197

Charansonney OL (2011) Physical activity and aging: a life-long story. Discov Med 12:177–185

Colman RJ, Anderson RM, Johnson SC, Kastman EK, Kosmatka KJ, Beasley TM, Allison DB, Cruzen C, Simmons HA, Kemnitz JW, Weindruch R (2009) Caloric restriction delays disease onset and mortality in rhesus monkeys. Science 325:201–204

Cotman CW, Berchtold NC (2002) Exercise: a behavioral intervention to enhance brain health and plasticity. Trends Neurosci 25:295–301

Farmer J, Zhao X, van Praag H, Wodtke K, Gage FH, Christie BR (2004) Effects of voluntary exercise on synaptic plasticity and gene expression in the dentate gyrus of adult male Sprague-Dawley rats in vivo. Neuroscience 124:71–79

Farooqui T, Farooqui AA (2009) Aging: an important factor for the pathogenesis of neurodegenerative diseases. Mech Aging Dev 130:203–215

Fontana L, Klein S, Holloszy JO (2010a) Effects of long-term calorie restriction and endurance exercise on glucose tolerance, insulin action, and adipokine production. Age 32:97–108.
Fontana L, Partridge L, Longo VD (2010b) Extending healthy life span--from yeast to humans. Science 328:321–326
Goto S, Takahashi R, Araki S, Nakamoto H (2002) Dietary restriction initiated in late adulthood can reverse age-related alterations of protein and protein metabolism. Ann N Y Acad Sci 959:50–56
Goyary D, Sharma R (2008) Late onset of dietary restriction reverses age-related decline of malate--aspartate shuttle enzymes in the liver and kidney of mice. Biogerontology 9:11–18
Gredilla R, Sanz A, Lopez-Torres M, Barja G (2001) Caloric restriction decreases mitochondrial free radical generation at complex I and lowers oxidative damage to mitochondrial DNA in the rat heart. FASEB J 15:1589–1591
Guarantee L (2006) Sit-ins as potential targets for metabolic syndrome. Nature 444:868–874
Haggis MC, Guarantee LP (2006) Mammalian sit-ins—emerging roles in physiology, aging, and calorie restriction. Genes Dev 20:2913–2921
Hamilton ML, Van Remmen H, Drake JA, Yang H, Guo ZM, Kiewit K, Walter CA, Richardson A (2001) Does oxidative damage to DNA increase with age? Proc Natl Acad Sci U S A 98:10469–74
Hepple RT, Baker DJ, McConkey M, Murynka T, Norris R (2006) Caloric restriction protects mitochondrial function with aging in skeletal and cardiac muscles. Rejuvenation Res 9:219–222
Howitz KT, Bitterman KJ, Cohen HY, Lamming DW, Lavu S, Wood JG, Zipkin RE, Chung P, Kisielewski A, Zhang LL, Scherer B, Sinclair DA (2003) Small molecule activators of sirtuins extend Saccharomyces cerevisiae lifespan. Nature 425:191–196
Jolliffe JA, Rees K, Taylor RS, Thompson D, Oldridge N, and Ebrahim S (2000) Exercise-based rehabilitation for coronary heart disease. Cochrane Database Syst Rev 4:CD001800
Katewa SD and Kapahi P (2010) Dietary restriction and aging. Aging Cell 9:105–112
Kaur M, Sharma S, Kaur G (2008) Age-related impairments in neuronal plasticity markers and astrocytic GFAP and their reversal by late-onset short term dietary restriction. Biogerontology 9:441–454
Kempermann G, Gast D, Gage FH (2002) Neuroplasticity in old age: sustained five fold induction of hippocampal neurogenesis by long-term environmental enrichment. Ann Neurol 52:135–143
Kitani K, Minami C, Yamamoto T, Kanai S, Ivy GO, Carrillo MC (2002) Pharmacological interventions in aging and age-associated disorders: potentials of propargylamines for human use. Ann N Y Acad Sci 959:295–307
Kumar S, Parkash J, Kataria H, Kaur G (2009) Interactive effect of excitotoxic injury and dietary restriction on neurogenesis and neurotrophic factors in adult male rat brain. Neurosci Res 65:367–374
Lappalainen Z (2011) Sirtuins: a family of proteins with implications for human performance and exercise physiology. Res Sports Med 19:53–65
Lee HC, Wei YH (2012) Mitochondria and aging. Adv Exp Med Biol 942:311–327
Lefevre M, Redman LM, Heilbronn LK, Smith JV, Martin CK, Rood JC, Greenway FL, Williamson DA, Smith SR, Ravussin E (2009) Caloric restriction alone and with exercise improves CVD risk in healthy nonobese individuals. Atherosclerosis 203:206–213
Liang H, Masoro EJ, Nelson JF, Strong R, McMahan CA and Richardson A (2003) Genetic mouse models of extended lifespan. Exp Gerontol 38:1353–1364
Lin SJ, Defossez PA, Guarente L (2000) Requirement of NAD and SIR2 for life-span extension by calorie restriction in Saccharomyces cerevisiae. Science 289:2126–2128
Lopez-Lopez C, LeRoith D, Torres-Aleman I (2004) Insulin-like growth factor I is required for vessel remodeling in the adult brain. Proc Natl Acad Sci U S A 101:9833–9888
López-Lluch G, Hunt N, Jones B, Zhu M, Jamieson H, Hilmer S, Cascajo MV, Allard J, Ingram DK, Navas P, de Cabo R (2006) Calorie restriction induces mitochondrial biogenesis and bioenergetic efficiency. Proc Natl Acad Sci U S A 103:1768–1773
Luo J, Nikolaev AY, Imai S, Chen D, Su F, Shiloh A, Guarantee L, Gu W (2001) Negative control of p53 by Sir2α promotes cell survival under stress. Cell 107:137–148

Matsumoto AM, Marck BT, Gruenewald DA, Wolden-Hanson T, Naai MA (2000) Aging and the neuroendocrine regulation of reproduction and body weight. Exp Gerontol 35:1251–1265
Mattson MP (2003) Gene--diet interactions in brain aging and neurodegenerative disorders. Ann Intern Med 139:441–444
Mattson MP, Duan W, Guo Z (2003) Meal size and frequency affect neuronal plasticity and vulnerability to disease: cellular and molecular mechanisms. J Neurochem 84:417–431
Mattson MP, Duan W, Lee J, Guo Z (2001) Suppression of brain aging and neurodegenerative disorders by dietary restriction and environmental enrichment: molecular mechanisms. Mech Aging Dev 122:757–778
Melov S, Ravenscroft J, Malik S, Gill MS, Walker DW, Clayton PE, Wallace DC, Malfroy B, Doctrow SR,Lithgow GJ (2000) Extension of life-span with superoxide dismutase/catalase mimetics. Science 289:1567–1569
Miwa S, Lawless C, von Zglinicki T (2008) Mitochondrial turnover in liver is fast in vivo and is accelerated by dietary restriction: application of a simple dynamic model. Aging Cell 7:920–923
Mitsui A, Hamuro J, Nakamura H, Kondo N, Hirabayashi Y, Ishizaki-Koizumi S, Hirakawa T, Inoue T, and Yodoi J (2002) Overexpression of human thioredoxin in transgenic mice controls oxidative stress and life span. Antioxid. Redox Signal 4:693–696
Motta MC, Divecha N, Lemieux M, Kamel C, Chen D, Gu W, Bultsma Y, McBurney, Guarente L (2004) Mammalian SIRT1 represses forkhead transcription factors. Cell 116:551–563
Munoz MJ (2003) Longevity and heat stress regulation in Caenorhabditis elegans. Mech Aging Dev 124:43–48
Nisoli E, Tonello C, Cardile A, Cozzi V, Bracale R, Tedesco L, Falcone S, Valerio A, Cantoni O, Clementi E, Moncada S, Carruba MO (2005) Calorie restriction promotes mitochondrial biogenesis by inducing the expression of eNOS. Science 310:314–317
O'Callaghan RM, Griffin EW, Kelly AM (2009) Long-term treadmill exposure protects against age-related neurodegenerative change in the rat hippocampus. Hippocampus 19:1019–1029
Omodei D, Fontana L. (2009) Calorie restriction and prevention of age-associated chronic disease. FEBS Lett 585:1537–1542
Park SY, Kim YW, Kim JE, Kim JY, (2006). Age-associated changes in fat metabolism in the rat and its relation to sympathetic activity. Life Sci 79:2228–2233
Piepoli MF, Davos C, Francis DP, and Coats AJ (2004) Exercise training meta-analysis of trials in patients with chronic heart failure (ExTra-MATCH). BMJ 328:189–195
Qiu G, Liu S, So KF (2010) Dietary restriction and brain health. Neurosci Bull 26(1):55–65
Radak Z, Takahashi R, Koriyama A, Nakamoto H, Ohno H, Ookawara T, Goto S (2002) Effect of aging and late onset dietary restriction on antioxidant enzymes and proteasome activities, and protein carbonylation of rat skeletal muscle and tendon. Exp Gerontol 37:1423–1430
Rogina B, Helfand SL (2004) Sir2 mediates longevity in the fly through a pathway related to calorie restriction. Proc Natl Acad Sci U S A. 101:15998–16003
Ripple MJ, Verweij M, Brand K, van de Ven M, Goemaere N, Van Den Engel S, Chu T, Forrer F, Müller C, de Jong M, van IJcken W, IJzermans JN, Hoeijmakers JH, de Bruin RW (2009) Short-term dietary restriction and fasting precondition against ischemia reperfusion injury in mice. Aging Cell 9:40–53
Sanz A, Caro P, Ibañez J, Gómez J, Gredilla R, Barja G (2005) Dietary restriction at old age lowers mitochondrial oxygen radical production and leak at complex I and oxidative DNA damage in rat brain. J Bioenergy Biomembr 37:83–90
Scali M, Baroncelli L, Cenni MC, Sale A, Maffei L (2012) A rich environmental experience reactivates visual cortex plasticity in aged rats. Exp Gerontol (Epub ahead of print).
Schwer B, Verdin E (2008) Conserved metabolic regulatory functions of sirtuins. Cell Metabol 7:104–112
Sharma S, Singh R, Kaur M, Kaur G (2010) Late-onset dietary restriction compensates for age-related increase in oxidative stress and alterations of HSP 70 and synapsin1 protein levels in male Wistar rats. Biogerontology 11:197–209
Shimokawa I, Chiba T, Yamaza H, Komatsu T (2008) Longevity Genes: Insights from Calorie Restriction and Genetic Longevity Models. Mol Cells 26:427–435

Shinmura K, Tamaki K, Saito K, Nakano Y, Tobe T, Bolli R (2007) Cardioprotective effects of short-term caloric restriction are mediated by adiponectin via activation of AMP-activated protein kinase. Circulation 116:2809–2817

Singh R, Lakhanpal D, Kumar S, Sharma S, Kataria H, Kaur M, Kaur G (2011) Late-onset intermittent fasting dietary restriction as a potential intervention to retard age-associated brain function impairments in male rats. Age (Dordr) (in press)

Solomon TP, Marchetti CM, Krishnan RK, Gonzalez F, Kirwan JP (2008) Effects of aging on basal fat oxidation in obese humans. Metabolism 57:1141–1147

Suttie AW, Dinse GE, Nyska A, Moser GJ, Goldsworthy TL, Maronpot RR (2005) An investigation of the effects of late-onset dietary restriction on prostate cancer development in the TRAMP mouse. Toxicol Pathol 33:386–397

Swain RA, Harris AB, Wiener EC, Dutka MV, Morris HD, Theien BE, Konda S, Engberg K, Lauterbur PC, GreenoughWT (2003) Prolonged exercise induces angiogenesis and increases cerebral blood volume in primary motor cortex of the rat. Neuroscience 117:1037–1046

Tatar M, Bartke A, Antebi A (2003) The endocrine regulation of aging by insulin-like signals. Science 299:1346–1351

Tissenbaum HA, Guarantee L (2001) Increased dosage of a sir-2 gene extends lifespan in Caenorhabditis elegans. Nature 410:227–230

Volkers KM, Scherder EJ (2011) Impoverished environment, cognition, aging and dementia. Rev Neurosci 22:259–266

Volk MJ, Pugh TD, Kim MJ, Frith CH, Daynes RA, Ershler WB, and Weindruch R (1994) Dietary restriction from middle age attenuates age-associated lymphoma development and interleukin 6 dysregulation in C57BL/6 mice. Cancer Res 54:3054–3061

Witte AV, Fobker M, Gillnet R, Knecht S, Floe A (2009) Caloric restriction improves memory in elderly humans. Proc Natl Acad Sci U S A 106:1255–1260

Wood JG, Regina B, Lavu S, Howitz K, Helfand SL, Tatar M, Sinclair D (2004) Sirtuin activators mimic caloric restriction and delay aging in metazoans. Nature 430:686–689

Yaffe K, Barnes D, Nevitt M, Lui LY, Covinsky K (2001) A prospective study of physical activity and cognitive decline in elderly women: women who walk. Arch Intern Med 161:1703–1708

Zhu M, Lee GD, Ding L, Hu J, Qiu G, de Cabo R, Bernier M, Ingram DK, Zou S (2007) Adipogenic signaling in rat white adipose tissue: modulation by aging and calorie restriction. Exp Gerontol 42:733–744

Chapter 11
Understanding Mechanism of Action of Herbal Drugs in Age Related Degenerative Brain Disorders

Maheep Bhatnagar, Ayushi Jain, Neha Jaiswal, Chavi Sharma and Pooja Suvalka

Abstract In this review, we will briefly introduce preventive strategies represented by selected plants which are also popularly used by different traditional medicines and have scientific evidences of possible alternative therapeutic value for neuroprotection. Among these commonly used in most traditional medicines of China and India are *Gingko biloba*, *Panax ginseng*, *Curcuma longa*, *Withania somnifera* (WS) etc. In addition, scientific evidences of usefulness of *Vitis vinifera* (Grapes) as red wine, Coffee sp and *Camelia sinensis* (Tea) will be discussed. Here, we will also discuss in detail the possible use of WS as potential candidate for treatment of AD. Clinical trials and animal research supported the use of WS for treatment of anxiety, cognitive and neurological disorders, senile dementia, Alzheimer's (AD) and Parkinson's disease (PD), and as antioxidant and anti-inflammatory agent. This might be important in suggesting therapeutic implications of WS in neurodegenerative disorders.

Keywords AChE • *Withania somnifera* • Co-localization • Neurodegeneration • NADPH-d • Alzheimer's • Parkinson's disease

11.1 Introduction

Aging is a complex physiological process that involves both morphological and biochemical changes occurring, with the passage of time, in single cells and the whole organism. Among the many theories proposed to explain the mechanism of aging at the molecular level, the oxidative stress or free radical hypothesis has received wide support. Biochemically, oxidative stress is defined as a disturbance in the cell oxidation/reduction (redox) status, leading to the production of partially reduced oxygen intermediates, more reactive than molecular oxygen in its ground state, termed as

M. Bhatnagar (✉) · A. Jain · N. Jaiswal · C. Sharma · P. Suvalka
Faculty of Science, University College of Science, MLS University,
Udaipur 313001, India
e-mail: mbhatnagar@yahoo.com

M. K. Thakur, S. I. S. Rattan (eds.), *Brain Aging and Therapeutic Interventions*,
DOI 10.1007/978-94-007-5237-5_11,

reactive oxygen species (ROS). ROS production and oxidative damage to biomacromolecules (nucleic acids, lipids and proteins) initiate the development of age-dependent degenerative diseases. This represents a condition in which the function and/or structure of affected tissues or organs progressively deteriorate over time, such as cardiovascular and neurodegenerative diseases. Neurodegenerative disease is mainly defined as a deterioration of the intellectual and cognitive faculties which are generally associated with aging and/or age associated disorders (AD, PD).

The human brain accounts for less than 2 % of the body weight, it consumes about 20 % of the oxygen available through respiration. Therefore, because of its high oxygen demand, the brain is the most susceptible organ to oxidative damage (Bajra 2004). Additionally, the high amount of polyunsaturated fatty acids (PUFAs) present in neuronal membranes makes the brain tissues particularly susceptible to lipid peroxidation reactions, resulting in the formation of cytotoxic aldehydes, such as malondialdhyde (MDA) and 4-hydroxynonenal (HNE) leading to cell degeneration.

11.2 Alzheimer's (AD) and Parkinson's (PD) Disease

Alzheimer's is today's the most prevalent disorder in the elderly population. It is characterized by progressive and irreversible memory loss, cognitive deterioration and personality changes, usually with an onset after 65 years of age. Though memory impairment appears in the early stages of the disease but motor and sensory functions are not affected until later stages. Parkinson's is the second most common age-related neurodegenerative disease. PD is a movement disorder characterized by resting tremors, bradykinesia, extrapyramidal rigidity and loss of postural reflexes i.e., disturbance in walking or equilibrium. Incidence rates of AD and PD increase exponentially with age. According to the World Health Organization (WHO), neurodegenerative diseases will become the world's second leading cause of death by the middle of this century, in fact overtaking cancer (Menken et al. 2000). It is also predicted that by 2050 the number of AD patients in the US only, could range from 11 to 16 million (Hebert et al. 2003). PD affects approximately 1 % of population aged 65–69 years and the prevalence increases to 3 % in the 80 year old or above group. According to an estimate, by 2030 in Western Europe, the number of PD cases will be double from 4.5 to 9 million and the prevalence varies in different ethnic and geographic groups (Dorsey et al. 2007).

11.3 Neuropathology of AD and PD

Although AD and PD differ in their clinical symptoms as well as disease course, but both are basically characterized by a progressive loss of neurons in different brain areas. Furthermore, they are characterized by the aggregation of intracellular proteins (Shastry 2003) as the presence of extracellular senile plaques and intracellular accumulation of neurofibrillary tangles (NFTs) in the brain of AD patients has been observed. Senile plaques are composed of fibrillar amyloid β (Aβ) peptides produced by cleavage of the Aβ precursor protein (APP), whereas NFTs consist of hyperphosphorylated microtubule associated tau protein (Pβ). Selective neuronal loss is particularly severe in specific cerebral areas—the neocortex, hippocampus, limbic system and subcortical areas (Selkoe 2001). On the contrary, PD is characterized by the selective degeneration of dopaminergic neurons located in the pars compacta of the substantia nigra. One of the main neuropathological hallmarks of PD is the aggregation of the intracellular protein β -synuclein, to form intracytoplasmic inclusions (Lewy bodies) in these neurons (Agorogiannis et al. 2004).

The etiology of both the diseases is multifactorial, with a complex combination of genetic and non-genetic components. Oxidative damage is believed to be one of the leading cause of neuronal degeneration in both AD and PD (Nikam et al. 2009a, b). Though the exact mechanism of AD is still unknown, several lines of evidence suggest that oxidative stress is implicated in Aβ -induced neurotoxicity, besides apoptosis and inflammation. Studies have suggested a close relationship between cerebral biometal (Fe, Cu, Zn) and AD pathology. These redox-active metals and Aβ peptides interact to elevate oxidative stress in brain tissues. In PD, the mechanisms involved in selective degeneration of dopaminergic neurons in the nigrostriatal system are not clearly known, though evidence suggests that oxidative stress may arise from the metabolism of dopamine, producing free radical species (Jenner 2004). Compared to the rest of brain, the subtantia nigra pars compacta is exposed to a higher rate of ROS formation and to higher levels of oxidative stress (Yuan et al. 2007).

11.4 Current Pharmacological Intervention for AD and PD

There is no cure for AD and PD and current therapies provide only symptomatic improvement by either replacing the levels or controlling the metabolism of neurotransmitters involved in the disease or to restore their imbalance. Cholinesterase inhibitors are still the first line prescript drug available for patients with mild to moderate AD. By inhibiting the hydrolysis of acetylcholine in the synaptic cleft, these drugs restore the levels of the neurotransmitter in the affected neurons (Persson et al. 2009). Memantine was approved for moderate to severe cases, which acts as a specific, non- competitive N-methyl-D-aspartate (NMDA) receptor antagonist, counteract the excitotoxicity of glutamate, the major excitatory neurotransmitter in the brain (Terriot et al. 2004). Anti-inflammatory and antioxidant therapies were also proposed as possible preventive strategies. In case of PD, current therapeutic approach for the symptomatic treatment includes Levodopa (L-DOPA) which is converted to dopamine in the body, thus replenish the decreased dopamine levels in affected tissues (Lewitt 2008; Olanow et al. 2009).

11.5 Neuroprotective Strategies

The term neuroprotection refers to the strategies to protect the central nervous system (CNS) against neuronal injury due to trauma, stroke or aging resulting into chronic neurodegenerative changes in the nervous system. Such age related changes are characteristic of the AD and PD. Oxidative damage is believed to be one of the leading causes of such neuronal degeneration in both AD and PD. Among various current strategies used, herbal medicines represent valuable resource for antioxidant defence that can counteract the imbalance of the cell redox homeostasis and keep the ROS levels under the cytotoxic threshold. Antioxidant defenses also comprise vitamins and nonenzymatic scavengers abundant in food and medicinal plants (Prior and Cao 2000). As complementary or alternative therapy, herbal medicine refers to the medical use of plant organs—leaves, stems, roots, flowers, fruits and seeds for their curative properties. Herbal preparations contain complex mixture of several active components (phytochemicals), including phenylpropanoids, isoprenoids and alkaloids, which have different biological activities and responsible for its medicinal properties. It is often difficult to determine which component of the herbs has such neuroprotective biological activity (Suk 2005; Mclatchey et al. 2009).

11.5.1 Ginkgo biloba L.

Chinese term Ginkgo meaning silver apricot. The use of this plant in traditional medicine can be traced back to approximately 5,000 years to the origins of traditional community medicines (TCM). Modern Chinese pharmacopoeia has also introduced Ginkgo leaves as treatment for vascular insufficiency and to improve longevity. Since 1965, German physicians have prescribed *G. biloba* for the treatment of cognitive dysfunctions, dementia and AD. In the early 1970s, the standardized extract of *G. biloba* leaves EGb 761 was isolated and was widely prescribed in Europe and US for the symptomatic treatment of AD, cerebral insufficiency (a nonspecific age related deterioration of mental functions), improvement of cerebral blood flow and memory (Birks and Grimley 2009). EGb 761 contains 24 % of flavonoids and 6 % of terpenic lactones. The flavonoid fraction is composed of three flavonols—quercetin, keampferol and isorhamnetin, whereas terpenic derivatives are represented by diterpenic lactones, the ginkgolides A, B, C, J and M, and a sesquiterpenic trilactone, the bilobalide. Bilobalide can reduce damage caused by global brain ischemia and excitotoxicity-induced neuronal death (Chandrasekaran et al. 2003).

Neuroprotective action of EGb 761 is due to combination of antioxidative, anti-amyloidogenic and anti-apoptotic activities, by virtue of the blend of its bioactive phytochemicals (Yao et al. 2001; Luo et al. 2002). The neuroprotective efficacy of the extract was assessed by different clinical studies. In a randomized, double-blind, placebo-controlled trial of patients, treatment groups received over a 24-week period an oral daily dose of 160 mg EGb 761 or 5 mg donepezil (a cholinesterase inhibitor), whereas the control group was treated with a placebo. Study (Syndrome Kurz Test, SKT, Mini-Mental State Examination, MMSE, and Clinical Global Impression, CGI) showed that both EGb 761 and donepezil were more effective in improving the cognitive function of patients with mild to moderate AD. In an analysis reviewing many randomized, double blind, placebo- controlled clinical studies, patients diagnosed with AD received 120–240 mg/day of EGb 761 for 3–6 months. Two phase III clinical trials, the GEM (Ginkgo Evaluation of Memory) study in US and the Guid Age study in France, focused on evaluation of EGb 761 efficacy in the prevention of AD in more than 3,000 patients older than 70 years. Both studies were randomized; double blind, placebo-controlled trials (DeKosky et al. 2006). In another study, EGb 761 was administered in a dose of 120 mg twice daily and the incidence of all-cause dementia was used as primary outcome. Secondary outcome included the rate of cognitive decline, the incidence of cardio- and cerebrovascular events and mortality. In another study, the efficacy of 240 mg daily dose of EGb 761 was evaluated, with the incidence of AD during a 5-year follow up period as primary outcome. This study was the largest clinical trial carried out in Europe on the prevention of AD (Vellas et al. 2006).

11.5.2 *Panax ginseng*

Panax ginseng (Ginseng) (Chinese rènshē n=man root) is another important herbal plant, refers to the shape of the root resembling the leg of a man. It is one of the most widely used herbs in TCM for boosting Qi (energy). It is an anti-aging herb, employed for thousands of years as a tonic and revitalizing agent. Several species within the Panax genus are growing in North- Eastern Asia. *P. ginseng* or Asian ginseng are among the most commonly used species in Korean traditional medicine and Japanese traditional medicine. Other important species are Vietnamese ginseng (*P. vietnamensis*), Siberian ginseng (*Eleutherococcus senticosus* Maxim. which is not a true ginseng) and American ginseng (*P. quinquefolius* L.) (Yun 2001). Ginseng root is characterized by the presence of ginsenosides (triterpenic saponin complexes). Ginseng is considered as an adaptogenic herb. Adaptogens are able to increase the body's resistance to stress, trauma, anxiety and fatigue by modulating the immune functions. Furthermore, it improves memory, learning performance and motor activity. Ginseng may provide protection against neurodegeneration by multiple mechanisms. In an experimental study, it was reported to attenuate Aβ and glutamate-induced toxicity, enhancing clearance of Aβ by stimulating the phagocytic activity of microglia and promoting neuron survival by increasing the levels of neurotrophic factors (Chen et al. 2006). These data show that ginseng acts on different stages of the neurodegenerative diseases. Studies in human subjects have also shown the efficacy of ginseng in treatment of AD. In a clinical trial, patients aged 50 years or older with mild to moderate AD related dementia were randomized into three groups, two treatment groups received an oral daily dose of 9 or 4.5 g of Korean red ginseng for 12 weeks. The high-dose ginseng group showed scores higher than the control group ones, while differences between low-dose ginseng and placebo were not significant (Joo et al. 2008, Heo et al. 2008). Apart from AD, Ginseng has also shown protective effects against PD in several cell culture and animal studies. Both ginsenosides and root extracts are able to promote neuronal cell survival by reducing the neurotoxicity induced by toxins or parkinsonism mimetics, such as 1-methyl-4-phenyl-1,2,3,6-tetra- hydropyridine (MPTP) and its active metabolite 1-methyl-4-phenylpyridinium (MPP+) in rodents. These neurotoxins induce oxidative stress and lead to cell death of dopaminergic neurons, as in PD (Van Kempen et al. 2003). In other studies, ginsenosides, besides protecting neuronal cells, have shown neurotrophic effects promoting neurite overgrowth (Rudakewich et al. 2001).

11.5.3 Curcuma longa L.

Curcuma longa or Turmeric is the dried rhizome. It's a spice used in curry, and widely used as flavouring agent in many food preparations, particularly in India. The bright yellow colour of turmeric is due to curcumin, the main bioactive constituent. Turmeric has been used for thousands of years in Ayurvedic and Chinese medicine as well. Curcuminoids is a group of polyphenols including mainly curcumin, demethoxycurcumin and bisdemethoxycurcumin. Components of turmeric are currently undergoing scientific evaluation for numerous potential benefits due to their anti-inflammatory, antiproliferative, pro-apoptotic, antioxidant, antiviral and antidiabetic activity. Numerous molecular targets of curcumin have been identified over the years, including cyclooxygenase (COX)-2 and lipoxygenase (LOX) (Strimpakos and Sharma 2008).

Based on epidemiological studies, a hypothesis has been raised that the wide use of Curcuma sp. among Indians may be responsible for the significantly lower prevalence of AD in India compared to US. In a transgenic animal model of AD, supplementation with a low dose of curcumin (160 ppm) for 6 months reduced indices of both inflammation and oxidative stress. In particular, the levels of pro-inflammatory cytokine IL-1β, of oxidized proteins and of Aβ peptide decreased significantly (Linn et al. 2001). Anti- amyloidogenic activity of curcumin was extensively reported in in vitro and animal models (Uno et al. 2004). The possible binding of curcumin to the redox-active metals iron and copper suggests alternative neuroprotective mechanism of the substance (Yang et al. 2005). The combination of non-steroidal anti-inflammatory drugs (NSADs) and curcumin attenuated oxidative damage, cognitive deterioration and Aβ peptide deposition in both cell culture and animal model. In the same study, anti-inflammatory activity of curcumin was observed, due to the inhibition of cytokine production and microglia activation and increase of phagocytosis index (Cole et al. 2004). Because the process of inflammation plays a major (detrimental) role in the pathogenesis of the most chronic illnesses including neurodegenerative diseases, the therapeutic potential of curcumin as anti-inflammatory agent in the prevention and treatment of chronic disorders has been recently highlighted (Aggarwal and Harikumar 2008). In fact, activation of microglial cells in CNS results in the production of pro-inflammatory mediators that propagate neuronal injury exacerbating neurodegenerative diseases. In rat, curcuminoid pigments suppressed NO production by LPS-activated microglia (Zhang et al. 2008). In a model of global cerebral ischemia, induced in Mongolian gerbils by transient occlusion of common carotid arteries, administration of curcumin by intraperitoneal injections (30 mg/kg body weight) for 2 months attenuated ischemia-induced neuronal death and glial activation. The decrease of lipid peroxidation, mitochondrial dysfunction and apoptotic indices were other biochemical responses mediated by curcumin.

11.5.4 Vitis vinifera L. (Grape) and Red Wine

Phytochemicals in Grape include phenylpropanoids, isoprenoids (responsible for the wine flavouring) and alkaloids (such as indolic compounds). Studies were recently focusing on the biological activity of selected grape polyphenols, such as the stilbene resveratrol and flavonoids (Pervaiz 2003). Population-based control studies have provided the substantial evidence that a regular (daily or possibly 3–4 times weekly) intake of moderate amounts (two glasses/day) of red wine (made from *V.vinifera*) is associated with a lower risk of developing dementia and AD (Pinder 2009). The Study evaluated the association between the type of alcoholic beverage and incidence of ischemic stroke, showing a protective effect of wine consumption among subject aged 60–69 years. In general, protective effects of grape polyphenols against neurodegenerative diseases can be ascribed to their anti-amyloidogenic, antioxidant and anti- inflammatory activity (Blanchet et al. 2008). The daily administration of resveratrol (50 or 100 mg/kg) for 1 or 2 weeks to adult male mice significantly prevented the nigrostriatal dopaminergic neuron depletion, after the acute treatment with the neurotoxin MPTP injected intraperitoneally (Rivière et al. 2008). In different cell lines stably transfected with human amyloid protein (APP), resveratrol was shown to promote the intracellular degradation of Aβ peptides via a mechanism that involves the proteasome, without direct inhibition of the enzymes β- and γ-secretases implicated in the Aβ protein synthesis. Neuroprotective effects of three major grape polyphenolic constituents (resveratrol, quercetin and catechin) were assessed in cultured mixed (glial/neuronal) cells of rat hippocampus. Treatment with polyphenols reduced the cytotoxicity induced by both the NO free radical donor sodium nitroprusside (SNP) and intracellular ROS accumulation (Bastianetto et al. 2000). In a mouse model of AD, the moderate consumption of Cabernet Sauvignon promoted the non-amyloidogenic processing of APP mediated by β-secretase, thereby preventing or delaying the generation of Aβ peptides. More recently, a grape seed polyphenolic extract significantly prevented Aβ protein oligomerization, by inhibiting the Aβ protein aggregation into high-molecular-weight oligomeric Aβ species, both in vitro and in Tg 2,576 mice. Besides, when orally administered to these animals, the extract attenuated the cognitive deterioration typical of AD.

11.5.5 Coffee (Coffea spp.)

Coffee is native to Yemen and Ethiopia. The genus Coffea (Rubiaceae family) includes two main species: *C. arabica* L., and *C. canephora* L. (syn. C. robusta L.). Caffeine, a methylxanthine, is the most important bioactive constituent of the coffee known to provide neuroprotection. Other structurally similar xanthine alkaloids are theophylline and theobromine, found primarily in tea and chocolate, respectively. As regards pharmacological activity, methylxanthines act as adenosine-receptor antagonists. In particular, caffeine is a nonspecific, competitive blocker of adenosine A1 and A2A receptors, distributed throughout the central nervous system (Cauli and Morelli 2005). According to human epidemiological studies, caffeine, as well as other adenosine A2A receptor antagonist, may play a role in preventing or delaying the onset of AD. A case control study involving subjects aged 50 years with probable diagnosis of AD and sex-matched controls found that individuals consuming two cups of coffee (approximately 200 mg of caffeine) per day for 20 years were at a significantly lower risk of developing the disease than those that consumed less caffeine (Maia and Mendonca 2002). These results were in accordance with previous studies in which coffee consumption was consistently protective against PD for men and women in the absence of estrogen therapy (Ascherio et al. 2001). It is noteworthy that acute intake of high doses of coffee (five cups of coffee, approximately 500 mg of caffeine, at one sitting) results in activation of stress responses, as demonstrated by increased plasma levels of cortisol, β -endorphin and epinephrine, in turn raising heart rate, blood pressure and releasing free fatty acids from storage.

11.5.6 Tea (Camellia sinensis Kuntze)

Three predominant types of tea: green, black and oolong are popular. Green tea is the least processed and thus provides the most antioxidant polyphenols, particularly catechins (epigallocatechin, epigallocatechin-3-gallate), flavonols (myricetin, quercetin, kaempherol) and proanthocyanidins (Khokhar and Magnusdottir 2002). Being catechins, particularly epigallocatechin- 3-gallate (EGCG), 10–20 times more concentrated than flavonols in normally brewed tea (Kuriyama et al. 2006), seem to be responsible for most of the health benefits of tea. Green tea drinkers appear to have lower risk for a wide range of diseases, from simple bacterial or viral infections to chronic degenerative conditions including cardiovascular disease, cancer and stroke (Coimbra et al. 2006). As regards protection against AD and PD, green tea catechins, until recently thought to work simply as antioxidants, are now known to invoke a wide spectrum of neuroprotective cellular mechanisms. These include iron chelation, scavenging of free radicals, activation of signaling pathways, and regulation of mitochondrial function to avoid excessive production of free radicals (Mandel and Youdim 2004). As reported above, iron accumulation in specific brain areas and free radical damage to brain cells are considered the major damaging factors responsible for a wide range of neurodegenerative disorders including AD and PD. In the brain, epigallocatechin-3-gallate (EGCG) has been shown to act as an iron chelator, binding to and removing iron, thus preventing it from contributing to the production of free radicals. In addition to removing iron, EGCG also increases the activity of two major antioxidant enzymes, superoxide dismutase (SOD) and catalase, further helping to decrease free radical damage (Weinreb et al. 2004). Another active compound in green tea, epicatechin (EC), reduces the formation of β -amyloid protein and of the consequent plaque-like deposits in the brain, characteristic of AD. The protective effects of black and green tea extracts and their main constituents, epigallocatechin gallate and epicatechin gallate have been shown in an in vitro system of cultured neurons. In the presence of these extracts, neurons survived to the toxic effect of β -amyloid protein. Green tea polyphenols have also demonstrated the ability to affect cell signaling pathways, in particular the MAPK pathways, which are triggered by oxidative stress. MAPK signaling pathways in brain cells are thought to play a critical role in neurodegenerative diseases.

Although no human studies on AD have yet reported benefit from tea consumption, population studies have shown that simply consuming two or more cups of green tea daily reduces the risk of cognitive decline and PD. A study at Japan's Tohoku University, using a Mini-Mental State Examination (a well-accepted standardized test for measuring cognitive function) on 1,003 subjects over age 70, researchers showed that drinking more than two cups per day of green tea reduces chances of cognitive impairment in both men and women by 64 % (Haque et al. 2006). Those drinking green tea experienced significantly less mental decline than those drinking the least. In particular, those drinking more than two cups a day had 54 % lower risk of age- related decline in memory, orientation, and ability to follow commands and attention as compared with elderly Japanese who drank less than three cups a week. Those drinking four to six cups of green tea a week (one cup a day) had a 38 % lower risk of decline in brain functions. As reported in the previous section, tea also contains caffeine, although half that found in coffee (Khokhar and Magnusdottir 2002). The amount of caffeine that ends up in a cup of green tea varies according to the amount of tea used and the length of time the leaves are infused (Perva-uzunalic et al. 2006). When green tea is brewed, its caffeine combines with catechins in the water, reducing the caffeine's activity compared to coffee or cocoa. In addition, L-theanine, which is only found in tea plants and some mushrooms, directly stimulates the production of alpha brain waves, calming the body while promoting a state of relaxed awareness.

11.5.7 Withania somnifera Dunal (WS)

Withania somnifera Dunal (WS) is known as Ashwagandha or Indian ginseng. It has been commonly used in Indian traditional medicines for over 3,000 years and categorized as Rasayana drug in Ayurveda. Rasayna drugs are known to augment defense against diseases, arrest aging, revitalize the body in debilitated condition, increase the capability of the individual to resist adverse environmental factors and create a sense of mental wellbeing. Animal research (Bhatnagar et al. 2005; Gupta and Rana 2007; Bhatnagar 2009) supported the use of WS for treatment of anxiety, cognitive and neurological disorders, senile dementia, Alzheimer's and Parkinson's disease and as antioxidant and anti-inflammatory agent. It has also been used to treat stress, insomnia and age related disorders including neurodegeneration (Gupta et al. 2003; Mishra et al. 2000). The biologically active constituents in WS are alkaloids (ashwagandhin, cuscohygrine, anahygrine, topine etc.), steroidal compounds, including ergostane type steroidallactones, withaferin A, withanolides A–Y, withasomniferin A, withasomnidienone, withasomnierose A–C, withanone etc. Other constituents include saponins containing an additional acyl group (Sitoindoside VII and VIII), and withanolides with a glucose at carbon 27 (sitoindoside IX and X) (Ganzera et al. 2003). It has been reported that phenolic compounds present in the root of WS contribute to the overall antioxidant activity of the plant (Prakash et al. 2007). Our laboratory (Jain et al. 2001, Bhatnagar et al. 2009), has reported neuroprotective actions of WS root extract which were correlated with its antioxidant property and ability to inhibit lipid peroxidation both in vitro and in vivo. Bhattacharya et al. (2000) suggested that glycowithanolides present in WS protect against lipid peroxidation due to its antioxidant action. In addition, withanolides and sitoindosides (VII–X) also enhance catalase and glutathione peroxidase activities in rat frontal cortex and straitum (Bhattacharya et al. 2001).

11.6 Neuroprotective Mechanism of *Withania somnifera*

In this review, we have mainly discussed possible neuroprotective mechanism of WS in the brain degenerative disorders. In the brain, peroxynitrite is a strong non radical prooxidant produced during metabolism of nitric oxide (NO), which mediates neuronal damage. NO, synthesized by the enzyme, neuronal nitric oxide synthase (nNOS) is a neuromodulator in hippocampus and cortex. nNOS forms NO from L-arginine in the presence of molecular oxygen. Several earlier reports have indicated that nNOS is identical to neuronal NADPH diaphorase (NADPH-d). Histochemical localization of NADPH-d staining in mouse hippocampus fully coincides with both histochemical NADPH-d and immunocytochemical nNOS staining in rat hippocampus. In the hippocampus, a number of NADPH-d positive cell bodies and dense fibers are present in CA1, CA2 and CA3 subfields and also in the oriens, pyramidal layer and stratum radiatum. In the dentate gyrus as well, number of NADPH-d positive neurons are found in polymorphic layer (Matsushita et al. 2001). Small amount of NO synthesized during neuronal activity mediates diverse physiological functions which include neuronal differentiation, neuronal survival, and synaptic plasticity. Excessive production of NO has also been implicated in a number of pathophysiological conditions including stress (Mcleod et al. 2001) and glutamate mediated neurotoxicity. De Oliveira et al. (2000) reported that exposure to stress can lead to enhanced nNOS expression, which is a glutamate mediated process. Neurotoxic effects of NO depend upon its redox state and are likely to be mediated by its free radical nature. NO reacts readily with superoxide (O2-) to produce peroxynitrite (ONOO-), which can oxidize iron–sulphur clusters, zinc fingers and protein thiols, thereby contributes to cellular energy depletion (Stamler 1994). In hippocampus, activity of nNOS is mainly regulated by glutamate and serotonin (Harwey et al. 2006). Release of glutamate and serotonin is modulated by glucocorticoids (GC); thus GC can activate nNOS by altering release of these two neurotransmitters. GC play defensive role during stress, but sustained elevated level of GC during chronic stress can lead to neurodegeneration. Hippocampus is most vulnerable to GC induced neurodegeneration because of presence of high concentration of GC receptors. Several studies suggest that inhibitors of the neuronal NO synthesizing enzyme (nNOS) may be useful as neuroprotective agents in treatment of neurodegenerative diseases. Considering the neuroactive properties of WS root extract and to understand the possible mechanism of neuroprotection, we studied the effects of WS root extract on NADPH-d activity, Choline acetyl transferase (ChAT) activity, serotonin level in hippocampus and serum GC level in mice exposed to chronic restraint stress. Results showed that exposure to restraint stress can lead to activation of significant proportion of NADPH-d positive neurons, decrease in ChAT activity and serotonin level in the hippocampus. Stress also elevated cortisone level. These effects of stress were significantly reversed in animals treated with WS root extract.

Hippocampus is known to mediate stress, learning and memory, LTP and antidepressant behavioral effects (Joca and Guimaraes 2006). Stress induced production of NO in hippocampus can negatively alter above functions. NO also facilitates the release of several neurotransmitters including gamma-aminobutyric acid (GABA), glutamate, biogenic amines and neuropeptides (Prast and Philipu 2001). Thus NO can modulate neuronal excitability, firing and neurotransmitter release. Excessive production of NO in brain and other tissues mediates injury in diverse disease states. NO toxicity is likely to be mediated by its free radical nature. NO can readily react with superoxide (O2-) to produce peroxynitrite (ONOO-) which mediates much of the toxic effects of NO. It is well reported that various physiological and physical stressors produce changes in the expression of nNOS in different brain areas. Bhatnagar et al. (2009) showed, a significant increase in nNOS positive neurons in hippocampus is shown in adult mice exposed to chronic restraint stress. The rational behind using restraint stress was the reported evidences that restraint stress can potentially stimulate nNOS in other brain regions as well viz., limbic region, hypothalamus and dorsal raphe nucleus (Echeverry et al. 2004; Masood et al. 2004; Okere and Waterhouse 2006). Generation of NO by nNOS is regulated directly or indirectly, by at least three other neurotransmitters i.e., glutamate, serotonin and acetylcholine. Glutamate by acting on NMDA receptor causes Ca^{++} influx and activates nNOS as NO generation is a Ca^{++}/Calmodulin dependent process. NMDA receptor and nNOS are found to be linked physically through a molecular scaffold protein PSD-95. Stress induces glutamate release in the brain and excitotoxic neurodegenerative effect of glutamate in chronic stress is mediated by increased expression of nNOS. It has been suggested that, in hippocampus, nNOS is under tonic inhibition by serotonergic neurons. An increased nNOS activity was observed when 5-HT2 receptor was inhibited by ritanserin in rats exposed to forced swimming (Harwey et al. 2006). Furthermore, serotonin depletion may result in excessive production of NO and neurodegeneration. Release of both, glutamate and serotonin is altered by glucocorticoids (corticosterone in rodents). Excessive production of glutamate during stress is associated with glucocorticoid release and stress induced elevation in extracellular glutamate release is attenuated by adrenalectomy. Hippocampal neurons are particularly sensitive to glucocorticoid level and are involved in termination of corticosterone secretion at the end of stress due to the presence of both type I and type II glucocorticoid receptors. Activity of glutamatergic neurons is also regulated by cholinergic neurons. In a study, exogenous ACh added to superfusion fluid inhibited the Ca^{++} dependent K^{+} evoked release of glutamate in a concentration dependent manner in rat hippocampus. It has been proposed that impaired serotonin level during stress is mediated by hypercortisolemia, acting on the high concentration of glucocorticoid receptors in the hippocampus (Campbell and Macqueen 2004). It has also been suggested that stress induced changes in hippocampal glutamate mechanism may precede changes in serotonin function (McEwen et al. 2002).Taking together these findings, we postulate that nNOS inhibitory property of WS is possibly mediated by suppression of glucocorticoid release and activation of cholinergic neurons and not by acting on glutamatergic or NOergic neurons. It has been reported that defined extract of WS do not directly affect the glutamatergic markers. Treatment with defined extract from WS does not affect NMDA and AMPA glutamate receptor subtypes in any cortical or sub cortical regions. Sitoindosides VII–X and withaferin A have been shown to modulate brain functions by binding with cholinergic receptors in the rat. WS extract can also reverse the reduction in cholinergic markers in rats (Bhattacharya and Muruganandam 2003). Schliebs et al. (1997) also suggested that defined extract from WS may affect preferentially, events in the cortical and basal forebrain cholinergic signal transduction cascade. Treatment with WS extract upregulates cortical muscarinic acetylcholine receptor expression. Both, low glucocorticoid level and acetylcholine release, in turn downregulates activity of glutamatergic neurons in the hippocampus while, stress induced impairment of serotonin release is attenuated by low glucocorticoid level. Modulation of release of these three neurotransmitters i.e., acetylcholine, glutamate and serotonin by WS in all probability contributes to inhibition of nNOS in extract treated stressed mice. Our results support this postulate as we have observed decreased glucocorticoid level and increased ChAT activity following WS treatment in stressed animals. These results confirm and extend previous findings and explain the nNOS inhibitory properties of WS. In summary, it is proposed that neuroprotective properties of WS are owing to neurochemical alterations of specific neurotransmitter systems. WS extract can also suppress glucocorticoid release in chronic stress. This purported new role of WS can be exploited for treatment of neurodegenerative disease like Alzheimer's, which is caused by a decline in ACh level as well as in oxidative stress. WS can inhibit the production of free radicals like peroxynitrite.

Bhatnagar et al. (2009) have investigated the effects of fresh leaf juice of WS on enzymes acetylcholinesterase (AChE) and nicotinamide adenine dinucleotide phosphate diaphorase (NADPH-d) activity in vivo and in vitro to support our earlier observations, and also to understand the potential therapeutic mechanism of WS in AD or related diseases. We reported that WS root extract can increase ACh level by increasing ChAT expression, and serotonin level in hippocampus (Bhatnagar et al. 2009). ACh in turn inhibits NO producing enzyme NADPH-d. The grey side of this study was that effect of WS extract on AChE was not studied. Also there was a lack of data on correlation between distribution of cholinergic neurons and NOergic neurons in various fore brain regions including hippocampus to support our hypothesis that ACh inhibits NADPH-d activity. Study revealed that WS fresh leaf juice significantly inhibits not only AChE activity but also NADPH-d activity which is clearly evident from histochemical, biochemical and in vitro observations. Counting of NADPH-d positive cell bodies in these areas also showed significant reduction in number of NADPH-d positive cell bodies in WS treated brain when compared with control brain. To prove that WS inhibits both AChE and NADPH-d, we attempted to co-localize both AChE and NADPH-d in same tissue sections. Results showed that AChE and NADPH-d cell bodies co-localizing both the enzymes not only showed reduced reactive enzyme intensity but also their number in forebrain areas after WS treatment as compared to cell bodies positive for either AChE or NADPH-d.

Reduced AChE activity thus suggested increased ACh, while reduced NADPH-d activity demonstrates decrease in NO. To further confirm that elevated ACh inhibits NO production, in vitro study was carried out. Primary hippocampal cell culture was exposed to glutamate in the presence and absence of ACh and then nitrite production was measured (Fig. 11.1).

Glutamate was used to elevate production of NO in cultured cells. It is well documented that nNOS is physically linked to NMDA glutamate receptors and activation of nNOS is positively correlated with NMDA receptor activation. Results showed significantly low nitrite level in glutamate treated cells which were incubated with ACh as compared to cell which were not. This confirms that NO production decreases in the presence of ACh.

One of the characteristics of AD is cholinergic deficit (Talesa 2001; Melo et al. 2003). Post-mortem studies have shown that AD brains are characterized by low ChAT, while AChE, a principal cholinesterase in brain which hydrolyzes endogenous neurotransmitter Ach (Talesa 2001), was shown to be increased within and around amyloid plaques to promote the assembly of amyloid beta peptides (Aβ) in the fibrils and to increase the toxicity of the peptides. Thus most accepted strategies for treatment of AD is the use of cholinesterase inhibitors. Inhibition of AChE results in increase in ACh level, which led to functional improvement of cholinergic synapses, reduced neuronal degeneration and enhanced regional synthesis of neurotrophic molecules. Thus many plant extracts—Ginkgo and Ashwagandha not names of the extracts but only plants which characteristically inhibit cholinesterase have been used as drug against early symptoms of AD in traditional medicinal system (Vinutha et al. 2007; Chowdhry et al. 2004).

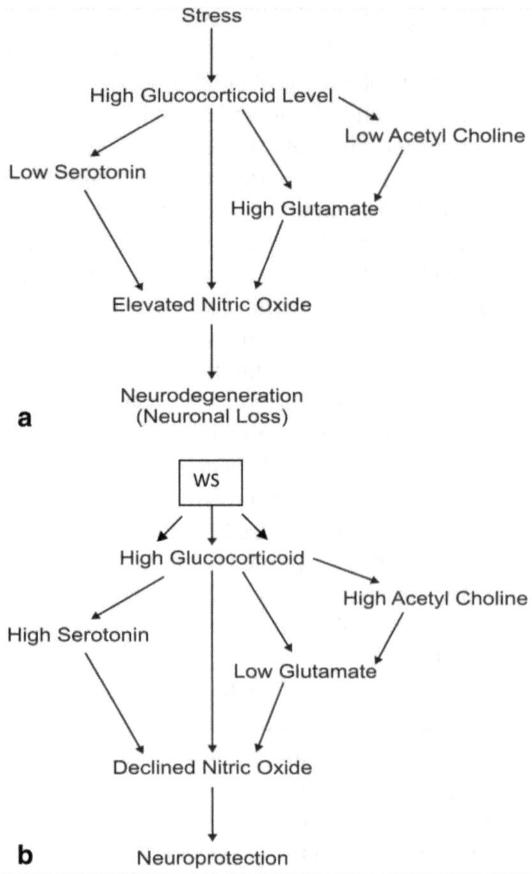

Fig. 11.1 Flow chart to explain possible mechanism of neuroprotective action of *Withania somnifera* (WS)

NO is also an intra and extra-cellular mediator of cell functions and is diffusible free radical cellular messenger. Kluchova et al. (2000) suggested that NO may play a role in control of cholinergic neuronal activity at synapses. Law et al. (2001a) have shown that aberrantly expressed nNOS in brain results in rise in NO that can be toxic due to its free radical properties. Law et al. (2001b) have also shown that Aβ increases NO release which decreases neuronal viability. In our study, as neurons showing co-localization of both the enzymes are less in WS treated brain as compared to control brain, a possible regulatory interaction of WS on AChE and NADPH-d can be envisaged. Based on these studies, we have suggested a mechanism of the inhibitory effects of WS.

11.7 Conclusions

Post-mortem studies in AD patient brain have shown clear links between the disease and deficiency of neurotransmitter Acetylcholine (ACh). In AD along with chronic shortage of ACh, high Nitric oxide (NO) was also reported. High NO is deleterious to neuronal cells and contributes to disease progression. Until recently, reversal of the deficiency by alleviating the level of neurotransmitters, use of agonists or the inhibition of the enzymes involved in the removal of the neurotransmitter at synapses, are the treatments used for AD and related diseases. But these treatments are not ideal and provide only symptomatic relief. A variety of natural products or their derivatives have shown the desired effects and some of these have been brought into clinical use to treat various degenerative disorders. Though the presence of receptors or transporters for phytochemicals in brain tissues remains to be ascertained, compounds with multiple targets appear as a potential and promising class of therapeutics for the treatment of CNS diseases. Our results are in agreement that WS inhibits AChE and thereby enhances cholinergic neurotransmission in cortical and basal forebrain areas. Study also suggests that WS directly inhibits AChE but inhibition of NADPH-d is indirect. WS mediated inhibition of both AChE and NADPH-d could have therapeutic implications in AD which is characterized by reduced ACh and elevated NO.

References

Aggarwal BB, Harikumar KB (2008) Potential therapeutic effects of curcumin, the anti-inflammatory agent, against neurodegenerative, cardiovascular, pulmonary, metabolic, autoimmune and neoplastic diseases. Int J Biochem Cell Biol 41:40–59

Agorogiannis EI, Agorogiannis GI, Papadimitriou A, Hadjigeorgiou GM (2004) Protein misfolding in neurodegenerative diseases. Neuropathol Appl Neurobiol 30:215–224

Ascherio A, Zhang SM, Hernan MA (2001) Prospective study of caffeine consumption and risk of Parkinson's disease in men and women. Ann Neurol 50:56–63

Barja G (2004) Free radicals and aging.Trends Neurosci 23:209–216

Bastianetto S, Zhang WH, Quirion R (2000) Neuroprotective abilities of resveratrol and other red wine constituents against nitric oxide toxicity in cultured hippocampal neurons. Br J Pharmacol 131:711–720

Blanchet, J. Longpré, F., Bureau, G., Morisette, M.; DiPaolo, T., Bronchti, G., Martinoli, M.G. (2008) Resveratrol, a red wine polyphenol, protects dopaminergic neurons in MPTP-treated mice. Progr Neuropsychopharmacol Biol Psych 32:1243–1250

Birks J, Grimley EJ (2009) Ginkgo biloba for cognitive impairment and dementia.Cochrane Database Syst Rev 1:CD003120

Bhattacharya SK, Muruganandam AV (2003) Adaptogenic activity of Withania somnifera: an experimental study using a rat model of chronic stress. Pharmacol Biochem Behav 75:547–55

Bhattacharya A, Ramanathan M, Ghosal S et al. (2000) Effect of Withania somnifera glycowithanolites on iron induced hepatotoxocity in rats. Phytother Res 14:568–570

Bhatnagar M (2009) Novel leads from herbal drugs for neurodegenerative diseases. In: Ramawat KG (ed) Herbal drugs: ethanomedicine to modern medicine. Springer, Berlin, pp 221–238

Bhatnagar M, Sisodia SS, Bhatnagar R (2006) Antiulcer and antioxidant activity of Asparagus racemosus WIILD and Withania somnifera DUNN in rats. Ann N Y Acad Sci 1056:261–278

Bhatnagar M, Sharma D, Salvi M (2009) Neuroprotective effects of Withania somnifera dunal.: a possible mechanism. Neurochem Res 34:1975–1983

Campbell S, Macqueen G (2004) The role of the hippocampus in the pathophysiology of major depression. J Psychiatry Neurosci 29:417–426

Cauli O, Morelli M (2005) Caffeine and the dopaminergic system. Behav Pharmacol 16:63–77

Chandrasekaran K, Mehrabian Z, Spinnewyn B, Chinopoulos C, Drieu K, Fiskum G (2003) Neuroprotective effects of bilobalide, a component of Ginkgo biloba extract (EGb 761) in global brain ischemia and in excitotoxicity-induced neuronal death. Pharmacopsychiatry 36:89–94

Chowdhry MT, Yousuf S, Nawajz SA, Ahmed S, Rahman AU (2004) Cholinesterase inhibiting withanolides from Withania somnifera. Chem Pharm Bull 52:1358–1361

Chen F, Eckman EA, Eckman CB (2006) Reductions in levels of the Alzheimer's amyloid β peptide after oral administration of ginsenosides. FASEB J 20:1269–1271

Coimbra S, Castro E, Rocha-Pereira P, Rebelo I, Rocha S, Santos-Silva A (2006) The effect of green tea in oxidative stress. Clin Nutr 25:790–796

Cole GM, Morihara T, Lim GP, Yang F, Begum A, Frautschy SA (2004) NSAID and antioxidant prevention of Alzheimer's disease: lessons from in vitro and animal models. Ann NY Acad Sci 1035:68–84

DeKosky ST, Fitzpatrick A, Ives DG, Saxton J, Williamson J, Lopez OL, Burke G, Fried L, Kuller LH, Robbins J, Tracy R, Woolard N, Dunn L, Kronmal R, Nahin R, Furberg C (2006) The Ginkgo evaluation of memory (GEM) study: design and baseline data of a randomized trial of Ginkgo biloba extract in prevention of dementia. Contemp Clin Trials 27:238–253

De Oliveira RMW, Deakin JF, Guimaraes FS (2000) Neuronal nitric oxide synthase (NOS) expression in the hippocampal formation of patients with schizophrenia and affective disorder. J Psychopharmacol 14:8

Dorsey ER, Constantinescu R, Thompson JP, Biglan KM, Holloway RG, Kieburtz K, Marshall FJ, Ravina BM, Schifitto G, Siderowf A, Tanner CM (2007) Projected number of people with Parkinson disease in the most populous nations, 2005 through 2030. Neurology 68:384–386

Echeverry MB, Guimarães FS, Del Bel EA (2004) Acute and delayed restraint stress-induced changes in nitric oxide producing neurons in limbic regions. Neuroscience 125:981–993

Ganzera M, Choudhary MI, Khan IA (2003) Quantitative HPLC analysis of withanolides in Withania somnifera. Fitoterapia 74:68–76

Gupta GL, Rana AC (2007) Withania somnifera (Ashwagandha): a review. Pharmacogn Rev 1:129–136

Gupta SK, Dua A, Vohra BP (2003) Withania somnifera (Ashwagandha) attenuates antioxidant defense in aged spinal cord and inhibits copper induced lipid peroxidation and protein oxidative modifications. Drug Metabol Drug Interact 19:211–222

Heo JH, Lee ST, Chu K, Oh MJ, Park HJ, Shim JY, Kim M (2008) An open-label trial of Korean red ginseng as an adjuvant treatment for cognitive impairment in patients with Alzheimer's disease. Eur J Neurol 15:865–868

Harwey BH, Retief R, Korff A et al. (2006) Increased hippocampal nitric oxide synthase activity and stress responsiveness after imipramine discontinuation: role of 5HT 2A/C receptors. Metab Brain Dis 21:211–220

Haque AM, Hashimoto M, Katakura M, Tanabe Y, Hara Y, Shido O (2006) Long-term administration of green tea catechins improves spatial cognition learning ability in rats. J Nut 136:1043–1047

Hebert LE, Scherr PA, Bienias JL, Bennett DA, Evans DA (2003) Alzheimer disease in the US population: prevalence estimates using the 2000 census. Arch Neurol 60:1119–1122

Jain S, Shukla SD, Sharma K et al. (2001) Neuroprotective Effects of Withania somnifera Dunn in hippocampal sub-regions of female albino rat. Phytother Res 15:544–548

Jenner P (2004) Preclinical evidence for neuroprotection with monoamine oxidase-B inhibitors in Parkinson's disease. Neurology 63:13–22

Joca SR, Guimaraes FS (2006) Inhibition of neuronal nitric oxide synthase in the rat hippocampus induces antidepressant like effects. Psychopharmacology (Berl) 185:298–305

Joo SS, Yoo YM, Ahn BW, Nam SY, Kim YB, Hwang KW, Lee DI (2008) Prevention of inflammation-mediated neurotoxicity by Rg3 and its role in microglial activation. Biol Pharm Bull 31:1392–1396

Kluchova D, Schmidtova K, Rybarova S, Lovasova K, Pomfy M, Prosbova T, Vatlak A (2000) Partial colocalization of NADPH-diphorase and acetylcholine esterase positivity in spinal cord neurons. Physiol Res 49:151–155

Khokhar S, Magnusdottir SG (2002) Total phenol, catachin and caffeine content of teas commonly consumed in the United Kingdom. J Agric Food Chem 50:565–570

Kuriyama S, Hozawa A, Ohmori K, Shimazu T, Matsui T, Ebihara S, Awata S, Nagatomi R, Arai H, Tsuji I (2006) Green tea consumption and cognitive function: a cross-sectional study from the Tsurugaya Project 1. Am J Clin Nutr 83:355–361

Law A, Gauthier S, Quirion R (2001a) Say NO to Alzheimer's disease: putative links between nitric oxide and dementia of Alzheimer's type. Brain Res Rev 1:73–96

Law A, Gauthier S, Quirion R (2001b) Neuroprotective and neurorescuing effects of isoform-specific nitric oxide synthatase inhibitors, nitric oxide scavengers and antioxidant against beta amyloid activity. Br J Pharmacol 133:1114–1124

Lewitt PA (2008) Levodopa for the treatment of Parkinson's disease. N Engl J Med 359:2468–2476

Linn GP, Chu T, Yang F, Beech W, Frautschy SA, Cole GM (2001) The curry spice curcumin reduces oxidative damage and amyloid pathology in an Alzheimer transgenic mouse. J Neurosci 21:8370–8377

Luo Y, Smith J, Paramasivam V, Burdick A, Curry K, Buford J, Khan I, Netzer W, Xu H, Butko P (2002) Inhibition of amyloid-β aggregation and caspase-3 activation by the Ginkgo biloba extract EGb761. Proc Natl Acad Sci U S A 99:12197–12202

Maia L, de Mendonca A (2002) Does caffeine intake protect from Alzheimer's disease? Eur J Neurol 9:377–382

Mandel S, Youdim MB (2004) Catechin polyphenols: neurodegeneration and neuroprotection in neurodegenerative diseases. Free Radic Biol Med 37:304–317

Masood A, Banerji B, Vijayan VK et al. (2004) Pharmacological and biochemical studies on the possible role of nitric oxide in stress adaptation in rats. Eur J Pharmacol 493:1111–1115

Matsushita H, Takeuchi Y, Kawata M et al. (2001) Distribution of NADPH Diaphorase positive neurons in the mouse brain: differences from previous finding in the rat brain and comparison with the distribution of serotonergic neurons. Acta Histochem Cytochem 34:235–257

Mclatchey WC, Mahady G, Bennett BC, Shiels L, Savo V (2009) Ethnobotany as a pharmacological research tool and recent developments in CNS-active natural products from ethnobotanical sources. Pharmacol Therapeut 12:239–254

McEwen BS, Magarinos AM, Reagan LP (2002) Structural plasticity and tianeptine: cellular and molecular targets. Eur Psychiatry 17:318–330

Mcleod TM, Lopez-Feguero AL, Lopez-Feguero MO (2001) Nitric oxide, stress and depression. Psychopharmacol Bull 35:24–41

Melo JB, Agostinho P, Oliveira CR (2003) Involvement of oxidative stress in the enhancement of acetylcholinesterase activity induced by amyloid beta peptide. Neurosci Res 45:117–127

Menken M, Munsat TL, Toole JF (2000) The global burden of disease study: implications for neurology. Arch Neuro 57:418–420

Mishra LC, Singh BB, Dagenais S (2000) Scientific basis for therapeutic use of Withania somnifera (ashwagandha): a review.Altern Med Rev 5:334–346

Nikam S, Nikam P, Ahaley SK, Sontakke AV (2009a) Oxidative stress in Parkinson's disease. Indian J Clin Biochem 24:98–101

Nikam S, Nikam P, Ahaley SK (2009b) Role of free radical and antioxidant imbalance in pathogenesis of Parkinson's disease. Biomed Res 20:55–58

Olanow CW, Stern MB, Sethi K (2009) The scientific and clinical basis for the treatment of Parkinson disease. Neurology 72:1–13.

Okere CO, Waterhouse BD (2006) A cute restraint increases NADPH-diaphorase staining in distinct subregions of the rat dorsal raphe nucleus: implications for raphe serotonergic and nitrergic transmission. Brain Res 1119:174–181

Persson CM, Wallin AK, Levander S, Minthon L (2009) Changes in cognitive domains during three years in patients with Alzheimer's disease treated with donepezil. BMC Neurol 9:7

Pervaiz S (2003) Resveratrol: from grapevines to mammalian biology. FASEB J 17:1975–1985

Pinder RM (2009) Does wine prevents dementia? Int J Wine Res 1:41–152

Prakash D, Suri S, Upadhyay G et al. (2007) Total phenol, antioxidant and free radical scavenging activities of some medicinal plants. Int J Food Sci Nutr 58:18–28

Prast H, Philippu A (2001) Nitric oxide as modulator of neuronal function. Prog Neurobiol 64:51–68

Prior RL, Cao G (2000) Antioxidant phytochemicals in fruits and vegetables: diet and health implications. Hortic Sci 35:588–592
Rivière C, Richard T, Vitrac X, Mérillon JM, Valls J, Monti JP (2008) New polyphenols active on β -amyloid aggregation. Bioorg Medic Chem Lett 18:828–831
Rudakewich M, Ba F, Benishin CG (2001) Neurotrophic and neuroprotective actions of ginsenoside Rb1 and Rg1. Planta Med 67:533–537
Schliebs R, Liebmann A, Bhattacharya SK et al. (1997) Systemic administration of defined extracts from Withania somnifera (Indian ginseng) and Shilajit differentially affects cholinergic but not glutamatergic and gabaergic markers in rat brain. Neurochem Int 30:181–190
Selkoe DJ (2001) Alzheimer's disease: genes, proteins, and therapy. Physiol Rev 81:741–766
Shastry BS (2003) Neurodegenerative disorders of protein aggregation. Neurochem Int 43:1–7
Strimpakos AS, Sharma RA (2008) Curcumin: preventive and therapeutic properties in laboratory studies and clinical trials. Antioxid Redox Signal 10:511–545
Suk K (2005) Regulation of neuroinflammation by herbal medicine and its implications for neurodegenerative diseases: a focus on traditional medicines and flavonoids. Neurosignals 14:23–33
Talesa VN (2001) Acetylcholineste in Alzheimer's disease. Mech Aging Dev 122:1961–1969
Terriot PN, Farlow MR, Grossberg GT, Graham SM, McDonald S, Gergel I (2004) Memantine treatment in patients with moderate to severe Alzheimer disease already receiving donepezil: a randomized controlled trial. JAMA 291:317–324
Uno K, Hasegawa K, Naiki H, Yamada M (2004) Curcumin has potent anti-amyloidogenic effects for Alzheimer's beta-amyloid fibrils in vitro. J Neurosci Res 75:742–750
Van Kampen J, Robertson H, Hagg T, Drobitch R (2003) Neuroprotective actions of the ginseng extracts G115 in two rodent models of Parkinson's disease. Exp Neurol 184:521–529
Vellas B, Andrieu S, Ousset PJ, Ouzid M, Mathiex-Fortunet H (2006) The GuidAge study.Methodological issues. A 5-year double-blind randomized trial of the efficacy of EGb 761® for prevention of Alzheimer disease in patients over 70 with a memory complaint. Neurology 67:6–11
Vinutha B, Prasantha HD, Salma K, Sreej SL, Pratiti D, Padmaja R, Radhika S, Amit A, Warulu KV, Deepak M (2007) Screening of selected Indian medicinal plants for acetylcholinesterase inhibitory activity. J Ethanopharmacol 109:359–363
Weinreb O, Mandel S, Amit T, Youdim MB (2004) Neurological mechanisms of green tea polyphenols in Alzheimer's and Parkinson's diseases. J Nutr Biochem 15:506–516
Yang F, Lim GP, Begum AN, Ubeda OJ, Simmons MR, Ambegaokar SS, Chen PP, Kayed R, Glabe CG, Frautschy SA, Cole GM (2005) Curcumin inhibits formation of amyloid β oligomers and fibrils, binds plaques, and reduces amyloid in vivo. J Biol Chem 280:5892–5901
Yao Z, Drieu K, Papadopoulos V (2001) The Ginkgo biloba extract EGb761 rescues the PC12 neuronal cells from beta-amyloid-induced cell death by inhibiting the formation of beta-amyloid-derived diffusible neurotoxic ligands. Brain Res 889:181–190
Yuan H, Zheng JC, Liu P, Zhang SF, Xu JY, Bai LM (2007) Pathogenesis of Parkinson's disease: oxidative stress, environmental impact factors and inflammatory processes. Neurosci Bull 23:125–130
Yun TK (2001) Brief introduction of Panax ginseng. J Korean Med Sci 16:3–5
Zhang LJ, Wu CF, Meng XL, Yuan D, Cai XD, Wang QL (2008) Comparison of inhibitory potency of three different curcuminoid pigments on nitric oxide and tumor necrosis factor production of rat primary microglia induced by lipopolysaccharide. Neurosci Lett 447:48–53

Chapter 12
Neurodegeneration in Hypoxia: Implications in Aging

Kalpana Barhwal Hota, Sunil Kumar Hota and Shashi Bala Singh

Abstract Hypoxia and ischemia resulting in reduced oxygen delivery to brain tissues is reported to cause neurodegeneration in both in vitro and in vivo models. Similar decrease in partial pressure of oxygen occurs on ascent to high altitude, a situation referred to as hypobaric hypoxia that limits oxygen availability to the brain. Our studies on human subjects reveal decrease in vigilance and response time along with decreased cerebral oxygenation which is both altitude and duration dependent. Alterations in evoked potentials and change in hedonic matrix were also observed following exposure to high altitude environment. Investigations in animal models exposed to simulated altitude showed occurrence of oxidative stress, neurodegeneration and memory impairment. This hypoxic response of neurons is multi-factorial and involves complex signaling pathways thereby limiting the therapeutic efficacy of several antioxidants in ameliorating hypobaric hypoxia–induced memory impairment. Animals exposed to hypobaric hypoxia show depletion in the antioxidant status along with increased free radical generation. Neuromorphological studies revealed neurodegeneration and dendritic atrophy in the hippocampus. Altered neurotransmitter synthesis, release and metabolism have also been observed along with occurrence of calcium overload in hypoxic neuronal cells. These changes in the hypoxic brain find an analogy with the aging related changes that include decreased conduction rate, generation of free radicals, protein oxidation and cellular apoptosis. Administration of N-acetyl cysteine to animals exposed to hypobaric hypoxia showed considerable improvement in memory functions along with decrease in free radical generation. Acetyl-L-Carnitine administration during hypobaric hypoxia also improved the cognitive capabilities in animal models. Our investigations revealed a multifactorial action of Acetyl-L-Carnitine that included

K. B. Hota (✉) · S. K. Hota
Department of Cognitive Sciences, High Altitude Physiology Division,
Defence Institute of High Altitude Research, C/o-56 APO, Leh, Ladakh, India
e-mail: drsunilhota@hotmail.com

S. B. Singh
Defence Institute of Physiology & Allied Sciences (DIPAS),
Defence R & D Organisation, Lucknow Road, Timarpur, Delhi 110054, India

M. K. Thakur, S. I. S. Rattan (eds.), *Brain Aging and Therapeutic Interventions*,
DOI 10.1007/978-94-007-5237-5_12,

improved mitochondrial bioenergetics, neurotrophin mediated signaling and antioxidant status. The implications of these compounds as anti aging and anti-senescence interventions, however, need to be investigated.

Keywords Hypoxia • Neurodegeneration • Aging • Acetyl-L-carnitine • Nrf-2 • Antioxidant • Stress • Cognitive impairment

12.1 Introduction

The brain is not only situated at the anterior most region of the body, but also regulates an array of physiological functions through its complex wired neuronal networks. It directly or indirectly influences the central, peripheral and autonomic responses which govern an individual's psychological, physical and physiological responses to internal and external stimuli. The brain comprises of billions of neurons and glial cells that work in unison to form complex circuits for storing and processing of information. These closely coordinated miniature electrical circuits operate through tightly regulated opening and closing of ion channels which could be ligand-gated or voltage-gated. Maintenance of a potential gradient across the neuronal membrane which is imperative for transmission of impulse through these neuronal circuits involves utilization of large amount of ATP. This high energy requirement makes brain metabolically the most active organ in human body. This probably also explains the reason why neurodegenerative disorders like Alzheimer's, Parkinson's, Amyotrophic Lateral Sclerosis are all associated with aging brain. Derailments in higher order cognitive functions and early dementia are considered to be preliminary symptoms of an aging brain. Interestingly, aging is often associated with vascular dementia and reduced oxygen supply to the brain. Several psychological, physiological and biochemical manifestations during aging appear to be similar to hypoxia and ischemia. However, aging related neurodegeneration is a slow and progressive phenomenon spanning over years, while hypoxia is a more severe insult on the neurons resulting in their immediate death. Hence, understanding the mechanisms of hypoxic neurodegeneration which is a much severe stress in comparison to aging could surely provide some valuable insights into strategies for preventing neurodegeneration during aging. Besides that, it could also help in understanding the effect of episodes of hypoxic stress during young and adult stages of an individual's life on neuronal aging at old age.

12.2 The Brain Function in Low Oxygen

The brain has the highest oxygen and glucose dependency and consumes 20 % of the total oxygen for generation of ATP through the aerobic mechanisms (Halliwell 1992). Decreased supply of oxygen to the brain during conditions of hypoxia and ischemia therefore results in neurodegeneration. A unique situation of global decrease in oxygen supply to the brain is encountered during ascent to high altitude. The reduction in partial pressure of oxygen on ascent to high altitude leads to decreased oxygen saturation of arterial blood and compromised oxygen delivery to tissues (Peacock and Jones 1997). This condition, referred to as hypobaric hypoxia, not only limits human performance (Pugh 1964; West 1988, 2002) but also triggers several physiological, sensory and neurobehavioral alterations (Houston et al. 1987; Hornbein 1992). The effects of hypoxia are greatly influenced by rate of ascent and duration of stay at high altitude. The range of altitude has been distinguished into: (1) Intermediate altitude (1,500–2,500 m), where physiological changes are detectable due to hypobaric hypoxia, but arterial oxygenation remains above 90 %. However, altitude illness is possible, (2) High altitude (2,500–3,500 m), where altitude illness is commonly observed due to rapid ascent above 2,500 m, (3) Very high altitude (3,500–5,800 m), where arterial oxygenation falls below 90 %. Altitude illness is common and marked hypoxemia can occur due to exercise, (4) Extreme altitude (> 5,800 m), where successful acclimatization cannot be achieved, progressive deterioration follows and hypoxemia occurs at rest. It is assumed that long term stay for humans is not possible above 5,500 m, although moderate altitudes can sometimes be tolerated without supplementary oxygen (Hackett and Roach 2001). Beginning with the balloon flights in the latter half of the nineteenth century, extensive literature has described the subtle effects of hypoxia on the brain and CNS (West 2004). Much early work by McFarland (1937) documented the effect of hypoxia on mental performance at high altitude. On the basis of observations and tests of sensory, motor and cognitive function, McFarland observed that individuals taken rapidly (hours) to 4,000–4,500 m exhibited impairment in both simple and complex psychological performance. Motor functions, such as handwriting, were also impaired but to a lesser extent, and sensory modalities were affected little if at all. Investigators have documented decrements in performance on a variety of neuropsychometric tests for cognitive and motor functions after sudden exposure to even relatively moderate hypoxia (2,000–4,500 m) (Stickney and Van Liere 1953; Ernsting 1978).

Changes in a visual-positioning test performed during light work have also been reported at an altitude as low as 1,500 m (Denison et al. 1966). A study in humans has shown that 15 adults (29–37 years old), tested under high altitude conditions (4,500 and 5,050 m), displayed difficulties in recalling word lists, specifically those words that came early in the list (primacy effect). In this study, memory recall remained impaired 45 days after descent from high altitude (Pelamatti et al. 2003). There is further evidence that memory impairment may last several months after returning to the lowlands. A number of other studies have shown that verbal and visual short-term memory capacity and recall is impaired at altitudes starting at 2,500 m (Cavaletti et al. 1987; Regard et al. 1989; Hopkins et al. 1995). Acute exposure to hypoxia (few minutes) at altitudes above 6,500 m is known to cause severe neurobehavioral dysfunctions and loss of consciousness in non-acclimatized individuals. These studies suggest that a critical impairment in higher cognitive functions is the earliest and most insidious consequence of exposure to high altitude.

12.3 Neuronal Response to Hypoxia

Various cell types in the brain and CNS show differential susceptibility to hypoxic insult, with the neurons dying of hypoxia long before glial cells and among glia, oligodendrocytes before astrocytes (Wang et al. 2002). Rats exposed to hypobaric hypoxia reveal occurrence of oxidative stress, neuronal degeneration and dendritic atrophy (Titus et al. 2007; Maiti et al. 2006). The mechanisms pertaining to hypobaric hypoxia induced neurodegeneration appear to be multi-factorial and may involve oxidative stress, neurotransmitter alterations, altered bioenergetics, altered neuromorphology and disturbed ionic homeostasis. Several studies have indicated towards the occurrence of glutamate excitotoxicity in hypoxic and ischemic stress (Won et al. 2002; Hemi et al. 2003). Hypoxia has been reported to cause robust calcium influx into neuronal cells through the NMDA receptors, thus mediating excitotoxic cell death (Khodorov et al. 1996; Hota et al. 2008). Calcium mediated free radical generation through activation of PhospholipaseA2 (PLA2), Xanthine Oxidase and Monoamine Oxidase by Calcium Calmodulin complex has also been reported in the hippocampus following hypoxic insult (Barhwal et al. 2009a). Exposure to hypobaric hypoxia also results in alterations in cholinergic transmission and altered corticosterone that could contribute to the memory impairment (Hota et al. 2009; Muthuraju et al. 2009).

12.4 The Aging Neuron

Aging has been classically considered as a process of slow deterioration of neuronal functions associated with degradation and altered recycling of long-lived proteins, macromolecular aggregates, and damaged intracellular organelles. Conversely, it is now evident that neuronal aging is a biological process tightly controlled by evolutionary highly conserved signaling pathways. Importantly, genetic mutations that enhance longevity significantly delay the loss of synaptic connectivity and, therefore, the onset of age-related brain disorders (Bano et al. 2011). The molecular mechanisms pertaining to neuronal degeneration are similar to hypoxic cell death in several aspects and involve dysregulation in calcium homeostasis, altered mitochondrial activity and cellular bioenergetics (Wang and Michaelis 2010) and alterations in cellular redox status such as increased generation of mitochondrial oxidants, altered GSH status, and increased protein oxidation. Cholinergic neurons of the basal forebrain complex have been described to undergo moderate degenerative changes during aging, resulting in cholinergic hypofunction that has been related to the progressing memory deficits with aging (Schliebs and Arendt 2006). Morphologically, both hypoxic insult and aging result in reduction of spine numbers and synaptic dysfunction (Hota et al. 2009; Bano et al. 2011). Aging however differs from hypoxic neurodegeneration on the basis of genetic determinants that serve as an internal trigger for cell death. Age-dependent accumulation of partially deleted mitochondrial DNA and altered transcriptome activity and synthesis of mitochondrial proteins have been suggested to contribute to aging and the development of age-associated diseases (Fukui and Moraes 2009).

12.5 Oxidative Stress in Hypoxia and Aging

The biological process of aging is associated with impairment of cellular bioenergetic function and increased oxidative stress (Escames et al. 2010; Floyd et al. 2002; Calabrese et al. 2001). The mitochondria is considered to be the most important cellular organelle to contribute to the aging process, mainly through respiratory chain dysfunction and formation of reactive oxygen species, leading to damage to mitochondrial proteins, lipids and mitochondrial DNA (Paradies et al. 2011; Calabrese et al. 2001). In addition to the changes in electron transport chain, ions like calcium and iron also play a key role in mediating free radical generation and oxidative stress. Alteration of calcium homeostasis in the aging brain results in calcium ion sequestration into the mitochondria. This calcium overload perturbs the redox state of mitochondria and causes oxidative stress (Foster 2007; Toescu and Verkhratsky 2007; Biessels and Gispen 1996). Several studies indicate that the sensitivity of mitochondria to Ca^{2+}-induced Permeability Transition Pore opening is greater in the aged compared to the young mature brain (Toman and Fiskum 2011). Post-translational modifications of proteins due to oxidative and nitrative stress have also been associated to the aging brain (Grimm et al. 2011).

Oxidative stress and related biochemical factors that play a major role in aging and related neurodegenerative disorders also appear to influence the neuronal survival in hypoxia. Free radical generation and oxidative damage to bio-molecules have been invariably associated to hypoxic exposure. Studies conducted in both in vitro and in vivo models of hypoxia and ischemia show increase in lipid peroxidation and DNA damage (Hota et al. 2007; Barhwal et al. 2008). This is also associated with decrease in antioxidant enzyme activities and depletion of cellular antioxidants (Blum and Fridovich 1985). The oxidative stress in hypoxic brain is primarily attributed to glutamate excitotoxicity and deregulation of calcium ion homeostasis. Increased release of glutamate in the excitatory synapses along with upregulation of N-methyl-D-aspartate (NMDA) receptors results in robust influx of calcium into the cells (Hota et al. 2008). Increased expression of L type calcium channels during hypoxic exposure has also been reported to exert an additive calcium overload in neuronal cells (Barhwal et al. 2009a). The calcium in turn activates several pro-oxidant enzymes viz., xanthine oxidases, monoamine oxidases, cytosolic phospholipase A2 and cyclooxygenase (COX-2) leading to generation of free radicals. Calcium also mediates leakage of electrons from the mitochondria and opening of the permeability transition pore (PTP) that triggers apoptosis.

Though the mechanisms pertaining to free radical generation and oxidative stress appear to be similar in both aging and hypoxia, a presumed difference between the two is that oxidative stress is considered to be a cause of aging but a consequence of hypoxia. There has been a growing consensus regarding acceleration of aging due to lipid peroxidation and post translational modification of proteins. On the other hand, hypoxia has been portrayed as a trigger for oxidative stress that in turn causes neurodegeneration. However, with the recent reports on role of free radicals as signaling molecules and regulation of the expression of transcription factors and protein activity through oxidation and carboxylation, the notion on oxidative stress being a consequence needs to be redefined. This is evident from the fact that subunits of NMDA receptor that contribute to the calcium overload in neuronal cells during hypoxia are themselves regulated by a free radical mediated mechanism (Hota et al. 2010). Besides that, the fact that there is an increase in lipid peroxidation, protein oxidation, DNA damage and accumulation of oxidized biomolecules in neurons exposed to hypoxia also raises a concern that hypoxic exposure could accelerate aging.

12.6 Nrf-2 Regulated Antioxidant Systems in Hypoxia and Aging

The fate of the neurons is dictated by an intricate balance between the oxidative stress and intracellular antioxidant systems in both hypoxia and aging. Overwhelming of the antioxidant defense systems by excess generation of free radicals acts as a trigger for the onset of aging and hypoxia mediated neurodegeneration. In recent years, it has been realized that peroxiredoxins may be the most important peroxide free radical removal systems (Rhee et al. 2005). They are a family of peroxidases that reduce H_2O_2 and organic peroxides. They are homodimers and contain no prosthetic group: the redox reactions are dependent on cysteine at the active sites. Thioredoxin-1 (Trx-1) is one such peroxiredoxin which is a small 12 kDa multifunctional protein having a redox-active disulfide/dithiol within its active site sequence, -Cys-Gly-Pro-Cys- and operates together with NADPH and thioredoxin reductase as a protein disulfide-reducing system (Holmgren 1985). In addition to peroxiredoxins, various phase II detoxification enzymes and antioxidants work together to reduce damage caused by oxidative stress. Many reports indicate that phase II detoxification enzymes and antioxidant genes are regulated by an antioxidant responsive element (ARE), which is located within the promoter regions of these genes (Huang et al. 2000; Lee et al. 2003). The ARE activity is regulated by an array of transcription factors including NF-E2-related factor2 (Nrf2). Nrf2, belonging to the basic leucine zipper family of proteins, is an important candidate involved in the transcriptional regulation of ARE motifs (Itoh et al. 1997). The genes regulated by ARE include glutathione-S-transferase (GST), NAD(P)H quinone oxidoreductase-1 (NQO1), Heme oxygenase-1 (HO-1), Glutamate-cysteine ligase (GCL), ferritin-L, metallothionin-1 and UDP-glucuronyl transferase (UGT) (Favreau and Pickett 1995).

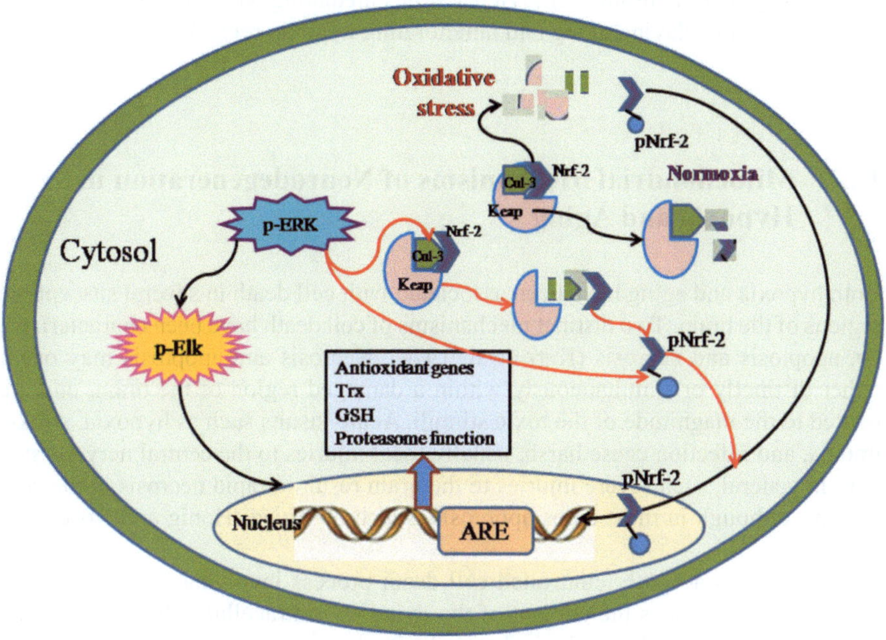

Fig. 12.1 Schematic diagram depicting regulatory role of Nrf2 during normoxic and oxidative stress. Supplmentation of ALCAR during hypoxia, results in degradation of Cul3 through pERK mediated mechanisms resulting in stabilization of Nrf2. (Barhwal et al. 2009)

In unstressed cells, Nrf2 is sequestered in the cytosol by Keap1 which is crucial for targeting Nrf2 for ubiquitination and degradation. However, Nrf2 may also exist in the nucleus under homeostatic resting conditions for basal transcription of Nrf2 mediated genes. When cells are exposed to oxidative or electrophilic stress, Nrf2 appears to be liberated from the Keap1-Nrf2 complex and translocates into the nucleus (Nakaso et al. 2003; Kobayashi et al. 2006), thereby activating Nrf2 dependent gene transcription. Thus, Keap1 negatively regulates Nrf2 stability by targeting Nrf2 for ubiquitination by Cul3 and subsequent degradation by the proteasome pathway (Fig. 12.1).

Several antioxidant compounds like Acetyl-L-Carnitine provide neuroprotection in hypoxia by eliciting Nrf2 mediated transcription of ARE regulated antioxidant genes through a pERK mediated mechanism (Barhwal et al. 2009b). Acetyl-L-Carnitine has also been found to be effective in ameliorating aging related neuronal death. Nrf2 mediated improvement in D1 receptor function of renal neurons has also been reported in old rats subjected to exercise (Asghar et al. 2007). Similarly, phytochemicals like plumbagin significantly reduce the amount of brain damage and ameliorate associated neurological deficits in focal ischemic stroke by activating Nrf2/ARE pathway. In addition to augmenting the antioxidant status in neuronal cells, Nrf2 also regulates expression of xenobiotic detoxifying (phase II) enzymes (Zhang et al. 2012). Removal of the xenobiotic compounds, on the other hand, slows the aging of neuronal cells. Hence drugs mediating Nrf-2 upregulation could be beneficial in delaying aging and ameliorating hypoxia related cognitive impairments.

12.7 Mitochondrial Mechanisms of Neurodegeneration in Hypoxia and Aging

Both hypoxia and aging have been associated with cell death in several susceptible regions of the brain. Two distinct mechanisms of cell death have been characterized, i.e. apoptosis and necrosis (Kerr et al. 1972). Necrosis and apoptosis may occur either distinctly or simultaneously within a damaged region of the brain, and are related to the magnitude of the toxic stimuli. Acute insults such as hypoxia, stroke, trauma, and infection cause harsh, usually focal injuries to the central nervous system. In general, such severe injuries to the brain result in rapid necrosis in the core regions, although in most cases apoptosis is also observed (Honig and Rosenberg 2000).

Apoptosis is a tightly controlled cell death process involving definite enzyme cascades, which keeps the content of the dying cell intracellular. It is initiated by both physiological and pathological stimuli. On the contrary, necrosis refers to relatively uncontrolled cell death and is generally correlated with injury (Sastry and Rao 2005). The cell's decision to die from necrosis or apoptosis is dictated at least in part by the abundance of intracellular energy stores. Whereas, apoptosis requires a minimal amount of intracellular ATP, necrosis is generally accompanied by its total depletion (Nicotera et al. 1998). Thus necrosis may be viewed as an accidental type of cell death. Necrosis is not genetically predetermined and normally occurs within a short period following a triggering insult (2–4 h). Necrosis has been invariably associated with immediate cell death following hypoxic or ischemic insult. Though it is not directly correlated to aging, necrotic cells can accelerate the aging process of neurons in their vicinity by causing neuroinflammation and oxidative stress.

Apoptosis, depending upon the origin of the activator molecule, is categorized into extrinsic and intrinsic pathways. In the extrinsic pathway (also known as "death receptor pathway"), apoptosis is triggered by an extracellular ligand-induced activation of death receptors at the cell surface. Such death receptors include the tumor necrosis factor (TNF) receptor-1, CD95/Fas (the receptor of CD95 L/FasL), as well as the TNF-related apoptosis inducing ligand (TRAIL) receptors-1 and -2. Several inflammatory cytokines belonging to the interlukin family also play a key role in mediating death receptor mediated apoptosis. Aging processes stimulate secretion of proinflammatory cytokines IL-1β and IL-18 that may contribute to age-related cognitive decline in the growing elderly population (Mawhinney et al. 2011). Besides that, the beneficial or detrimental transcriptional response of the inflammatory mediator TNFα, that activates a signaling cascade involving NFκB translocation to the nucleus, is also governed by the age of the neurons (Patel and Brewer 2008).

In the intrinsic pathway (also called "mitochondrial pathway"), apoptosis results from an intracellular cascade of events in which mitochondrial permeabilization plays a crucial role (Scaffidi et al. 1998). Activation of a specific class of proteases, the caspases ("cysteine protease cleaving after Asp"), is required for the rapid and complete manifestation of apoptotic features. However, not all caspases are required for apoptosis and the process generally results from the activation of a limited subset of caspases, in particular, caspases-3, -6, and -7 (Fuentes-Prior and Salvesen 2004). These are the "executioner" caspases that mediate their effects by cleavage of specific substrates in the cell.

The release of pro-apoptotic factors occurs through the permeabilization of the mitochondrial membrane. The opening of the permeability transition pore causes swelling of the mitochondrial matrix, which results in mitochondrial uncoupling, rupturing of the mitochondrial outer membrane, and release of pro-apoptotic proteins into the cytosol leading to apoptosis (Yang and Cortopassi 1998). Altered calcium ion homeostasis resulting due to robust influx of extracellular calcium during hypoxic insult is known to play a key role in opening of the permeability transition pore. Aging and aging related neurodegenerative disorders have also been associated with calcium mediated toxicity and cellular apoptosis. The entry of calcium ion into the mitochondria occurs through an electrogenic uniporter, now known to be a channel, and is pumped out again by a Na^+/Ca^{2+} antiporter (Gunter et al. 2000). The activity of the Na^+/Ca^{2+} antiporter saturates as mitochondrial matrix calcium increases, whereas the uniporter acts as a channel and is thus not saturated with increasing extramitochondrial calcium concentration. Consequently, as the extramitochondrial calcium concentration increases beyond a certain value, the mitochondria can no longer regulate their matrix calcium concentration, and mitochondrial calcium overload ensues (Gunter et al. 2000). When the overload is accompanied by a combination of other factors, most notably oxidative stress, high phosphate concentrations and low adenine nucleotide concentrations, the mitochondria undergo a permeability transition i.e. a pore opens in their inner membrane, known as the 'mitochondrial permeability transition pore' (MPTP), causing the membrane to become nonspecifically permeable to any molecule less than 1.5 kDa in size. This results in proton leak, and thus the mitochondria become uncoupled and are no longer able to maintain a pH gradient or membrane potential. As a result, mitochondria not only become incapable of ATP synthesis, but also now actively degrade ATP, as the proton-translocating ATPase reverses. Left unchecked, this inevitably leads to a loss of metabolic and ionic integrity of the cells, and ultimately to cell death (Halestrap 2004). Altered cellular bioenergetics in aging related neurodegeneration is attributed to the decreased activity of Complexes I, II and IV leading to chronic inflammation and triggering of apoptotic cell death pathways (Menardo et al. 2012). Hypoxic stress has also been associated with reduced Complex I and Complex IV activity. Interestingly, supplementation of Acetyl-L-Carnitine that is known to improve mitochondrial biogenesis and ATP generation has been found to be beneficial in both hypoxia and aging.

12.8 Role of Antioxidant Supplementation in Preventing Hypoxic Neurodegeneration

Antioxidant supplementation has been a widely accepted prophylactic strategy for both hypoxia and aging. Antioxidants like carnosine, melatonin and herbal extracts of gingko have been reported to reduce aging related changes in the brain. Antioxidants like N-Acetyl Cysteine and Acetyl-L-Carnitine, on the other hand, have been reported to ameliorate hypoxia induced neurodegeneration. Studies carried out by Barhwal et al. (2007) have shown improved working and reference memory of hypoxic rats supplemented with Acetyl-L-Carnitine. The nootrophic effect of Acetyl-L-Carnitine is due to its ability to augment NGF-TrkA mediated neurotrophin signaling mechanisms and stabilization of Nrf-2 through ERK mediated mechanisms. This probably explains the role of Acetyl-L-Carnitine as an antioxidant despite its inability to directly quench the free radicals. Besides that, Acetyl-L-Carnitine also mediates mitochondrial biogenesis resulting in buffering of calcium ions into nonfunctional mitochondria during hypoxic stress. Alpha lipoic acid and ascorbic acid supplementation also protect neurons from oxidative stress mediated cell death by directly quenching the free radicals. However, the efficacy of these antioxidants in delaying aging related cognitive impairment and prevention of age related neurodegenerative disorders remains to be conclusively proved for human population.

12.9 Implications of Hypoxic Research for Aging Related Cognitive Impairment

Though the causative factors for hypoxia and aging related cognitive impairment appear to differ distinctly, the down stream events resulting in compromised neuronal activity during both these conditions are similar to a great extent. The pathophysiology in both these conditions is invariably associated with oxidative stress, altered calcium ion homeostasis and mitochondrial dysfunction. Inflammatory responses and activation of microglia play a key role in both aging and hypoxic neuronal damage. At the molecular level, the hypoxia inducible factor (HIF) is the master regulator for hypoxia-induced gene expression. Recent studies displayed age-related changes in the HIF system that might explain reduced ability to cope with hypoxia in elderly. Conversely, oxidative damage to sub cellular components following hypoxic insult could accelerate aging and age associated neurodegenerative disorders. Future research on the effect of hypoxia on genomic and proteomic changes in the neuronal cells and the effect of these changes on aging could surely help in identifying prophylactic and therapeutic targets for delaying aging and age related cognitive impairment.

References

Asghar M, George L, Lokhandwala MF (2007) Exercise decreases oxidative stress and inflammation and restores renal dopamine D1 receptor function in old rats. Am J of Physiol Renal Physiol, 293:F914–9

Bano D, Agostini M, Melino G, Nicotera P (2011) Aging, neuronal connectivity and brain disorders: an unsolved ripple effect. Mol Neurobiol 43:124–130

Barhwal K, Hota SK, Baitharu I, Prasad D, Singh SB, Ilavazhagan G (2009a) Isradipine antagonizes hypobaric hypoxia induced CA1 damage and memory impairment: complementary roles of L-type calcium channel and NMDA receptors. Neurobiol Dis 34:230–244

Barhwal K, Hota SK, Jain V, Prasad D, Singh SB, Ilavazhagan G (2009b) Acetyl-l-carnitine prevents hypobaric hypoxia--induced spatial memory impairment through extracellular related kinase--mediated nuclear factor erythroid 2-related factor 2 phosphorylation. Neuroscience 161:501–514

Barhwal K, Hota SK, Prasad D, Singh SB, Ilavazhagan G (2008) Hypoxia induced deactivation of NGF mediated ERK ½ signaling in hippocampal cell culture: neuroprotection with Acetyl-L-Carnitine. J Neurosci Res 86:2705–2721

Barhwal K, Singh SB, Hota SK, Jayalakshmi K, Ilavazhagan G (2007) Acetyl-L-Carnitine ameliorates hypobaric hypoxic impairment and spatial memory deficits in Rats. Eur J Pharmacol 570:97–107

Biessels G, Gispen WH (1996) The calcium hypothesis of brain aging and neurodegenerative disorders: significance in diabetic neuropathy. Life Sci 59:379–387

Blum J, Fridovich I (1985) Inactivation of glutathione peroxidase by superoxide radical. Arch Biochem Biophys 240:500–508

Calabrese V, Scapagnini G, Giuffrida Stella AM, Bates TE, Clark JB (2001) Mitochondrial involvement in brain function and dysfunction: relevance to aging, neurodegenerative disorders and longevity. Neurochem Res 26:739–64

Cavaletti G, Moroni R, Garavaglia P, Tredici G (1987) Brain damage after high-altitude climbs without oxygen. Lancet 10:101

Denison DM, Ledwith F, Poulton EC (1966) Complex reaction times at simulated cabin altitudes of 5,000 feet and 8,000 feet. AeMed 37:1010–1013

Ernsting J (1978) Prevention of hypoxia--acceptable compromises. Aviat Space Environ Med, 49:495–502

Escames G, López A, García JA, García L, Acuña-Castroviejo D, García JJ, López LC (2010) The role of mitochondria in brain aging and the effects of melatonin. Curr Neuropharmacol 8:182–93

Favreau LV, Pickett CB (1995) The rat quinone reductase antioxidant response element. Identification of the nucleotide sequence required for basal and inducible activity and detection of antioxidant response element-binding proteins in hepatoma and non-hepatoma cell lines. J Biol Chem 270:24468–24474

Floyd RA, Hensley K (2002) Oxidative stress in brain aging. Implications for therapeutics of neurodegenerative diseases. Neurobiol Aging 23:795–807

Foster TC (2007) Calcium homeostasis and modulation of synaptic plasticity in the aged brain. Aging Cell 6:319–325. (Review)

Fuentes-Prior P, Salvesen GS (2004) The protein structures that shape caspase activity, specificity, activation and inhibition. J Biochem (Tokyo) 384:201–232

Fukui H, Moraes CT (2009) Mechanisms of formation and accumulation of mitochondrial DNA deletions in aging neurons. Hum Mol Genet 18:1028–1036

Grimm S, Hoehn A, Davies KJ, Grune T (2011) Protein oxidative modifications in the aging brain: consequence for the onset of neurodegenerative disease. Free Radic Res 45:73–88

Gunter TE, Buntinas L, Sparagna G, Eliseev R, Gunter K (2000) Mitochondrial calcium transport: mechanisms and functions. Cell Calcium 28:285–296

Hackett PH, Roach RC (2001) High-altitude illness. N Engl J Med 345:107–114

Halestrap AP (2004) Mitochondrial permeability: dual role for the ADP/ATP translocator? Nature 430:1

Halliwell B (1992) Reactive oxygen species and the central nervous system. J Neurochem 59:1609–1623

Hemi T, Ikeda M, Yasuhara T, Murota S (2003) Oxidative neuronal death caused by glutamate uptake inhibition in cultured hippocampal neurons. J Neurosci Res 71: 679–688

Holmgren A (1985) Thioredoxin. Annu Rev Biochem 54:237–271

Honig LS, Rosenberg RN (2000) Apoptosis and neurologic disease. Am J Med 108:317–330

Hopkins RO, Kesner RP, Goldstein M (1995) Item and order recognition memory in subjects with hypoxic brain injury. Brain Cogn 27:180–201

Hornbein TF (1992) Long term effects of high altitude on brain function. Int J Sports Med 1: S43–S45

Hota SK, Hota KB, Prasad D, Ilavazhagan G, Singh SB (2010) Oxidative-stress-induced alterations in Sp factors mediate transcriptional regulation of the NR1 subunit in hippocampus during hypoxia. Free Radic Biol Med 49:178–191

Hota SK, Barhwal K, Baitharu I, Prasad D, Singh SB, Ilavazhagan G (2009) Bacopa monniera leaf extract ameliorates hypobaric hypoxia induced spatial memory impairment. Neurobiol Dis 34:23–39

Hota SK, Barhwal K, Singh SB, Sairam M, Ilavazhagan G (2008) NR1 and GluR2 expression mediates excitotoxicity in chronic hypobaric hypoxia. J Neurosci Res 86:1142–1152

Hota SK, Barhwal K, Singh SB, Ilavazhagan G (2007) Differential temporal response of hippocampus, cortex and cerebellum to hypobaric hypoxia: a biochemical approach. Neurochem Int 51:384–390

Houston CS, Sutton JR, Cymerman A, Reeves JT (1987) Operation Everest II: man at extreme altitude. J Appl Physiol 63:877–882

Huang HC, Nguyen T, Pickett CB (2000) Regulation of the antioxidant response element by protein kinase C-mediated phosphorylation of NF-E2-related factor 2. Proc Nat Acad Sci U S A 97:12475–12480

Itoh K, Chiba T, Takahashi S, Ishii T, Igarashi K, Katoh Y, Oyake T, Hayashi N, Satoh K, Hatayama I, Yamamoto M, Nabeshima Y (1997) An Nrf2/small Maf heterodimer mediates the induction of phase II detoxifying enzyme genes through antioxidant response elements. Biochem Biophys Res Commun 236:313–22

Kerr J F, Wyllie A H Currie A R (1972) Apoptosis: a basic biological phenomenon with wide-ranging implications in tissue kinetics. Br J Cancer 26: 239–257

Khodorov B, Pinelis V, Vergun O, Storozhevykh T, Vinskaya N (1996) Mitochondrial deenergization underlies neuronal calcium overload following a prolonged glutamate challenge. FEBS Letters 397:230–234

Kobayashi A, Kang MI, Watai Y, Tong KI, Shibata T, Uchida K, Yamamoto M (2006) Oxidative and electrophilic stresses activate Nrf2 through inhibition of ubiquitination activity of Keap1. Mol Cell Biol 26:221–229

Lee JM, Shih AY, Murphy TH, Johnson JA (2003) NF-E2-related factor-2 mediates neuroprotection against mitochondrial complex I inhibitors and increased concentrations of intracellular calcium in primary cortical neurons. J Biol Chem 278:37948–37956

Menardo J, Tang Y, Ladrech S, Lenoir M, Casas F, Michel C, Bourien J, Ruel J, Rebillard G, Maurice T, Puel JL, Wang J (2012) Oxidative stress, inflammation, and autophagic stress as the key mechanisms of premature age-related hearing loss in SAMP8 mouse cochlea. Antioxid Redox Signal 16:263–74

Maiti P, Singh SB, Sharma AK, Muthuraju S, Ilavazhagan G, Banerjee PK (2006) Hypobaric hypoxia induces oxidative stress in rat brain. Neurochem Int 49:709–716

Mawhinney LJ, de Vaccari Rivero JP, Dale GA, Keane RW, Bramlett HM (2011) Fischer 344 rats. BMC Neurosci 1(12):123

McFarland RA (1937) Pscycho-physiological studies at high altitude in the Andes II: sensory and motor responses during acclimatization. Comp Psychol 23:227–258

Muthuraju S, Maiti P, Solanki P, Sharma AK, Amitabh, Singh SB, Prasad D, Ilavazhagan G (2009) Acetylcholinesterase inhibitors enhance cognitive functions in rats following hypobaric hypoxia. Behav Brain Res 203:1–14
Nakaso K, Yano H, Fukuhara Y, Takeshima T, Wada-Isoe K, Nakashima K (2003) PI3K is a key molecule in the Nrf2-mediated regulation of antioxidative proteins by hemin in human neuroblastoma cells. FEBS Lett 546:181–184
Nicotera P, Leist M, Ferrando-May E (1998) Intracellular ATP, a switch in the decision between apoptosis and necrosis. Toxicol Lett 102:139–142
Paradies G, Petrosillo G, Paradies V, Ruggiero FM (2011) Mitochondrial dysfunction in brain aging: role of oxidative stress and cardiolipin. Neurochem Int 58:447–57
Patel JR, Brewer GJ (2008) Age-related differences in NFkappaB translocation and Bcl-2/Bax ratio caused by TNFalpha and Abeta42 promote survival in middle-age neurons and death in old neurons. Exp Neurol 213:93–100
Peacock AJ, Jones PL (1997) Gas exchange at extreme altitude: results from the British 40th Anniversary Everest Expedition. Eur Respir J 10:1439–1444
Pelamatti G, Pascotto M, Semenza C (2003) Verbal free recall in high altitude: proper names vs. common names. Cortex 39:97–103
Pugh LG (1964) Man at high altitude: studies carried out in the Himalaya. Sci Basis Med Annu Rev 32–54
Regard M, Oelz O, Brugger P, Landis T (1989) Persistent cognitive impairment in climbers after repeated exposure to extreme altitude. Neurology 39:210–213
Rhee SG, Yang KS, Kang SW, Woo HA, Chang TS (2005) Controlled elimination of intracellular H2O2: regulation of peroxiredoxin, catalase, and glutathione peroxidase via post-translational modification. Antioxid Redox Signal 7:619–626
Sastry PS, Rao KS (2000) Apoptosis and the nervous system. J Neurochem 74:1–20
Scaffidi C, Fulda S, Srinivasan A, Friesen C, Li F, Tomaselli KJ, Debatin KM, Krammer PH, Peter ME (1998) Two CD95 (APO-1/Fas) signaling pathways. EMBO J 17:1675–1687
Schliebs R, Arendt T (2006) The significance of the cholinergic system in the brain during aging and in Alzheimer's disease. J Neural Transm 113:1625–1644
Stickney JC, Van Liere EJ (1953) Acclimatization to low oxygen tension. Physiol Rev 33:13–34
Titus AD, Shankaranarayana Rao BS, Harsha HN, Ramkumar K, Srikumar BN, Singh SB, Chattarji S, Raju TR (2007) Hypobaric hypoxia-induced dendritic atrophy of hippocampal neurons is associated with cognitive impairment in adult rats. Neuroscience 145:265–278
Toescu EC, Verkhratsky A (2007) The importance of being subtle: small changes in calcium homeostasis control cognitive decline in normal aging. Aging Cell 6:267–273 (Review)
Toman J, Fiskum G (2011) Influence of aging on membrane permeability transition in brain mitochondria. J Bioenerg Biomembr 43:3–10
Wang X, Michaelis EK (2010) Selective neuronal vulnerability to oxidative stress in the brain. Front Aging Neurosci 30:2–12
Wang JY, Shum AY, Wang JY (2002) Hypoxia/reoxygenation induces cell injury via different mechanisms in cultured rat cortical neurons and glial cells. Neurosci Lett 322:187–191
West JB (1988) High points in the physiology of extreme altitude. Adv Exp Med Biol 227:1–15
West JB (2002) Unexplained severe fatigue and lassitude at high altitude. High Alt Med Biol 3:237–241
West JB (2004) Paralysis and blindness during a balloon ascent to high altitude. High Alt Med Biol 5:453–456
Won SJ, Kim DY, Gwag BJ (2002) Cellular and molecular pathways of ischemic neuronal death. J Biochem Mol Biol 35:67–86
Yang JC, Cortopassi GA (1998) Induction of the mitochondrial permeability transition causes release of the apoptogenic factor cytochrome c. Free Radic Biol Med 24:624–631
Zhang H, Liu H, Davies KJ, Sioutas C, Finch CE, Morgan TE, Forman HJ (2012) Nrf2-regulated phase II enzymes are induced by chronic ambient nanoparticle exposure in young mice with age-related impairments. Free Radic Biol Med [Epub ahead of print]

Chapter 13
Stress and Memory: from Mechanisms to Long-Lasting Consequences

Harmen J. Krugers and Marian Joels

Abstract Memories for emotionally arousing and fearful events are remembered well in general. This memory enhancing effect is mediated by stress hormones which are released during and shortly after exposure to the events and reflects a highly adaptive process that enables the retention of relevant information. However, in susceptible individuals, exposure to stressful events may result in post-traumatic stress disorder (PTSD) where traumatic memories are vividly expressed. Stress also has an important influence on the brain throughout the lifespan. For instance, stress during the early postnatal period impairs spatial learning and memory processes but enhances emotional memory formation later in life. Prolonged exposure to corticosteroids is also thought to promote hippocampal aging and the onset of Alzheimer's disease. Understanding how stress affects memory is therefore crucial to understand the development of stress-related psychopathology. In this chapter, mechanisms that underlie the effects of (early life) stress on memory formation as well as potential approaches to target the effects of stress on memory formation will be addressed.

Keywords Stress • Memory • Spatial learning • Fear conditioning • Synapses • Hippocampus

13.1 Introduction

In our daily life, we are regularly exposed to emotionally arousing and stressful experiences that can range from small displeasures to major life events such as the loss of relatives. Exposure to stressful events activates several systems that help to

H. J. Krugers (✉)
Swammerdam Institute of Life Sciences, Center for Neuroscience,
University of Amsterdam, Science Park 904, 1098 XH, Amsterdam, The Netherlands
e-mail: h.krugers@uva.nl

M. Joels
Department of Neuroscience and Pharmacology, Division of Neuroscience,
UMC Utrecht, Rudolf Magnus Institute, Utrecht, The Netherlands

M. K. Thakur, S. I. S. Rattan (eds.), *Brain Aging and Therapeutic Interventions*,
DOI 10.1007/978-94-007-5237-5_13,

respond to these challenging conditions (Kim and Diamond 2002; De Kloet et al. 2005). Ultimately, these actions are aimed to restore the disturbed equilibrium. The response to a stressful experience is therefore highly adaptive and might even be beneficial for the survival of individuals. Exposure to stressful experiences in vulnerable individuals, on the other hand, can increase the risk to develop psychopathological diseases across the lifespan such as depression and post-traumatic stress disorder (PTSD) (Yehuda 2009). In depression and PTSD, the mechanisms that can promote behavioral adaptation to stressful events are often dysregulated (De Kloet et al. 2005).

The ability to acquire, store and retrieve information (i.e. learning and memory) can be considered as one of the most important forms of behavioral adaptation. As such, remembering emotionally arousing and fearful events can be viewed as a highly adaptive process. In this chapter, the mechanisms that promote the memory of (acute) stressful events will be addressed. Second, the persistent effects of stress during early life on learning and memory processes will be summarized. We will briefly address the relationship between stress and aging. Since effects of stress may have detrimental effects on learning and memory processes, potential therapeutic approaches will be discussed that might potentially restore or normalize learning and memory processes. The focus of this chapter will be on animal studies, unless stated otherwise.

13.2 Neuro-endocrine Responses to Stress

Upon exposure to stressful events, the locus coeruleus (LC) becomes rapidly activated. In the LC, the majority of noradrenergic neurons are located, which project to other brain areas, such as prefrontal cortex, cerebellum, amygdala and hippocampus all of which are critically involved in learning and memory processes (Foote et al. 1983; Roozendaal et al. 2009). Noradrenergic projections affect neuronal function via activation of α-adrenergic and β-adrenergic receptors. In addition, stressful events stimulate the hypothalamus–pituitary–adrenal (HPA) axis which leads to a slow increase in the release of glucocorticoid hormones from the adrenal cortex (corticosterone in most rodents; cortisol in humans). These hormones enter the brain and bind to two subtypes of discretely localized receptors, i.e. the mineralocorticoid receptor (MR) and glucocorticoid receptor (GR), which (like adrenergic receptors) are expressed in regions that are critical for memory formation such as hippocampus, amygdala and prefrontal cortex. Mineralocorticoid receptors are occupied when hormone levels are low and exert their effects classically via the genome. Glucocorticoid receptors have a tenfold lower affinity for corticosterone, become substantially activated when hormone levels rise after stress and exert slow genomic actions in cells carrying the receptor (De Kloet et al. 2005). Importantly, recent evidence has revealed that corticosteroid hormones can also regulate synaptic function via non-genomic effects, both via activation of MRs and GRs (Orchinik et al. 1991; Karst et al. 2005; Groc et al. 2008; Karst et al. 2010; Di et al. 2005;

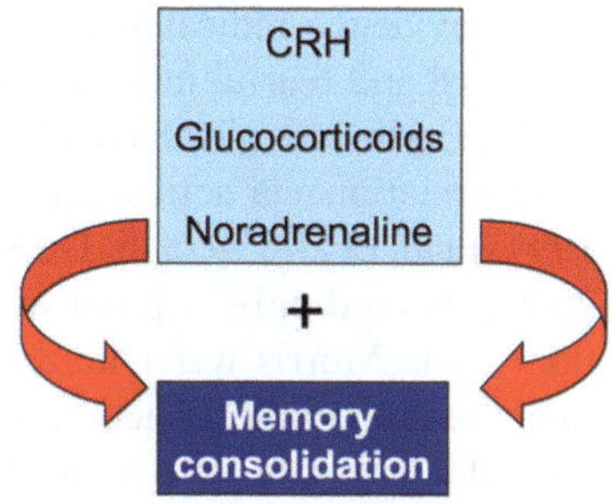

Fig. 13.1 Exposure to stressful events results in the release of several neuromodulators such as corticotrophin releasing hormone (CRH), glucocorticoids and noradrenaline. Together, they promote the consolidation of relevant information

Venero and Borrell 1999; Wiegert et al. 2006). This yields a completely new picture how glucocorticoids can regulate cellular function: the resultant cellular responses to the surge of corticosterone after exposure to a stressful event are determined by the dynamic interaction between corticosteroid hormones binding to MRs and GRs, via their coordinated genomic and non-genomic actions.

From the functional point of view, it is important to realize that there is an overlap in the time domains during which neurotransmitters and hormones—such as noradrenaline and corticosteroid hormones—are released after exposure to stressful experiences (Joëls and Baram 2009). This is particularly relevant since these compounds can interact to modulate behavioral responses and neuronal activity (Joëls et al. 2011). In interaction with a number of other compounds—such as (nor) adrenaline, corticotropin releasing hormone, endocannabinoids—corticosteroid hormones via their receptors alter neuronal activity in areas that play central roles in the storage of relevant information and promote behavioral adaptation (Roozendaal et al. 2006; Roozendaal et al. 2008; Campolongo et al. 2009) (Fig. 13.1).

13.3 Acute Stress and Memory Formation

Numerous studies have shown that the most vivid memories tend to be of emotionally arousing events (Cahill and McGaugh 1998; McGaugh 2000). This may be beneficial from the evolutionary point of view since it promotes the memory formation of potentially relevant events. Noradrenaline and corticosteroid hormones, via their receptors, play an important role in the memory enhancing effects of stress and emotion. Noradrenaline enhances memory formation of emotional events via the brain β-adrenergic receptors (β-ARs) both in humans and rodents: post-training applications of noradrenaline or β-ARs agonists promote memory consolidation in various memory tasks such as inhibitory avoidance task, fear conditioning and in Morris water-maze learning (Hu et al. 2007; Roozendaal et al. 2009). Activation of α-adrenergic receptors also enhances memory, presumably by enhancing the actions of β-adrenergic actions (Ferry et al. 1999a, b).

Corticosteroid hormones, via MRs have been implicated in the appraisal process and response selection (Oitzl and de Kloet 1992; Sandi and Rose 1994). However, recent evidence indicates that activation of MRs is also important for the storage of spatial and fearful information (Berger et al. 2006; Zhou et al. 2010; Zhou et al. 2011). Corticosteroids have also been reported to promote long-term consolidation of information via activation of GRs (Oitzl and De Kloet 1992; Sandi and Rose 1994; Pugh et al. 1997a, b; De Kloet et al. 1999; Joëls et al. 2006; Roozendaal et al. 2009). Accordingly, a point mutation in the mouse GR impairs memory formation in the Morris water maze task (Oitzl et al. 2001). While these studies point to a genomic mode of action, recent evidence suggests that membrane-associated GRs also promote long-term memory in an object recognition task via chromatin modification (Roozendaal et al. 2010). Thus, it is likely that both non-genomic as well as genomic actions of corticosteroid hormones promote the storage of relevant information. Besides these well-described effects of stress and glucocorticoids on consolidation processes, these hormones also affect memory retrieval mechanisms (de Quervain et al. 1998; de Quervain et al. 2000) and extinction processes (Brinks et al. 2009) which ultimately favor consolidation of relevant information and facilitate behavioral adaptation (De Kloet et al. 2005; Schwabe et al. 2010).

Several lines of evidence indicate that corticosteroids and noradrenaline work in concert for optimal memory performance both in humans and rodents (De Quervain et al. 2009; Roozendaal et al. 2009). In rodents, the presence of noradrenaline is crucial for facilitation of emotional memory (Quirarte et al. 1997) and corticosterone can enhance noradrenergic effects on memory formation. For example, post-training corticosterone administration enhances spatial and aversive memory formation, which can be blocked by administration of a β-adrenergic receptor antagonist (Roozendaal et al. 2006). Similarly, corticosterone administered to naive (aroused) rats enhances object recognition, an effect that can be blocked by the β-adrenergic receptor antagonist propranolol. In agreement, corticosterone was ineffective in animals which were extensively habituated (Okuda et al. 2004). Conversely, corticosterone is only effective in enhancing memory formation in well-habituated rats when the release of endogenous noradrenaline is enhanced (Roozendaal et al. 2006).

Also at the mechanistic level, corticosterone and noradrenaline interact. For example, they rapidly regulate AMPA receptor function which is critical for memory formation (Kessels and Malinow 2009). More specifically, there are optimal combinations at which noradrenaline and corticosterone interact to regulate AMPAR function, AMPA receptor surface expression and AMPA receptor phosphorylation (Krugers et al. 2010; Zhou et al. 2011). Finally, activation of β-adrenergic receptors and corticosterone interact at the network level (Pu et al. 2007). For instance, in the dentate gyrus, application of the β-adrenergic receptor agonist isoproterenol just prior to and during high-frequency stimulation causes robust synaptic potentiation. The onset of synaptic facilitation is increased by co-application of corticosterone to isoproterenol. This indicates that synaptic potentiation is most prominent when both stress hormones are present at the time when synaptic activation occurs. Taken together, emotionally arousing events are remembered well, and the release of stress hormones during these events promotes the formation of emotional memories, and facilitates cellular and molecular mechanisms that underlie learning and memory formation.

13.4 Early Life Stress and Memory Formation

While remembering emotionally arousing and fearful events may be beneficial, exposure to stress may also have negative impact on individuals. In particular, exposure to stressful experiences during the early postnatal period i.e. when the brain is still developing—may result in altered brain development, affect cognitive performance and alter the risk to develop psychopathology such as seen in depression and anxiety (Hackman et al. 2010). These studies indicate that negative exposures during the early life period can persistently affect brain development, brain function and learning and memory processes. In animal models, the consequences of early life experience can be examined in detail. Here we will address how maternal care and maternal deprivation affect brain development, synaptic plasticity and spatial and emotional learning and memory processes.

In rodents, early postnatal stress is usually induced by disturbing the mother (dam)–infant relationship during the first 2 weeks of life. Throughout this period, the presence of the mother is the most important environmental factor for the pup, and disturbing the mother-pup interaction provides a major stress experience. During approximately the first two weeks after birth, the hypothalamo-pituitary-adrenal axis is still developing and mild to moderate stressors usually do not result in elevated corticosterone levels in the offspring. This period is called the stress hyporesponsive period (SHRP) and lasts between postnatal day 0–12 (mice) or 3–14 (rats). For the SHRP, the presence of the dam is essential (Levine 2002). The SHRP is thought to serve a protective function, preventing high glucocorticoid levels during early postnatal development and results from a decreased sensitivity of the pituitary to CRH and of the adrenal cortex to ACTH (Dent et al. 2000).

Handling pups during the early postnatal period results in lower stress-induced corticosterone levels due to an enhanced negative feedback of the HPA-axis (Plotsky and Meaney 1993; Meaney et al. 1993). This beneficial effect of early handling is attributed to increased levels of maternal care in response to nest disturbance (Francis and Meaney 1999) and is accompanied by increased spatial cognitive performance later in life (Meaney et al. 1988). Subsequent studies revealed that also natural variations in the amount of licking and grooming (LG) and active "arch-back" nursing (ABN) by the dam during the first postnatal week tightly regulate activation of the HPA-axis, brain development and cognitive processes (Hackman et al. 2010). When compared to animals that received high levels of maternal care (high-LG/ABN), adult animals which received low levels of LG/ABN display (i) enhanced activation of the HPA-axis upon exposure to a stressful experience, (ii) enhanced anxiety, and (iii) impaired spatial learning (Liu et al. 1997; Francis et al. 2000; Liu et al. 2000; Weaver et al. 2006).

Recent studies have shown that dendritic complexity and spine number are reduced in several hippocampal subfields of young-adult low-LG/ABN animals when compared to high-LG/ABN animals, and that synaptic potentiation in the hippocampal formation is reduced in offspring of low-LG/ABN animals (Champagne et al. 2008; Bagot et al. 2010). Similar findings were observed in young-adult offspring that was exposed to maternal deprivation for 24 h on postnatal day 3 (Oomen et al. 2010). These studies suggest that early life adversity has negative consequences for hippocampal development and spatial cognitive processes, which is in agreement with other observations in rodents (e.g. Brunson et al. 2005; Rice et al. 2008; Wang et al. 2011).

Interestingly, cognitive processes are not necessarily impaired by negative early life experiences per se. For example, animals which are exposed to early life adversity (either less maternal care or maternal deprivation) display enhanced contextual fear conditioning responses (Champagne et al. 2008; Bagot et al. 2009). In addition, synaptic potentiation in deprived as well as low-LG/ABN animals is greatly enhanced by application of stress hormones (noradrenaline and/or corticosterone). These observations may point to a possible adaptive programming of early life adversity, i.e. animals which were raised in a stressful environment develop the ability to remember stressful events better later in life (Champagne et al. 2008; Bagot et al. 2009; Oomen et al. 2010). At this moment, it remains to be investigated exactly how negative early life experiences enhance memory formation of emotional events.

13.5 Stress in Relation to Aging

Dysregulation of the HPA-axis has also been observed in relation to aging, both in rodents and humans (Lupien et al. 2009). More specifically, aged rats show elevated basal corticosteroid levels (Landfield et al. 1978; Issa et al. 1990) and in humans mean diurnal levels of cortisol become higher with aging (Raskind et al. 1994). Interestingly, both in rodents and humans, there are large variations among subjects. In general, elevated corticosteroid levels correlate negatively with hippocampal volume and cognitive performance of the individual (Lupien et al. 1998).

It was proposed that the dysregulated HPA-axis function results from a self-propelling cascade (Sapolsky et al. 1986). In this view, small aberrations in corticosteroid level negatively impact on the survival of hippocampal neurons, so that the inhibitory tone that these cells normally exert on the HPA-axis activity is disturbed. As a consequence, the HPA-axis will be disinhibited, causing even higher levels of corticosteroid hormone levels which threaten the survival of hippocampal cells even more. The way in which corticosteroids could increase vulnerability of hippocampal principal cells is by their effect on calcium influx (Joëls and Karst 2012). Phil Landfield and colleagues proposed that L-type calcium currents, which cause considerable calcium influx into hippocampal cells upon depolarization are enhanced with aging (Campbell et al. 1996; Thibault and Landfield 1996; Toescu et al. 2004). Similarly, L-type channels are also a target for glucocorticoids (Kerr et al. 1992; Chameau et al. 2007), so that the over-exposure to corticosteroid hormones may accelerate the process of aging (Fig. 13.2). Most of the available data on calcium currents and glutamate signaling support this, although in some cases corticosteroid actions may also deviate from the natural aging process (Landfield et al. 2007).

13.6 Potential Therapeutic Approaches to Target Memory Formation

As mentioned earlier, the capacity to remember emotionally arousing events so well may be a highly adaptive process. On the other hand, it might also increase the risk to develop psychopathology, such as in post-traumatic stress disorder (PTSD) - where these memories are vividly expressed - and anxiety. Recent evidence emerged that retrieval and re-activation of fearful events renders these memories labile and protein synthesis is required after reactivation to re-consolidate the memory trace (Nader et al. 2000). Reconsolidation has been demonstrated in various tasks and species (Eisenberg et al. 2003; Nader et al. 2000; Sangha et al. 2003), including humans (Kindt et al. 2009; Schiller et al. 2010). Evidence that stored memories can be turned into a labile state has opened new avenues to reduce excessive fears. For example, in healthy individuals, it was shown that extinction training in the reconsolidation window persistently attenuates the expression of fear, both in animals (Monfils et al. 2009) and humans (Schiller et al. 2010).

The notion that stress hormones such as noradrenaline and corticosterone regulate the formation of these memories might open therapeutic approaches to reduce the expression of fearful memories using pharmacological approaches. Several studies have now examined whether targeting stress hormones and their receptors affect retrieval of emotional information. Pharmacological treatment with β-adrenergic receptor antagonists during re-exposure has been reported to affect the subsequent expression of fear for a considerable period of time in rodents and humans (Debiec and Ledoux 2004; Kindt et al. 2009; Soeter et al. 2011). Moreover, blockade of MRs prior to reactivation of memories strongly reduces the expression of contextual fear, implying that MRs in particular play an important role in retrieval of emotional information and subsequent fear expression (Zhou et al. 2011). Interestingly, a recent study reported that blocking GRs after reactivation was effective in suppressing fear (Pitman et al. 2011). This suggests that both corticosteroid receptor types could be targeted when trying to interfere with emotional memories.

As discussed before, exposure to negative life experiences during the early postnatal period has persistent negative consequences for spatial learning and memory processes. There is evidence that these effects can also be modulated. For example, the reduction in spatial memory performance in animals that received less maternal care during the first postnatal week, can be prevented by raising pups from low-LG mothers by high LG-mothers (Liu et al. 2000) as well as by environmental enrichment (Bredy et al. 2003). Whether these treatments also affect the memory formation of fearful events is currently not known. With respect to the age-associated hippocampal damage and cognitive impairment, it was shown that keeping glucocorticoid levels of rats low during middle-age effectively protects against the presumed glucocorticoid-dependent exacerbation of the aging process (Landfield et al. 1978). Anti-glucocorticoids are therefore interesting candidate-drugs to be tested for their efficacy in attenuating age-related cognitive decline.

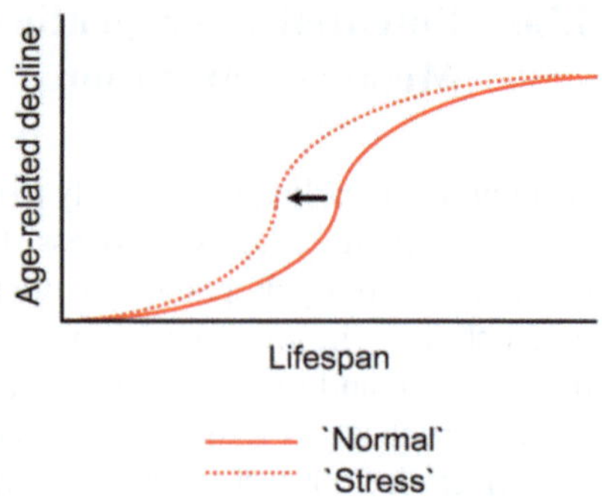

Fig. 13.2 The incidence to develop age-related cognitive deficits increases over lifespan. Exposure to stress (early life stress or chronic stress later in life) may enhance the vulnerability to develop cognitive decline

Taken together, there is substantial evidence that emotionally arousing events can be facilitated by the release of stress-hormones. Targeting these hormones and their receptors may prevent the expression of excessive fearful memories. Stressful experiences during the early postnatal period can persistently (and negatively) affect spatial memories; effects which can also (at least in part) be reversed by post-stress manipulations.

References

Berger S, Wolfer DP, Selbach O, Alter H, Erdmann G, Reichardt HM, Chepkova AN, Welzl H, Haas HL, Lipp HP, Schütz G (2006) Loss of the limbic mineralocorticoid receptor impairs behavioral plasticity. Proc Natl Acad Sci U S A 103:185–200

Bagot RC, van Hasselt FN, Champagne DL, Meaney MJ, Krugers HJ, Joëls M (2009) Maternal care determines rapid effects of stress mediators on synaptic plasticity in adult rat hippocampal dentate gyrus. Neurobiol Learn Mem 92:292–300

Bredy TW, Humpartzoomian RA, Cain DP, Meaney MJ (2003) Partial reversal of the effect of maternal care on cognitive function through environmental enrichment. Neuroscience 118:571–576

Brinks V, de Kloet ER, Oitzl MS (2009) Corticosterone facilitates extinction of fear memory in BALB/c mice but strengthens cue related fear in C57BL/6 mice. Exp Neurol 216:375–382

Brunson KL, Kramár E, Lin B, Chen Y, Colgin LL, Yanagihara TK, Lynch G, Baram TZ (2005) Mechanisms of late-onset cognitive decline after early-life stress. J Neurosci 25:9328–9238

Cahill L, McGaugh JL (1998) Mechanisms of emotional arousal and lasting declarative memory. Trends Neurosci 21:294–299

Campbell LW, Hao SY, Thibault O, Blalock EM, Landfield PW (1996) Aging changes in voltage-gated calcium currents in hippocampal CA1 neurons. J Neurosci 16:6286–6295

Campolongo P, Roozendaal B, Trezza V, Hauer D, Schelling G, McGaugh JL, Cuomo V (2009) Endocannabinoids in the rat basolateral amygdala enhance memory consolidation and enable glucocorticoid modulation of memory. Proc Natl Acad Sci U S A 106:4888–4893

Champagne DL, Bagot RC, van Hasselt F, Ramakers G, Meaney MJ, de Kloet ER, Joëls M, Krugers H (2008) Maternal care and hippocampal plasticity: evidence for experience-dependent structural plasticity, altered synaptic functioning, and differential responsiveness to glucocorticoids and stress. J Neurosci 28:6037–6045

Chameau P, Qin Y, Spijker S, Smit AB, Joëls M (2007) Glucocorticoids specifically enhance L-type calcium current amplitude and affect calcium channel subunit expression in the mouse hippocampus. J Neurophysiol 97:5–14
Debiec J, Ledoux JE (2004) Disruption of reconsolidation but not consolidation of auditory fear conditioning by noradrenergic blockade in the amygdala. Neuroscience 129:267–272
Dent GW, Okimoto DK, Smith MA, Levine S (2000) Stress-induced alterations in corticotropin-releasing hormone and vasopressin gene expression in the paraventricular nucleus during ontogeny. Neuroendocrinol 71:333–342
Di S, Malcher-Lopes R, Halmos KC, Tasker JG (2003) Nongenomic glucocorticoid inhibition via endocannabinoid release in the hypothalamus: a fast feedback mechanism. J Neurosci 23:4850–4857
Eisenberg M, Kobilo T, Berman DE, Dudai Y (2003) Stability of retrieved memory: inverse correlation with trace dominance. Science 301:1102–110415
Ferry B, Roozendaal B, McGaugh JL (1999a) Involvement of alpha1-adrenoceptors in the basolateral amygdala in modulation of memory storage. Eur J Pharmacol 372:9–1616
Ferry B, Roozendaal B, McGaugh JL (1999b) Basolateral amygdala noradrenergic influences on memory storage are mediated by an interaction between beta- and alpha1-adrenoceptors. J Neurosci 19:5119–5123
Foote SL, Bloom FE, Aston-Jones G (1983) Nucleus locus ceruleus: new evidence of anatomical and physiological specificity. Physiol Rev 63:844–914
Francis DD, Meaney MJ (1999) Maternal care and the development of stress responses. Curr Opin Neurobiol 9:128–134
Francis D, Diorio J, Liu D, Meaney MJ (2000) Nongenomic transmission across generations of maternal behavior and stress responses in the rat. Science 286:1155–1158
Groc L, Choquet D, Chaouloff F (2008) The stress hormone corticosterone conditions AMPAR surface trafficking and synaptic potentiation. Nat Neurosci 11:868–870
Hackman DA, Farah MJ, Meaney MJ (2010) Socioeconomic status and the brain: mechanistic insights from human and animal research. Nat Rev Neurosci 11:651–659
Hu H, Real E, Takamiya K, Kang M, Ledoux JE, Huganir RL, Malinow R (2007) Emotion enhances learning via norepinephrine regulation of AMPA-receptor trafficking. Cell 131:160–173
Issa AM, Rowe W, Gauthier S, Meaney MJ (1990) Hypothalamic-pituitary-adrenal activity in aged, cognitively impaired and cognitively unimpaired rats. J Neurosci 10:3247–3254
Joëls M, Baram TZ (2009) The neuro-symphony of stress. Nat Rev Neurosci 10:459–466
Joels M, Karst H (2012) Corticosteroid effects on calcium signaling in limbic neurons. Cell calcium 51:277-283
Joëls M, Karst H Joels M, Pu Z, Wiegert O, Oitzl MS, Krugers HJ (2006) Learning under stress: how does it work? Trends Cogn Sci 10:152–158
Joëls M, Fernandez G, Roozendaal B (2011) Stress and emotional memory: a matter of timing. Trends Cogn Sci 15:280–288
Karst H, Berger S, Turiault M, Tronche F, Schutz G, Joels M (2005) Mineralocorticoid receptors are indispensable for nongenomic modulation of hippocampal glutamate transmission by corticosterone. Proc Natl Acad Sci U S A 102:19204–19207
Karst H, Berger S, Erdmann G, Schütz G, Joëls M (2010) Metaplasticity of amygdalar responses to the stress hormone corticosterone. Proc Natl Acad Sci U S A 107:14449–14454
Kerr DS, Campbell LW, Thibault O, Landfield PW (1992) Hippocampal glucocorticoid receptor activation enhances voltage-dependent Ca2+ conductances: relevance to brain aging. Proc Natl Acad Sci U S A 89:8527–8531
Kessels HW, Malinow R (2009) Synaptic AMPA receptor plasticity and behavior. Neuron 61:340–350
Kim JJ, Diamond DM (2002) The stressed hippocampus, synaptic plasticity and lost memories. Nat Rev Neurosci 3:453–462
Kindt M, Soeter M, Vervliet B (2009) Beyond extinction: erasing human fear responses and preventing the return of fear. Nat Neurosci 12:256–258

de Kloet ER, Oitzl MS, Joels M (1999) Stress and cognition: are corticosteroids good or bad guys? Trends Neurosci 22:422–426
de Kloet ER, Joels M, Holsboer F (2005) Stress and the brain: from adaptation to disease. Nat Rev Neurosci 6:463–475
Krugers HJ, Hoogenraad CC, Groc L (2010) Stress hormones and AMPA receptor trafficking in synaptic plasticity and memory. Nat Rev Neurosci 11:675–681
Landfield PW, Waymire JC, Lynch G (1978) Hippocampal aging and adrenocorticoids: quantitative correlations. Science 202:1098–10102
Landfield PW, Blalock EM, Chen KC, Porter NM (2007) A new glucocorticoid hypothesis of brain aging: implications for Alzheimer's disease. Curr Alzheimer Res 4:205–212
Levine S (2002) Regulation of the hypothalamic-pituitary-adrenal axis in the neonatal rat: the role of maternal behavior. Neurotox Res 4:557–564
Liu D, Diorio J, Tannenbaum B, Caldji C, Francis D, Freedman A, Sharma S, Pearson D, Plotsky PM, Meaney MJ (1997) Maternal care, hippocampal glucocorticoid receptors, and hypothalamic-pituitary-adrenal responses to stress. Science 277:1659–1662
Liu D, Diorio J, Day JC, Francis DD, Meaney MJ (2000) Maternal care, hippocampal synaptogenesis and cognitive development in rats. Nat Neurosci 3:799–806
Lupien SJ, McEwen BS, Gunnar MR, Heim C (2009) Effects of stress throughout the lifespan on the brain, behaviour and cognition. Nat Rev Neurosci 10:434–445
Lupien SJ, de Leon M, de Santi S, Convit A, Tarshish C, Nair NP, Thakur M, McEwen BS, Hauger RL, Meaney MJ (1998) Cortisol levels during human aging predict hippocampal atrophy and memory deficits. Nat Neurosci 1:69–73
McGaugh JL (2000) Memory—a century of consolidation. Science 287:248–251
Meaney MJ, Aitken DH, van Berkel C, Bhatnagar S, Sapolsky RM (1988) Effect of neonatal handling on age-related impairments associated with the hippocampus. Science 239:766–768
Meaney MJ, Bhatnagar S, Diorio J, Larocque S, Francis D, O'Donnell D, Shanks N, Sharma S, Smythe J, Viau V (1993) Molecular basis for the development of individual differences in the hypothalamic-pituitary-adrenal stress response. Cell Mol Neurobiol 13:321–347
Monfils MH, Cowansage KK, Klann E, LeDoux JE (2009) Extinction-reconsolidation boundaries: key to persistent attenuation of fear memories. Science 324:951–955
Nader K, Schafe GE, Le Doux JE (2000) Fear memories require protein synthesis in the amygdala for reconsolidation after retrieval. Nature 406:722–726
Okuda S, Roozendaal B, McGaugh JL (2004) Glucocorticoid effects on object recognition memory require training-associated emotional arousal. Proc Natl Acad Sci U S A 101:853–858
Oitzl MS, de Kloet ER (1992) Selective corticosteroid antagonists modulate specific aspects of spatial orientation learning. Behav Neurosci 106:62–71
Oitzl MS, Reichardt HM, Joëls M, de Kloet ER (2001) Point mutation in the mouse glucocorticoid receptor preventing DNA binding impairs spatial memory. Proc Natl Acad Sci U S A 98:12790–12795
Orchinik M, Murray TF, Moore FL (1991) A corticosteroid receptor in neuronal membranes. Science 252:1848–1851
Oomen CA, Soeters H, Audureau N, Vermunt L, van Hasselt FN, Manders EM, Joëls M, Lucassen PJ, Krugers H (2010) Severe early life stress hampers spatial learning and neurogenesis, but improves hippocampal synaptic plasticity and emotional learning under high-stress conditions in adulthood. J Neurosci 30:6635–6645
Pitman RK, Milad MR, Igoe SA, Vangel MG, Orr SP, Tsareva A, Gamache K, Nader K (2011) Systemic mifepristone blocks reconsolidation of cue-conditioned fear; propranolol prevents this effect. Behav Neurosci 125;632–638
Pu Z, Krugers HJ, Joëls M (2007) Corticosterone time-dependently modulates beta-adrenergic effects on long-term potentiation in the hippocampal dentate gyrus. Learn Mem 14:359–367
Pugh CR, Fleshner M, Rudy JW (1997a) Type II glucocorticoid receptor antagonists impair contextual but not auditory-cue fear conditioning in juvenile rats. Neurobiol Learn Mem 67:75–79
Pugh CR, Tremblay D, Fleshner M, Rudy JW (1997b) A selective role for corticosterone in contextual-fear conditioning. Behav Neurosci. 111:503–511

Quirarte GL, Roozendaal B, McGaugh JL (1997) Glucocorticoid enhancement of memory storage involves noradrenergic activation in the basolateral amygdala. Proc Natl Acad Sci U S A 94:14048–14053
de Quervain DJ, Roozendaal B, McGaugh JL (1998) Stress and glucocorticoids impair retrieval of long-term spatial memory. Nature 394:787–790
de Quervain DJ, Roozendaal B, Nitsch RM, McGaugh JL, Hock C (2000) Acute cortisone administration impairs retrieval of long-term declarative memory in humans. Nat Neurosci 3:313–314
de Quervain DJ, Aerni A, Schelling G, Roozendaal B (2009) Glucocorticoids and the regulation of memory in health and disease. Front Neuroendocrinol (Epub ahead of print)
Rice CJ, Sandman CA, Lenjavi MR, Baram TZ (2008) A novel mouse model for acute and long-lasting consequences of early life stress. Endocrinology 149:4892–4900
Roozendaal B, Okuda S, Van Der Zee EA, McGaugh JL (2006) Glucocorticoid enhancement of memory requires arousal-induced noradrenergic activation in the basolateral amygdala. Proc Natl Acad Sci U S A 103:6741–676
Roozendaal B, Castello NA, Vedana G, Barsegyan A, McGaugh JL (2008) Noradrenergic activation of the basolateral amygdala modulates consolidation of object recognition memory. Neurobiol Learn Mem 90:576–579
Roozendaal B, McEwen BS, Chattarji S (2009) Stress, memory and the amygdala. Nat Rev Neurosci 10:423–433
Roozendaal B, Hernandez A, Cabrera SM, Hagewoud R, Malvaez M, Stefanko DP, Haettig J, Wood MA (2010) Membrane-associated glucocorticoid activity is necessary for modulation of long-term memory via chromatin modification. J Neurosci 30:5037–5046
Sandi C, Rose SP (1994) Corticosteroid receptor antagonists are amnestic for passive avoidance learning in day-old chicks. Eur J Neurosci 6:1292–1297
Sangha S, Scheibenstock A, Lukowiak K (2003) Reconsolidation of a long-term memory in Lymnaea requires new protein and RNA synthesis and the soma of right pedal dorsal 1. J Neurosci 23:8034–8040
Sapolsky RM, Krey LC, McEwen BS (1986) The neuroendocrinology of stress and aging: the glucocorticoid cascade hypothesis. Endocr Rev 7:284–301
Schiller D, Monfils MH, Raio CM, Johnson DC, Ledoux JE et al (2010) Preventing the return of fear in humans using reconsolidation update mechanisms. Nature 463:49–53
Schwabe L, Wolf OT, Oitzl MS (2010) Memory formation under stress: quantity and quality. Neurosci Biobehav Rev 34:584–591
Soeter M, Kindt M (2011) Disrupting reconsolidation: pharmacological and behavioral manipulations. Learn Mem 18:357–366
Thibault O, Landfield PW (1996) Increase in single L-type calcium channels in hippocampal neurons during aging. Science 272:1017–10120
Toescu EC, Verkhratsky A, Landfield PW (2004) Ca2+ regulation and gene expression in normal brain aging. Trends Neurosci 27:614–620
Venero C, Borrell J (1999) Rapid glucocorticoid effects on excitatory amino acid levels in the hippocampus: a microdialysis study in freely moving rats. Eur J Neurosci 11:2465–2473
Wang XD, Rammes G, Kraev I, Wolf M, Liebl C, Scharf SH, Rice CJ, Wurst W, Holsboer F, Deussing JM, Baram TZ, Stewart MG, Müller MB, Schmidt MV (2011) Forebrain CRF1 modulates early-life stress-programmed cognitive deficits. J Neurosci 31:13625–13634
Weaver IC, Meaney MJ, Szyf M (2006) Maternal care effects on the hippocampal transcriptome and anxiety-mediated behaviors in the offspring that are reversible in adulthood. Proc Natl Acad Sci U S A 103:3480–3485
Wiegert O, Joëls M, Krugers H (2006) Timing is essential for rapid effects of corticosterone on synaptic potentiation in the mouse hippocampus. Learn Mem 13:110–113
Yehuda R (2009) Status of glucocorticoid alterations in post-traumatic stress disorder. Ann N Y Acad Sci 1179:56–69
Zhou M, Kindt M, Joëls M, Krugers HJ (2011) Blocking Mineralocorticoid receptors prior to retrieval reduces contextual fear memory in mice. PLoS One e26220

Zhou M, Bakker EH, Velzing EH, Berger S, Oitzl M, Joëls M, Krugers HJ (2010) Both mineralocorticoid and glucocorticoid receptors regulate emotional memory in mice. Neurobiol Learn Mem 94:530–537
Zhou M, Bakker EH, Velzing EH, Berger S, Oitzl M, Joëls M, Krugers HJ (2010) Both mineralocorticoid and glucocorticoid receptors regulate emotional memory in mice. Neurobiol Learn Mem 94:530–537

Chapter 14
Estrogen-Mediated Neuroprotection: Hope to Combat Neuronal Degeneration and Synaptic Plasticity Post-menopause

Raj D. Mehra, Mukesh K. Varshney and Pavan Kumar

Abstract Recent decade has seen a surge in identifying modifiable risk and protective factors for cognitive decline associated with natural aging and with common dementing disorders such as Alzheimer's disease (AD). Ovarian steroid hormone estrogen is extensively studied among these factors with profound effects on many tissues and organs, including the brain. Brain aging in female is also accompanied with decline in estrogen levels. In women, it is characterized by natural depletion of hormone levels and menopause, whereas in rodents, it results in estropause. A decent amount of evidence associates the estrogen (E2, 17β estradiol) with hippocampal activity, an area of brain related to cognition and memory. Presence of estrogen receptors (ER) in the hippocampus gives further evidence to it being one of the target brain regions for the hormone activity. Our findings have revealed that ovariectomy or natural aging leads to decreased synaptic activity, degenerative cytoarchitectural changes and altered protein levels in hippocampal neurons. Further, it was seen that long-term estrogen therapy maintains the synaptic plasticity, regulates apoptotic proteins and affords neuroprotection to the hippocampal neurons through both the nuclear and membrane estrogen receptor mediated pCREB and MAPK activation. Interestingly, normal aging also exhibits immune activation and cell infiltration in the brain. Neuroprotective effects of estrogen may include its anti-inflammatory response via regulating the neuro-immune response and levels of pro-inflammatory cytokines. However, the exact mechanism of anti-inflammatory actions of estrogen in senescent female brain is not yet fully characterized and needs to be undertaken to fully embark on neuro-immune processes in female brain aging. Attention is now largely focused on collective and beneficial approach of estrogen replacement therapy that shall not only support the cognitive function but also prevent neurodegenerative pathologies.

Keywords Estrogen • Synaptic plasticity • Neurodegeneration • Inflammatory • Neuroprotection • SERM

R. D. Mehra (✉) · M. K. Varshney · P. Kumar
Department of Anatomy, All India Institute of Medical Sciences, New Delhi 110029, India
e-mail: rdmehra98@hotmail.com

M. K. Thakur, S. I. S. Rattan (eds.), *Brain Aging and Therapeutic Interventions*,
DOI 10.1007/978-94-007-5237-5_14,

14.1 Introduction

Prevention and treatment of age-related brain disorders require deeper understanding of the basic neurological processes behind the normal and pathological brain aging. Growing evidence suggests that gonadal hormones exert different effects in male and female subjects, perhaps because of underlying dimorphism in some brain processes. These processes are closely related to brain regions involved in memory, cognition and affective state, such as the hippocampus, amygdala, cerebral cortex (Baron-Cohen et al. 2005; McCarthy and Konkle 2005; Cahill 2006; Cosgrove et al. 2007; Wilson and Davies 2007), and regions controlling sensorimotor and reward systems (Dewing et al. 2006; Cantuti-Castelvetri et al. 2007; McArthur et al. 2007a). The loss of gonadal steroid hormones during normal aging increases the risk of disease and dysfunction in hormone-responsive tissues (Baumgartner et al. 1999; Morley 2001). Age-related hormone depletion likely results in diminished neuroprotective actions of hormones in brain and an increased risk to neurodegenerative diseases such as Alzheimer's disease (AD) (Pike et al. 2006; Rosario and Pike 2008). In case of humans, the decline of estrogen production in female is fast and generally accompanied by slow progression of cognitive disturbances, and in some cases by dementia (Henderson 2008). In AD, postmenopausal women have a greater toll than men (Swaab 2004). Estrogen has been identified as a vital protective factor in women in providing them the benefit against the diseases which are prevalent in men. However, a rapid decline in estrogen after menopause leads to the loss of this advantage. The knowledge of the significance of physiological and pharmacological actions of estrogen in brain is indispensable for realizing the full translational prospective role of this ubiquitous female steroid hormone in maintaining the health and wellbeing. This chapter is focused to deliver current knowledge of neuroprotective effects of estrogen in the context of cognitive decline and neurodegeneration in postmenopausal women. To study the impact of estrogen loss on brain plasticity and cognitive functions, the ovariectomized rat is a suitable experimental model for clinical representation of menopause in animals. We will discuss pleiotropic nature of estrogen, mechanism of action in brain and its role in ameliorating cognitive decline and neurodegeneration. This information is essential to understand the nature of estrogen and its translational value for future use to combat neurological disorders in aging female brain.

14.2 Estrogen, Menopause and Brain Aging

Women now live a larger part of their lives in estrogen deprived state (menopause) which predisposes them to cognitive decline, memory disturbances and neurodegeneration. AD is one of the most debilitating diseases of the central nervous system following progressive brain aging and results in the formation of beta-amyloid plaques, neurofibrillary tangles and neuronal loss. Estradiol is biologically most prevalent and active compound of a class of steroids called estrogens (Behl et al. 2000) and exerts potent and wide-ranging effects on the development, growth, differentiation and function of various tissues throughout the body. It is mainly synthesized in the ovaries and to a lesser extent in testes and placenta. Estrogen is known to occur in mammals in several forms, i.e. estrone (E1), 17β estradiol (E2), estriol (E3), and 17α estradiol (17α). Recent results of experimental and clinical studies have indicated that estrogen acts not only on the hypothalamus-hypophysis axis, but also on other brain regions to name a few like amygdala, hippocampal formation, cerebellum etc., thus influencing brain functions not related to reproductive activity. In these brain areas, estrogen modulates memory, cognition, postural stability, fine motor activity and mood. Age related decline of estrogen in postmenopausal women poses a great risk of cognitive deficits and progressive AD in comparison to the same age group men. Extensive work in the field of steroid hormones and their actions in brain have led us to the remarkable but partial understanding of estrogen's neuroprotective role in certain brain areas involved in learning, memory and cognition.

Estrogen has been investigated for its neuroprotective effects in a variety of systems and experimental models of neurodegenerative disorders and cerebral ischemia (Dubal et al. 1998; Green and Simpkins 2000). The association between memory and estrogen was first clinically reported when menopausal women frequently expressed complaints of memory disturbance and concentration problems (Sherwin 2000). Indeed alterations in cognitive performance have long been linked with menopause (Neurgaren and Kraines 1965). These clinical observations led to the beginning of scientific human study in the 1980s and thereafter Sherwin and colleagues accomplished a systematic analysis of the influence of estrogen loss and replenishment on memory functions. Results of these investigations established deterioration of verbal memory with estrogen loss and estrogen replacement therapy immediately after menopause restored the memory alterations to premenopausal state (Sherwin 1988). These findings prompted Fillit and colleagues (1986) to investigate the effect of estrogen replacement therapy on cognitive tasks in women with AD. The results of this small clinical trial proved to be pivotal to establish the role of estrogen in memory mechanisms in female brain. Several in vivo and in vitro studies suggest that estrogen exerts a protective effect in various brain disorders by influencing the inflammatory response. This anti-inflammatory hypothesis also stems from the evidence that menopause, which is characterized by the drastic drop in estrogen levels, results in an increased incidence of inflammatory pathologies of brain and other tissues. Treatment with physiological doses of estrogen before the onset of disease downregulates the expression of inflammatory factors, including cytokines, chemokines and their receptors (Matsuda et al. 2001; Matejuk et al. 2001), apolipoprotein E and other modulators of leukocyte migration (Horsburgh et al. 2002; Vegeto et al. 2003).

Results of basic science, clinical science, and epidemiological analyses need more data to demonstrate and understand the neuroprotective potential of estrogen and certain other compounds with estrogen-like activity against age-related risk factors of developing AD and other neurodegenerative disorders.

14.3 Mechanism of Action of Estrogen

Estrogen produces its actions through binding to specific receptors known as estrogen receptors (ERs). ERs are cis-acting transcription factors which are members of steroid receptors super family (Giguère et al. 1988). ERs contain three main structural and functional domains, a highly conserved DNA-binding domain, C-terminal ligand-binding domain and hyper variable N-terminal transactivation domain (Mangelsdorf et al. 1995). After binding to its ligand, two molecules of ER dimerize and bind to the specific DNA sequence, estrogen response element (ERE) inside the nucleus and lead to the activation of target gene transcription factors (Tsai and O'Malley 1994). The mechanism of action of estrogen has been reviewed considerably following the discovery of the novel member of the steroid receptor super family i.e. ERβ (Kuiper et al. 1996) with high degree of sequence homology (95 %) with the classical ERα (Giguère et al.1988). Each receptor shows high affinity binding with estrogen and may bind to each other as homodimers or heterodimers. This receptor-ligand dimer then binds with ERE or associate with AP1 transcription factors c-jun/c-fos to regulate the transcription of responsive genes (Kuiper et al. 1996, 1997; Paech et al. 1997). Several studies have also established that estrogen rapidly (within seconds to a few minutes) influences cellular physiology in different cell types of estrogen responsive tissues via activating a multitude of intracellular signaling mechanisms (Belcher and Zsarnovsky 2001). In addition to regulation of gonadal functions, ERα and ERβ are also present in both female and male brains, specifically in brain areas involved in memory and cognition (McEwen 2001). Among the brain regions, major interest is focused on hippocampus and neocortex (Mehra et al. 2005). In rat and mouse, different regions and cell-populations in the brain, including hypothalamus, hippocampus, cerebellum and pituitary appear to express ERα and ERβ (Mitchner et al. 1998; Osterlund et al. 1998). While the protein sequences of ERα and ERβ are highly homologous, they represent two distinct gene products. In humans, the gene for ERα is located on chromosome 6 while that for ERβ is on chromosome 14 (Couse and Korach 1999).

Since estrogen is a potent neuroprotective hormone, to reveal its exact molecular and cellular mechanisms of action would offer putative drug target points. Gonadal steroids act on both genomic and nongenomic pathways related to nuclear as well as membrane and cytoplasmic receptors, respectively. Extensive research activity is going on worldwide, including our recent research work, to define both genomic and intracellular signaling pathways in order to determine the molecular actions of estrogens. For example: (1) Activation of Src/ERK/CREB/Bcl-2 signaling pathways by estrogen triggers neuroprotective mechanism (Sharma and Mehra 2008), (2) Estradiol (E2)-induced formation of dendritic spines in hippocampus acts via Akt (protein kinase B)-mediated signaling events (Zhou et al. 1996), and (3) modulation of cyclic AMP response element binding protein (CREB) pathway (Szegõ et al. 2006; Wappler et al. 2009) provides an insight into the existence of the 'nongenomic' action of the ovarian hormone. According to Falkenstein et al. (2000), estrogen rapidly activates adenylate cyclase, ERK 1 and 2, and MAPK pathways. Activation of adenylate cyclase is known to result in increased cAMP concentration and downstream activation of protein kinase A (PKA) through a well described cAMP-PKA signal transduction pathway (Gu and Moss 1996). Estradiol increases cAMP accumulation in hypothalamic neurons (Weissman et al. 1975) and human neuroblastoma cells (Watters and Dorsa 1998) and exerts cellular effects in neurons consistently with increased cAMP levels (Gu and Moss 1996; Minami et al. 1996) and increased phosphorylation of CREB protein (Gu and Moss 1996; Sharma et al. 2007). Further in this regard, a rapid estrogen induction of phosphorylated CREB was found in the periventricular nucleus (Gu and Moss 1996), preoptic area and the bed nucleus of striaterminalis in rat brain (Zhou et al. 1996). Extensive studies in this research area are being conducted worldwide revealing estrogenic actions in rat hippocampus which occur via nuclear and membrane receptors associated with the synaptic plasticity and neuroprotection. In this course, we have shown that increased phosphorylation of CREB results in i) increased synaptophysin activity, ii) higher Bcl2:Bax ratio (attenuates apoptosis) (Sharma et al. 2007; Sharma and Mehra 2008) and iii) regulates mitochondrial cellular energy balance which plays a prominent role (Toulmond et al. 1996) in estrogen mediated neuroprotection. Estrogen induced increase in dendritic spine density in the hippocampus has been reported to be dependent on CREB phosphorylation (Segal and Murphy 1998; Sharma et al. 2007). Our planned studies will continue to search for the involvement of E2-induced additional remarkable signaling molecules with a significance to find potent therapeutic targets.

14.4 Estrogen and Neuroprotection

Estrogen mediated neuroprotection has been described in several neuronal culture models of neuronal toxicity including that of the serum deprivation (Gollapudi and Oblinger 1999), β amyloid-induced toxicity (Behl et al. 1997; Gridley et al. 1997) and excitotoxicity systems (Weaver et al. 1997; Singer 1999). It has also been demonstrated in experimental models of oxidative stress (Moosmann and Behl 1999). Estrogen has a large number of cellular effects including the modulation of apoptotic factors, which has been shown to enhance neuronal survival (Green and Simpkins 2000). The Bcl-2 family of proteins are important modulators of neuronal apoptosis and include both inhibitors (Bcl-2 and Bcl-XL) as well as promoters (Bax and Bad). A marked increase in the Bcl-2 immunoreactivity has been observed in NT2 neuronal cell cultures (Singer et al. 1998) and in the neurons of the arcuate nucleus of rat following 17α estradiol administration (Gollapudi and Oblinger 1999). Similarly, 17β estradiol increased i) Bcl-XL mRNA levels in PC 12 cells transfected with ERα (Gollapudi and Oblinger 1999) and ii) Bcl-XL immunoreactivity in primary rat hippocampal neurons (Pike 1999). 17β estradiol exposure also caused a marked decrease in the levels of pro-apoptotic protein BAD in ERα transfected PC 12 cells (Gollapudi and Oblinger 1999). The expression of a member of Bcl-2 binding proteins family (BNIP) was significantly reduced by treatment with 17β estradiol in neural cell culture (Balcredito et al. 2001). It may be postulated that the activation of cAMP signaling and/or increased CREB phosphorylation could contribute to the neuroprotective effects of estradiol in these above mentioned studies as activation of cAMP pathway is associated with decreased susceptibility of neuronal cells to apoptotic signals (Kobayashi and Shinozawa 1997). Further, activation of cAMP-PKA-CREB pathway has been postulated to be associated with enhanced neuronal survival following an increase in the expression of anti-apoptotic protein Bcl-2. Recent studies of Wappler et al. (2010) have reported that a single high dose of estradiol (4 mg/kg b.w.) pre-treatment results in significant neuroprotection against hippocampal cell loss in ischemic gerbils of various age groups. All relevant behavioral tests of hippocampal memory functions offered evidence of improved memory in these animals. Wappler and colleagues (2011) have also reported that a single pre-treatment dose of estradiol exerts varying effects on hippocampal synaptic plasticity in different age groups at both shorter (4 postoperative days) and longer (25 post-operative days) time points. It increased hippocampal synaptic density in both age groups, however, this increase was more pronounced in younger animals. Thus it is clear from these studies that with aging there is a lower tendency of synaptogenesis.

In our laboratory, to understand the neuroprotective potential of estrogen and other estrogen-like compounds, we have systematically examined the protein chemistry of various brain areas by using immunohistochemical and proteomic approaches. The functional outcome has been assessed with behavioral tests of experimental learning and memory paradigms in ovx and aging female rats. Our experimental results have so far revealed that estrogen decline following ovariectomy in adult female rats leads to degenerative changes in hippocampal neurons. Following ovariectomy or aging, there appeared cytoplasmic vacuolation and Nissl substance was unevenly distributed, rarefied and juxtaposed against the cell membrane in the pyramidal neurons of the CA3-CA1 (Fig. 14.1b). Nuclear changes observed with DAPI staining also confirmed the juxtamembranous condensation of chromatin material in hippocampal neurons of OVX and aged animals (Fig. 14.2b, c). Estradiol therapy (0.1 mg/kg body wt. for 30 days) given to ovx rats seemed to reverse the effects of ovariectomy, such that the uniformity of Nissl staining patterns, position of nucleoli and cytoplasmic consistency were seen to be very much like that in the ovary-intact hippocampus (Fig. 14.1e). Nuclear morphology of hippocampal neurons of E2 treated ovx rats was more or less comparable to that of the ovary intact rat hippocampal neurons (Fig. 14.2d). These results were further substantiated by results on the expression of anti-apoptotic Bcl2 and pro-apoptotic Bax proteins in the hippocampii of various experimental groups. Hormonal depletion (ovx or aging) resulted in downregulation of Bcl-2 and increased Bax expression in CA1-CA3 and dentate gyrus, while E2 treatment to ovx rats resulted in the reversal (near to ovary intact levels) of these markers of cell death and survival (Fig. 14.3a). Hormone treatment led to an increased Bcl-2:Bax ratio indicative of a shift towards neuronal survival. Neuronal cell death in various subfields of hippocampus was further confirmed by TUNEL assay where percentage of TUNEL positive neurons was increased following ovariectomy or aging, while E2 therapy decreased the percent TUNEL positive neurons (Fig. 14.3b).

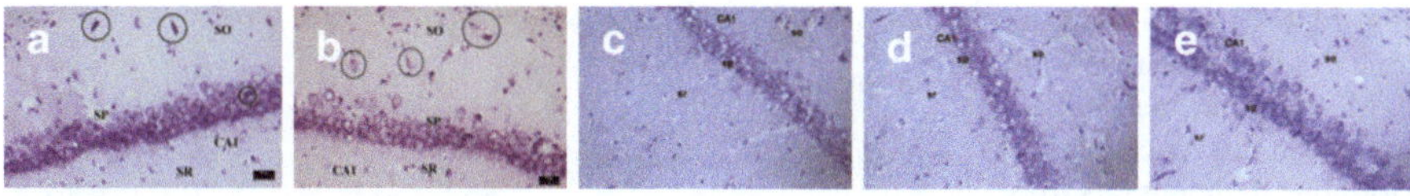

Fig. 14.1 Cresyl violet stained coronal sections of **a** Ovary intact adult, **b** OVX adult, **c** OVX aged (24 months), **d** OVX+E2 aged (24 months), **e** OVX+E2 adult rat hippocampus CA1 neuronalcytoarchitecture. Note the cytoplasmic vacuolation and reduced Nissl staining (**b**, **c**, **d**) following ovariectomy and aging and reversal of ovariectomy-induced changes (**e**) following E2 therapy. (*SO* stratum oriens; *SR* stratum radiatum; *SP* stratum pyramidale; Scale bars –25 μm)

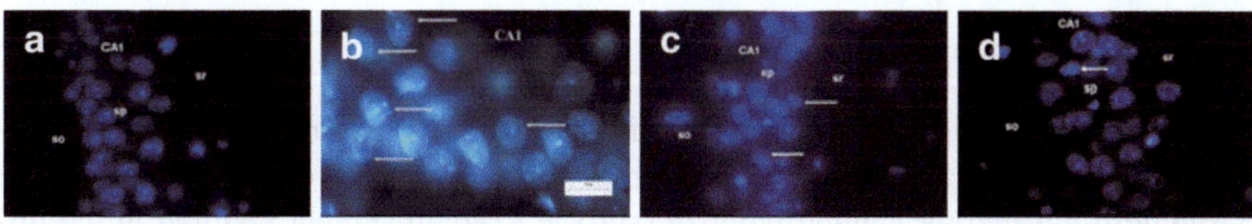

Fig. 14.2 High power photomicrographs of DAPI stained coronal sections of **a** Ovary intact adult; **b** OVX adult; **c** aged (24 months), and **d** OVX+E2 adult rat hippocampus CA1 showing the nuclear morphology of CA1 pyramidal neurons. Certain cardinal features of apoptosis like juxtamembranous condensation and clumping of chromatin material (*arrows*), membrane 'blebbing' etc., were displayed by the nuclei of some of the pyramidal neurons of experimental groups. (*SO* stratum oriens; *SR* stratum radiatum; *SP* stratum pyramidale; Scale bars –25 μm (**b**) and 50 μm (**a, c, d**))

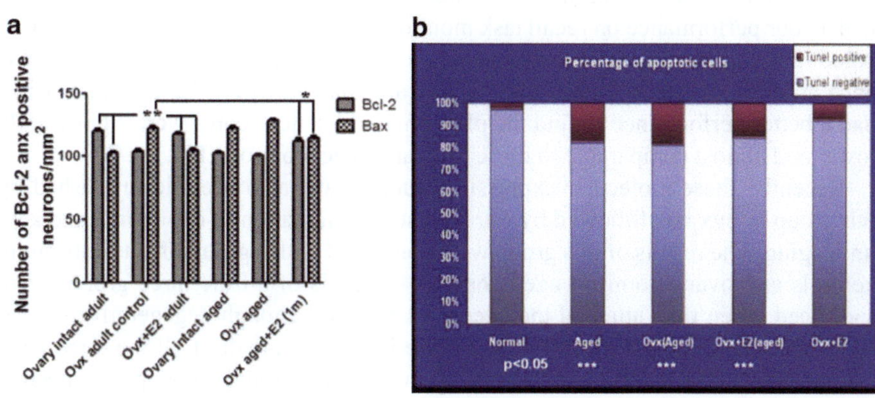

Fig. 14.3 Bar diagrams depicting **a** the number of Bcl-2 and Bax positive neurons/mm^2 and **b** percentage of apoptotic cells (TUNEL positive) in CA1-3 of hippocampus from various experimental groups. Ovariectomy or aging decreased the number of Bcl-2 positive neurons which led to a shift towards apoptotic side. 17β-estradiol (E2) treatment increased the Bcl-2 positive neurons which led to the reversal of Bcl-2:Bax ratio towards neuronal survival. Percentage of TUNEL positive cells was also increased following ovariectomy or aging. A decrease in percent apoptotic cells can be seen following E2 therapy

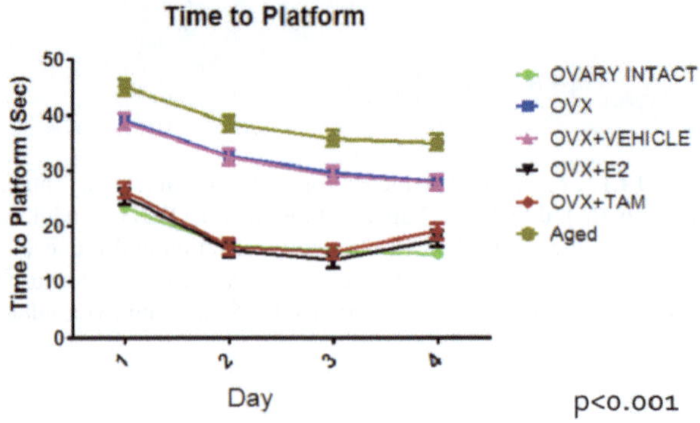

Fig. 14.4 Graph showing the time to find hidden platform in Morris water maze task for spatial reference memory. Hormone deficient rats (ovx or aged) required more time to find the platform than ovary intact or E2/TAM supplemented ovx rats

Also, the synaptic activity in estrogen deficit (ovx or naturally aged) rat hippocampus was significantly decreased as observed with the expression of presynaptic nerve terminal marker synaptophyysin (syp). E2 replenishment resulted in the up-regulation of synaptophysin activity in ovx rat hippocampus. We have also investigated the p-CREB expression in the hippocampus of these experimental animals and observed a decrease in CREB phosphorylation after ovariectomy or aging, while increased CREB phosphorylation was observed in E2 supplemented ovx rats (Sharma et al. 2007). These observations are consistent with other findings where p-CREB is reported to have increased dendritic spine density (Murphy and Segal 1997) and enhanced neuronal survival in hippocampus (Jin et al. 2001). Our studies have further been substantiated by behavioral assessment of hippocampal learning and memory through Morris-water maze task performed by these experimental animals. Ovx rats had a poor performance on recall task monitored as latency to find hidden platform. Aged rats also performed in the same way and did not show any significant difference in platform latency time vis-à-vis ovx animals. However, E2 treated ovx rats had a better performance to find the platform and latency scores were significantly lower and almost comparable to those of ovary intact controls (Fig. 14.4).

Recently, these molecular expression studies have also been accomplished by our group in ovx rats followed by estrogen supplementation of one month and kept until aging. The results of this group were compared with a group of naturally aging controls and ovariectomized aged controls. Animals of all the three groups were sacrificed when they attained the age of 24 months. Though degenerative changes in neuronal cytoarchitecture were visible in hippocampaii of all the three aged groups (Fig. 14.1c, d and 14.2c), but the changes were certainly more pronounced in the ovx aged group (Fig. 14.1c). The synaptophysin, p-CREB and Bcl-2 expression was greatly downregulated in ovx aged rats than in their naturally aging counterparts or the ones with one month E2 therapy in adulthood (Fig. 14.3a). However, this treatment schedule did not seem to be of great help in fully restoring the synaptic activity and neuronal health. Results of the ovx aged control group explain the view that abrupt cessation of estrogen production may have an adverse outcome on age-related neurodegeneration and AD type dementia and that short-term estrogen

Table 14.1 Summary of the changes observed in ER expression, synaptic activity (synaptophysin expression), recall memory (Morris water maze task) and neuronal degeneration (Bcl2:Bax ratio/TUNEL positive cells) following ovaricetomy, aging and estrogen therapy in female rat hippocampus

Experimental Group (female wistar rat)	ERα–ERβ expression	Synaptic activity (synaptophysin expression)	Morris water maze task (recall memory/latency to find platform)	Bcl2:Bax ratio	Degenerative changes (cyto-architectural/nuclear morphology)
Ovx adult	↑↑	↓↓	↑↑	↓↓	++
Ovx+E2 (0.1 mg/kg, 1 month)	↓↓	↑↑	↓↓	↑↑	––
Aged	↑↑	↓↓	↑↑	↓↓	++
Ovx aged	↑↑	↓↓↓	↑↑	↓↓↓	+++
Ovx+E2 (1 month) aged[a]	↑	↓	↑	↓	+

[a] One month therapy following ovariectomy and allowed to age thereafter

replenishment after ovariectomy may not support the hormone`s neuroprotective effects for a longer period in due course of aging. These findings raise a need to formulate a long-term estrogen therapy to obtain consistent neuroprotective effects of the hormone throughout aging of the female brain. These observations from the experimental animal model of postmenopausal aging are summarized in Table 14.1.

Wappler et al. (2010) have also investigated neuroprotective efficacy of a single high dose of estradiol (4 mg/kg b.w.) pre-treatment in young (4 months), middle-aged (9 months) and old (18 months) female gerbils following 10 min global brain ischemia. In this study, both apoptotic and necrotic cells were quantified and a battery of behavioral tests were done for functional assessment of efficacy of a single dose of estradiol in ischemic gerbil hippocampus. Estradiol pre-treatment ensued in significant neuroprotection against hippocampal cell loss in all experimental age groups. Estrogen improved memory performances in all the behavioral tests at each of the experimental ages. However, age-related differences were observed in behavioral tests. It is thus obvious that age of the experimental animals may affect the outcome of E2 therapy following brain ischemia.

14.5 Neurodegeneration, Immune Response and Estrogen

Acute and chronic inflammation in brain areas is supposed to play an important role in a number of brain functions including learning and memory and also in age related neurodegenerative processes underlying the progress of brain disorders. Brain aging and neurodegeneration are closely related to immune processes originating either in the central nervous system or invading the brain from the periphery. Microglia and astrocytes in the brain also produce different interleukins and cytokines, which respond to injury and degenerative pathologies. Many of the inflammatory cytokines generally associated with the peripheral immune system are found and produced within the central nervous system (Pan et al. 1998;Toulmond et al. 1996). Neurons can also endogenously produce cytokines in the brain apart from their primary originating source of immune system (Gahring et al 1996). The production of cytokines in CNS can be stimulated by peripheral cytokines. In the CNS, cytokines instigate their effects through both the cross-talk with their receptors (expressed by both glial and neuronal cells) and modulation of neurotransmitter receptor function. For instance, IL-1 modulates GABA receptors and enhances the inhibitory response. Synaptic plasticity is modulated by both IL-1 and IL-6 through inhibiting long-term potentiation. Moreover, TNF-α has been reported to modulate the neuronal response of NMDA activated glutamate receptors (GluR). Excessive NMDA receptor activation results in neuronal death through excitotoxicity. Neuronal cell death in ischemia, trauma, and neurodegenerative diseases is largely a result of excitotoxicity. Antioxidants, growth factors and certain cytokines protect against excitotoxicity, either through directly modulating receptor function or indirectly through inhibiting key metabolic steps subsequent to GluR activation. Further, TNF-α receptor deficient mice have greater vulnerability to ischemic brain damage following arterial occlusion, indicating the neuroprotective role of TNF-α in brain (Carlson et al 1999). Post-menopausal decline of estrogen has been postulated to lead to elevation of proinflammatory cytokines and estrogen replacement therapy restores the cytokine to normal levels in blood serum (Porter 2001; Fahlman 2000). Although mechanisms responsible for this beneficial effect of estrogen have not been completely elucidated, certain studies suggest that estrogen replacement therapy (ERT) lowers the production of proinflammatory cytokines such as IL-6 in postmenopausal women (Saucedo 2002). In rodents also, estropausal aging has been associated with increased secretion of pro-inflammatory cytokines such as interleukin-6 (Ye and Johnson 2001; Godbout and Johnson 2004) and decreased secretion of anti-inflammatory cytokines, such as interleukin-10 (Ye and Johnson 2001). The mechanism of neuroprotective effects augmented by estrogen may include anti-inflammatory responses and may change i) the levels of various cytokines (interferonγ, tumor necrosis factorα, different types of interleukins) and ii) the function of microglia as the only immune competent cells housed in the central nervous system. Varying levels of cytokines in brain areas between ovx state, aging and following hormone therapy will serve as an approach to systematically address inflammatory pathophysiological changes in age related neurodegenerative disorders. Comparison of various signaling molecules, receptor proteins and cytokines in specified brain areas in the course of aging and followed by estrogen and other drug therapies may provide evidence and explanations of changes in behavioral, cognitive and motor functions. This will serve as an approach to systematically address pathophysiological changes at the protein level in age related neurodegenerative disorders.

14.6 Selective Estrogen Receptor Modulators (SERMs)

It is now known that most of the cellular effects of E2 are mediated through its binding to ERs. Furthermore, the action of E2 is inhibited by certain synthetic chemical analogs as they avidly bind to the ERs and thereby preventing their activation. This class of chemical compounds (anti-estrogens) has been successfully used in the treatment and prevention of breast cancer in women (Halbreich and Kahn 2000). Among the list of anti-estrogens, tamoxifen (TAM) is the most widely and commonly used therapeutic agent. However, its anti-estrogenic property is not seen in uterus and bone; instead, it behaves as an agonist in these tissues. This bimodal characteristic of TAM can be explained by the fact that it selectively modulates ER in the body. Such a drug that mimics the activity of the natural hormone, 17β-estradiol in some tissues (e.g. skeletal tissue) while opposing the action of the hormone in other tissues (e.g. breast tissue) is known as Selective Estrogen Receptor Modulator (SERM). TAM has been widely employed in the treatment of breast cancer, but its bio-character in brain remains largely unknown, particularly in context of its neuroprotective role. Before one takes a look at the biological effects of SERMs, it is imperative to know why an estrogen-agonist behaves as an agonist and why an estrogen-antagonist behaves as an antagonist following its binding to ligand-binding domains of ER. The most important information regarding this phenomenon has been made available from the 3-Dimensional (3D) crystallographic studies (Littleton-Kearney et al. 2002). However, factors that make the ER to adopt certain tissue specific structural differences, thereby exhibiting mixed agonist/antagonist responses following the coupling of TAM to ER still remains elusive. Besides being used as a therapeutic agent for breast cancer, the biological character of TAM in the central nervous system is not yet fully understood. Recently, the role of TAM as a neuroprotectant in experimental model systems of neurodegeneration and ischemic insults has received a lot of attention. It has been shown that TAM administration prevents neuronal loss in the hilar region of the hippocampus following cytotoxic insults (kainic acid induction) to OVX rats (Ciriza et al. 2004). Moreover, partial reversal of hippocampal damage (revealed by bilateral cell count) was observed in four vessels occluded (global ischemia) male Wistar rats following TAM administration (Bagetta et al. 2004). The same bio-character of TAM has been observed in our experiments on ovx rats where synaptic plasticity and neuroprotection was restored (Sharma et al. 2007, Sharma and Mehra 2008). Furthermore, TAM has still not been investigated in brain aging especially at different stages of menopause (viz. perimenopause, middle age and aged). It can also provide greater understanding on the role of chronic E2 or TAM therapy influencing hippocampal function.

14.7 Where to Go

Extensive review of the estrogenic actions in female brain areas involved with learning, memory and cognition has so far provided understanding of its mechanism of action in female brain. Age associated effects of this hormone are still not clear as to how it could behave postmenopausally where no therapy is initiated at perimenopause phase. These assumptions may put some light on the varying effects of diverse doses of estrogen at different stages during aging. Future studies should be planned to explore the effects and mechanism of action of different doses of various estrogenic ligands, because of their varying potency, in middle aged (perimenopausal) and aged (postmenopause) female brain. This approach will further help to identify designer estrogenic ligands of tissue specific nature and strength and their targeted delivery where outweighing risk factors will be insignificant for institution of a better estrogen therapy for age related neurological disorders in postmenopausal women.

References

Baron-Cohen S, Knickmeyer RC, Belmonte MK (2005) Sex differences in the brain: implications for explaining autism. Science 310:819–823

Bagetta G, Chiappetta O, Amantea D, Iannone M, Rotiroti D, Costa A, Nappi G, Corasaniti MT (2004) Estradiol reduces cytochrome c translocation and minimizes hippocampal damage caused bytransient global ischemia in rat. Neurosci Lett 368:87–91

Baumgartner RN, Waters DL, Gallagher D, Morley JE, Garry PJ (1999) Predictors of skeletal muscle mass in elderly men and women. Mech Aging Dev 107(2):123–136

Behl C, Skutella T, Lezoualc'h F, Post A, Widmann M, Newton CJ, Holsboer F (1997) Neuroprotection against oxidative stress by estrogens: structure-activity relationship. Mol Pharmacol 51(4):535–41

Behl C, Moosmann B, Manthey D, Heck S (2000) The female sex hormone oestrogen as neuroprotectant: activities at various levels. Novartis Found Symp 230:221–234

Belcher SM, Zsarnovszky A (2001) Estrogenic actions in the brain: estrogen, phytoestrogens, and rapid intracellular signaling mechanisms. J Pharmacol Exp Ther 299(2):408–414

Belcredito S, Vegeto E, Brusadelli A, Ghisletti S, Mussi P, Ciana P, Maggi A (2001) Estrogen neuroprotection: the involvement of the Bcl-2 binding protein BNIP2. Brain Res Brain Res Rev 37(1–3):335–342

Cahill L (2006) Why sex matters for neuroscience. Nat Rev Neurosci 7:477–484

Carlson NG, Wieggel WA, Chen J, Bacchi A, Rogers SW, Gahring LC (1999) Inflammatory cytokines IL-1α, IL-1β, IL-6, and TNF-α impart neuroprotection to an excitotoxin through distinct pathways1. J Immunol 163(7):3963–3968

Ciriza I, Carrero P, Azcoitia I, Lundeen SG, Garcia-Segura LM (2004) Selective estrogen receptor modulators protect hippocampal neurons from kainic acid excitotoxicity: differences with the effect of estradiol. J Neurobiol 61:209–221

Cantuti-Castelvetri I, Keller-McGandy C, Bouzou B, Asteris G, Clark TW, Frosch MP, and Standaert DG (2007) Effects of gender on nigral gene expression and parkinson disease. Neurobiol Dis 26:606–614

Cosgrove KP, Mazure CM, and Staley JK (2007) Evolving knowledge of sex differences in brain structure, function, and chemistry. Biol Psychiatry 62:847–855

Couse JF, Korach KS (1999) Estrogen receptor null mice: what have we learned and where will they lead us. Endocr Rev 20(3):358–417

Dewing P, Chiang CW, Sinchak K, Sim H, Fernagut PO, Kelly S, Chesselet MF, Micevych PE, Albrecht KH, Harley VR, et al. (2006) Direct regulation of adult brain function by the male-specific factor SRY. Curr Biol 16:415–420

Dubal DB, Kashon ML, Pettigrew LC, Ren JM, Finklestein SP, Rau SW, Wise PM (1998) Estradiol protects against ischemic injury. J Cereb Blood Flow Metab 18(11):1253–1258

Fahlman MM, Boardley D, Flynn MG, Bouillon LE, Lambert CP, Braun WA (2000) Effects of hormone replacement therapy on selected indices of immune function in postmenopausal women. Gynecol Obstet Invest 50(3):189–193

Falkenstein E, Tillmann HC, Christ M, Feuring M, Wehling M (2000) Multiple actions of steroid hormones--a focus on rapid, nongenomic effects. Pharmacol Rev 52(4):513–556

Fillit H, Weinreb H, Cholst I, Luine V, McEwen B, Amador R, Zabriskie J (1986) Observations in a preliminary open trial of estradiol therapy for senile dementia-Alzheimer's type. Psychoneuroendocrinology 11:337–345

Gahring LC, Carlson NG, Kulmar RA, Rogers SW (1996) Neuronal expression of tumor necrosis factor a in the murine brain. Neuroimmunomodulation 3:289

Giguère V, Yang N, Segui P, Evans RM (1988) Identification of a new class of steroid hormone receptors. Nature 331(6151):91–94

Godbout JP, Johnson RW (2004) Interleukin-6 in the aging brain. J Neuroimmunol 147(1-2):141–144

Gollapudi L, Oblinger MM (1999) Estrogen and NGF synergistically protect terminally differentiated, ERalpha-transfected PC12 cells from apoptosis. J Neurosci Res 1;56(5):471–481

Green PS, Simpkins JW (2000) Neuroprotective effects of estrogens: potential mechanisms of action. Int J Dev Neurosci 18:347–358

Gridley KE, Green PS, Simpkins JW (1997) Low concentrations of estradiol reduce beta-amyloid (25-35)-induced toxicity, lipid peroxidation and glucose utilization in human SK-N-SH neuroblastoma cells. Brain Res 778(1):158–165

Gu Q, Moss RL (1996) 17 beta-Estradiol potentiates kainate-induced currents via activation of the cAMP cascade. J Neurosci 16(11):3620–3629

Halbreich U, Kahn LS (2000) Selective oestrogen receptor modulators--current and future brain and behaviour applications. Expert Opin Pharmacother 1:1385–1398

Henderson VW (2008) Cognitive changes after menopause: influence of estrogen. Clin Obstet Gynecol 51(3):618–626

Horsburgh K, Macrae IM, Carswell H (2002) Estrogen is neuroprotective via an apolipoprotein E-dependent mechanism in a mouse model of global ischemia. J Cereb Blood Flow Metab 22(10):1189–1195

Jin K, Mao XO, Simon RP, Greenberg DA (2001) Cyclic AMP response element binding protein (CREB) and CREB binding protein (CBP) in global cerebral ischemia. J Mol Neurosci 16(1):49–56

Kobayashi Y, Shinozawa T (1997) Effect of dibutyrylcAMP and several reagents on apoptosis in PC12 cells induced by a sialoglycopeptide from bovine brain. Brain Res 778(2):309–317

Kuiper GG, Enmark E, Pelto-Huikko M, Nilsson S, Gustafsson JA (1996) Cloning of a novel receptor expressed in rat prostate and ovary. Proc Natl Acad Sci U S A 93(12):5925–5930

Littleton-Kearney MT, Ostrowski NL, Cox DA, Rossberg MI, Hurn, PD (2002) Selective estrogen receptor modulators: tissue actions and potential for CNS protection. CNS Drug Rev 8:309–330

Mangelsdorf DJ, Thummel C, Beato M, Herrlich P, Schütz G, Umesono K, Blumberg B, Kastner P, Mark M, Chambon P, Evans RM (1995) The nuclear receptor superfamily: the second decade. Cell 83(6):835–839

Matejuk A, Adlard K, Zamora A, Silverman M, Vandenbark AA, Offner H (2001) 17 beta-estradiol inhibits cytokine, chemokine, and chemokine receptor mRNA expression in the central nervous system of female mice with experimental autoimmune encephalomyelitis. J Neurosci Res 65(6):529–542

Matsuda J, Vanier MT, Saito Y, Suzuki K, Suzuki K (2001)Dramatic phenotypic improvement during pregnancy in a genetic leukodystrophy: estrogen appears to be a critical factor. Hum Mol Genet 10(23):2709–2715

McArthur S, McHale E, and Gillies GE (2007a) The size and distribution of midbrain dopaminergic populations are permanently altered by perinatal glucocorticoid exposure in a sex- region- and time-specific manner. Neuropsychopharmacology 32:1462–1476

McCarthy MM and Konkle AT (2005) When is a sex difference not a sex difference? Front Neuroendocrinol 26:85–102

McEwen BS (2001) Estrogens effects on the brain: multiple sites and molecular mechanisms. J Appl Physiol 91(6):2785–2801

Mehra RD, Sharma K, Nyakas C, Vij U (2005) Estrogen receptor alpha and beta immunoreactive neuron in normal adult and aged female rat hippocampus: a qualitative and qunatitative study. Brain Research 1056:22–35

Mitchner NA, Garlick C, Ben-Jonathan N (1998) Cellular distribution and gene regulation of estrogen receptors alpha and beta in the rat pituitary gland. Endocrinology 139(9):3976–3983

Moosmann B, Behl C (1999) The antioxidant neuroprotective effects of estrogens and phenolic compounds are independent from their estrogenic properties. Proc Natl Acad Sci U S A 96(16):8867–8872

Morley JE (2001) Androgens and aging. Maturitas 38(1): 61–71

Murphy DD, Segal M (1997) Morphological plasticity of dendritic spines in central neurons is mediated by activation of cAMP response element binding protein. Proc Natl Acad Sci 94(4):1482–1487

Neurgaren BL, Kraines RJ (1965) Menopausal symptoms in women of various ages. Psycho Med 27:266–273

Osterlund M, Kuiper GG, Gustafsson JA, Hurd YL (1998) Differential distribution and regulation of estrogen receptor-alpha and -beta mRNA within the female rat brain. Brain Res Mol Brain Res 54(1):175–180

Paech K, Webb P, Kuiper GG, Nilsson S, Gustafsson J, Kushner PJ, Scanlan TS (1997) Differential ligand activation of estrogen receptors ERalpha and ERbeta at AP1 sites. Science 277(5331):1508–1510

Pan W, Zadina JE, Harlan RE, Weber JT, Banks WA, Kastin AJ (1998) Tumor necrosis factor-α: a neuromodulator. Endocrinology 139(9):3976–3983

Pike CJ (1999) Estrogen modulates neuronal Bcl-xL expression and beta-amyloid-induced apoptosis: relevance to Alzheimer's disease. J Neurochem 72(4):1552–1563

Pike CJ, Rosario ER, Nguyen TV (2006) Androgens, aging, and Alzheimer's disease. Endocrine 29(2): 233–241

Porter VR, Greendale GA, Schocken M, Zhu X, Effros RB (2001) Immune effects of hormone replacement therapy in post-menopausal women. Exp Gerontol 36(2):311–326

Rosario ER, Pike CJ (2008) Androgen regulation of beta-amyloid protein and the risk of Alzheimer's disease. Brain Res Rev 57(2): 444–453

Saucedo R, Rico G, Basurto L, Ochoa R, Zárate A (2002) Transdermal estradiol in menopausal women depresses interleukin-6 without affecting other markers of immune response. Gynecol Obstet Invest 53(2):114–117

Segal M, Murphy DD (1998) CREB activation mediates plasticity in cultured hippocampal neurons. Neural Plast 6(3):1–7

Sharma K, Mehra RD. (2008) Long-term administration of estrogen or tamoxifen to ovariectomized rats affords neuroprotection to hippocampal neurons by modulating the expression of Bcl-2 and Bax. Brain Res 1204:1–15

Sharma K, Mehra RD, Dhar P, Vij U (2007) Chronic exposure to estrogen and tamoxifen regulates synaptophysin and phosphorylated cAMP response element-binding (CREB) protein expression in CA1 of ovariectomized rat hippocampus. Brain Res 1132(1):10–19

Sherwin BB (1988) Estrogen and/or androgen replacement therapy and cognitive functioning in surgically menopausal women. Psychoneuroendocrinology 13:345–357

Sherwin BB (2000) Oestrogen and cognitive function throughout the female lifespan. Novartis Found. Symp 230:188–196

Singer CA, Rogers KL, Dorsa DM (1998) Modulation of Bcl-2 expression: a potential component of estrogen protection in NT2 neurons. Neuroreport 9(11):2565–2568

Singer CA, Figueroa-Masot XA, Batchelor RH, Dorsa DM (1999) The mitogen-activated protein kinase pathway mediates estrogen neuroprotection after glutamate toxicity in primary cortical neurons. J Neurosci 19(7):2455–2463

Swaab DF (2004) Sexual differentiation of the human brain: relevance for gender identity, transsexualism and sexual orientation. Gynecol Endocrinol 19:301–312

Szegõ EM, Barabás K, Balog J, Szilágyi N, Korach KS, Juhász G, Abrahám IM (2006) Estrogen induces estrogen receptor alpha-dependent cAMP response element-binding protein phosphorylation via mitogen activated protein kinase pathway in basal forebrain cholinergic neurons in vivo. J Neurosci 26(15):4104–4110

Tsai MJ, O'Malley BW (1994) Molecular mechanisms of action of steroid/thyroid receptor superfamily members. Annu Rev Biochem 63:451–486

Toulmond S, Parnet P, Linthorst AC (1996) When cytokines get on your nerves: cytokine networks and CNS pathologies. Trends Neurosci 19:409

Vegeto E, Belcredito S, Etteri S, Ghisletti S, Brusadelli A, Meda C, Krust A, Dupont S, Ciana P, Chambon P, Maggi A (2003) Estrogen receptor-alpha mediates the brain antiinflammatory activity of estradiol. Proc Natl Acad Sci U S A 100(16):9614–9619

Wappler EA, Szilágyi G, Gál A, Skopál J, Nyakas C, Nagy Z, Felszeghy K (2009) Adopted cognitive tests for gerbils: Validation by studying aging and ischemia. Physiol Behav 97:107–114

Wappler EA, Felszeghy K, Szilágyi G, Gál A, Skopál J, Mehra RD, Nyakas C, Nagy Z (2010) Neuroprotective effects of estrogen treatment on ischemia-induced behavioural deficits in ovariectomized gerbils at different ages. Behav Brain Res 209(1):42–48

Wappler EA, Felszeghy K, Varshney M, Mehra RD, Nyakas C, Nagy Z (2011) Brain plasticity following ischemia: effect of estrogen and other cerebroprotective drugs. In: Balestrino M (ed) Brain ischemia: Book 2. InTech – Open Access Publisher, ISBN 979-953-307-734-4

Watters JJ, Dorsa DM (1998) Transcriptional effects of estrogen on neuronal neurotensin gene expression involve cAMP/protein kinase A-dependent signaling mechanisms. J Neurosci 18(17):6672–6680

Weaver CE Jr, Park-Chung M, Gibbs TT, Farb DH (1997) 17beta-Estradiol protects against NMDA-induced excitotoxicity by direct inhibition of NMDA receptors. Brain Res 761(2):338–341

Weissman BA, Daly JW, Skolnick P (1975) Diethylstilbestrol-elicited accumulation of cyclic AMP in incubated rat hypothalamus. Endocrinology 97(6):1559–1566

Wilson CA and Davies DC (2007) The control of sexual differentiation of the reproductive system and brain. Reproduction 133:331–359

Ye SM, Johnson RW (2001) An age-related decline in interleukin-10 may contribute to the increased expression of interleukin-6 in brain of aged mice. Neuroimmunomodulation 9(4):183–192

Zhou Y, Watters JJ, Dorsa DM (1996) Estrogen rapidly induces the phosphorylation of the cAMP response element binding protein in rat brain. Endocrinology 137(5):2163–2166

Chapter 15
Potential Therapeutic Targets for Improving Memory Impairments and Dementia: Clues Obtained from Memory-Enhanced Mice

Shogo Endo

Abstract Memory, the basis for behaviours and thoughts, has been a major research subject in philosophy and psychology for centuries. The presence of memory, however, was scientifically proved to be the fruits of brain functions only a half century ago. Since then, memory and central nervous system have become a focal subject of biological research; however, it was a few decades ago when flexibility of brain function (i.e., neuronal plasticity) was demonstrated electrophysiologically. The rapid development of molecular biology has provided important tools, such as genetically modified mice, to elucidate the molecular mechanisms underlying learning and memory and neuronal plasticity in the central nervous system. In this review, a brief history of memory research and the basic concept of memory in psychology are presented. Then, current research on memory mechanisms using genetically modified mice including our ICER mutant mice, is discussed. Finally, based on the developments emerging from research using genetically modified mice, potential molecular targets are proposed for ameliorating memory impairments and dementia.

Keywords: Alzheimer's disease • cAMP • CREB • CREM • Gene regulation • Genetically modified mice • ICER • Learning • Memory • PKA

15.1 Introduction

Memory is the essential basis for higher cognitive functions. Thoughts, emotions, and languages supported by memory are involved in our daily behaviour in many ways and contribute to the formation of our personality. Memory, therefore, is an indispensable function of the central nervous system for a biological human to become a human being. Diseases that compromise this biology compromise one's

S. Endo (✉)
Aging Regulation Research Team, Tokyo Metropolitan Institute of Gerontology, Itabashi, Tokyo 173-0015, Japan
e-mail: sendo@tmig.or.jp

M. K. Thakur, S. I. S. Rattan (eds.), *Brain Aging and Therapeutic Interventions*,
DOI 10.1007/978-94-007-5237-5_15,

very being. Thus, dementia and memory impairments associated with a variety of diseases and brain injuries have a huge impact on the lives of patients with these disorders. Decline in memory also occurs with normal aging.

As aging populations continue to grow around the world, overcoming and delaying the onset of memory impairment through therapeutic interventions are an ongoing task for biomedical research. To tackle this problem, a huge amount of basic research on learning and memory is aimed at identifying the molecular targets for future memory-enhancing drugs. Despite major advances in this arena, there are still no clear answers to several basic questions: How is sensory information acquired? How and where is information stored? Once stored, how is stored information recalled or how does it become inaccessible or lost?

Memory has been an important subject of inquiry since the days of the Greek philosopher Socrates (Plato 2004, 2007, 2010a, b). The experimental characterization of memory systems had its start in modern psychology with Herman Ebbinghaus (1885). Nearly 65 years later, Donald Hebb (1949) posited that flexibility (plasticity) of the nervous system underlies cellular mechanisms for memory. However, it was not until the 1970s and 1980s that discoveries of neuronal plasticity (Bliss and Lømo 1973; Ito 2011) ignited the explosion of investigations of molecules involved in neuronal plasticity and memory (Milner et al. 1998; Kandel 2001).

Neurological diseases—including schizophrenia, bipolar disorders, Alzheimer's disease and Parkinson's disease—not only impair cognitive functions (Kidd 2008; Danion et al. 2007; Pfennig et al. 2007; Tröster 2008), but also significantly affect learning and memory (for reviews, see Kidd 2008; Danion et al. 2007; Pfennig et al. 2007; Tröster 2008). Modern research on diseases that affect the central nervous system has developed in order to identify the causal relationships between a particular disease and gene(s), protein(s), neurotransmitter(s), and brain region(s) (neuronal circuitry). A series of studies provided not only basic information on several diseases but also revealed the mechanisms underlying memory. Furthermore, based on these results, a variety of genetically modified animal models, such as mice, *Drosophila* and *C. elegans*, have been generated and studied in detail to elucidate the mechanisms underlying higher cognitive functions including learning and memory.

During the course of research using genetically modified animals, researchers discovered animals that display enhanced cognitive functions. Among these discoveries were memory-enhanced mice, which have become valuable tools, not only for basic memory research but also for the development of therapeutic strategies geared toward enhancing memory.

In this review, first, memory as viewed through the lenses of philosophy and psychology will be discussed. This presentation will include a brief summary of memory classification in psychological terms and neuronal plasticity as a cellular substrate for memory. Second, recent research on genetically modified mice will be discussed. Our recent findings on memory-enhanced inducible cAMP early repressor (ICER) mutant mice will also be discussed. Finally, novel approaches will be discussed for treating memory impairment and dementia.

15.2 The Past—Memory Research in Philosophy and Psychology

15.2.1 Memory in Philosophy

In the fourth century B.C., Socrates made the bold claim that the recording of facts and thoughts in written documents was destroying our memory. He believed that thoughts in written words were "dead words because words do not allow an objection ... [and] written words lack flexibility. Thoughts and discussion need memory in individuals." According to Socrates, it was dangerous to rely on written records of thoughts rather than on one's own memory (Plato 2010b). Because he abhorred written documents, Socrates did not record his own works in written form. It is ironic that Socrates' students, who apparently did not subscribe to his ideas, documented his words in writing, providing us with a tangible record of his thoughts on memory.

Plato, a student of Socrates, defined sensation as the simultaneous movement of the soul and the physical body (Plato 2004). He believed that the purpose of memory is to retain the movement of sensation and that memory belongs to the soul (Plato 2010a). Memory is recorded by stamping the sensation on the wax tablet of our soul (Plato 2007). As long as the sensation is embedded within the wax tablet, we are able to recall the memory of that sensation.

Aristotle, a student of Plato, used memory to judge the superiority of an animal to another animal: "By nature animals are born with the faculty of sensation, and from sensation, memory is produced in some of them, though not in others. And, therefore, the former is more intelligent and apt at learning than those which cannot remember" (Aristotle 2012b). Aristotle further discussed memory in his relatively short work "On Memory and Reminiscence" (Aristotle 2012a).

Regarding Aristotle's superior-inferior hypothesis of animals, we now know that all animal species, from *C. elegans* to human, can form memories, and we know that memory is an essential function if animals are to survive in an ever-changing environment. Although the essential and important role of memory has been studied in philosophical terms for centuries, our understanding of the scientific nature of memory emerged relatively recently with the advent of modern psychology.

15.2.2 Memory in Psychology

Psychology, as with philosophy, considers memory to be an important basis for behaviour. Hence, memory has been a major subject of psychological research since the dawn of modern psychology in late nineteenth century. In 1885, German psychologist Hermann Ebbinghaus (1885) published the first scientific report on memory. Since Ebbinghaus' seminal research, new research methods for studying memory have been developed. Psychological steps comprising memory were char-

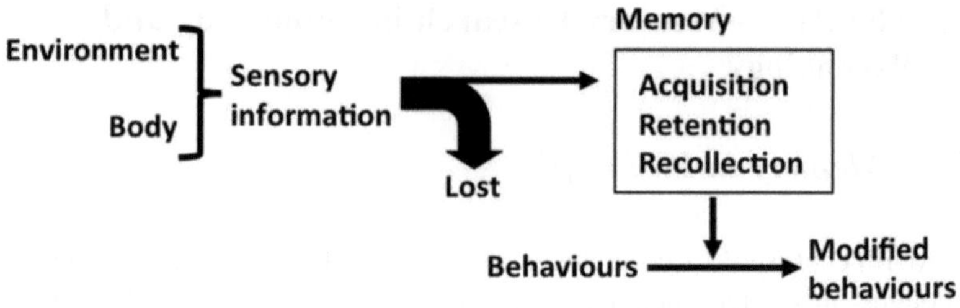

Fig. 15.1 Sensory information, memory, and behaviorus. Huge amounts of sensory information flow through our nervous system to the brain, although most are lost within a second, a fraction of the sensory information is stored as memory. Memory comprises three steps: the acquisition of sensory information, the retention of information in a storable form, and the recollection of the stored information. As memory modifies behaviorus, memory can be examined by observing modified behaviours

acterized. Then, classifications and definitions of memory were proposed. There are several ways to define memory. One definition is: "A relatively long-lasting change in behaviour brought about by experience." The evaluation of memory is possible only by observing modified "behaviours."

Sensory information from inside and outside of our body is received by peripheral sensory receptors, which transmit this information through the nervous system to the brain. The brain processes this information so that we can adapt to our environment. Although most sensory information is lost quickly after reception, a small fraction is retained as memory (Fig. 15.1). For memory to occur, three steps are necessary: (1) the acquisition of sensory information, (2) the retention of acquired information, and (3) the recollection of stored information. Loss of any one of these three steps prevents memory formation.

15.2.3 Classification of Memory

Psychologists have classified memory in several ways. Two typical ways of memory classification are: (1) Classification according to the period of memory retention, and (2) classification according to the content of memory. These two types of classification are described below.

15.2.3.1 Long-Term Memory and Short-Term Memory

A huge amount of sensory information from inside and outside of our body flows constantly into the sensory system (Fig. 15.1). The information is utilized for physiological responses such as maintaining body temperature and posture, avoiding hot objects, etc. The specific sensations that we attend to are then stored as short-term memory. Short-term memory is formed readily. Thus, the neuronal plasticity under-

Table 15.1 Classification of memory according to its retention duration

Retention duration	Acquisition	Capacity	Interference after memory acquisition	Gene regulation	Responsible mechanisms
Seconds to minutes (short-term memory)	Easy	Small	Fragile	Not required	Protein modifications, altered receptor and channel activity, changes in cellular pH, changes in ion concentration
Hours to lifetime (long-term memory)	Difficult	Large	Resistant	Required	Morphological changes in neurons and synapses

lying short-term memory is supported in neurons by rapidly unfolding biochemical alterations, such as equilibrium of protein modifications, alteration of protein synthesis and degradation, oxide-reduction state, and pH. A series of cellular changes may induce, for example, changes in the numbers, activity, sensitivity, and distribution of channels and receptors for neurotransmitters in synapses (Milner et al. 1998; Kandel 2001; Malenka and Bear 2004; Newpher and Ehlers 2008).

On the other hand, long-term memory can be retained for several hours and up to the lifetime of an animal. Long-term memory cannot be stored by means of biological molecules, which turnover at a high rate. Thus, the leading hypothesis for the formation of long-term memory posits that memory is stored and maintained through structural changes in neurons, such as altered numbers of synapses and/or structural changes of dendritic spines (Milner et al. 1998; Kandel 2001). These morphological changes depend on new protein synthesis (de novo protein synthesis), accomplished through gene regulation (Milner et al. 1998; Kandel 2001; Govindarajan et al. 2006). Another hypothesis posits that long-term memory is supported mainly by prolonged post-translational modification (for review, see Routtenberg 2008). As we discuss research findings on transcription factors from genetically modified mice later in this chapter, we will see how gene regulation plays an important role in long-term memory.

The conversion of sensory information or short-term memory into long-term memory is called memory consolidation. During memory consolidation, information is "fixed" as long-term memory through its connection with the pre-existing body of knowledge in the brain. Another difference between short-term and long-term memories is that long-term memory requires gene transcription and translation, whereas short-term memory does not (Milner et al. 1998; Kandel 2001). Table 15.1 summarizes other characteristics of short-term and long-term memory.

One of the obstacles we face in memory research using mammalian models is the absence of a model with an identified memory storage site (engram or memory trace). As a result, no experimental evidence exists to associate a localized structural change in mammalian brain with experimentally induced long-term memory. On the other hand, in the marine mollusc *Aplysia californica*, remarkable localized structural changes occur in association with a specific long-term memory, such as

Table 15.2 Classification of memory according to its contents

Memory	Acquisition	Description in words	Effort needed to recall
Declarative memory (semantic memory, episodic memory)	Quick	Possible	Necessary
Non-declarative memory (reflex, skills, movement, habits, procedural memory)	Slow	Difficult	Not necessary

long-term sensitization of the defensive gill withdrawal reflex (Milner et al. 1998; Kandel 2001; Bailey and Chen 1988; Bailey et al. 2004).

15.2.3.2 Declarative and Non-Declarative Memory

The second classification of memory has been done according to content, most prominently by Larry Squire. He has classified memory into declarative and non-declarative types, based on the types of behaviours influenced by acquisition of memory (Table 15.2) (Squire and Zola 1996; Milner et al. 1998; Gazzaniga 2002; Squire 2009). In simplified terms, declarative memory in humans is memory that can be described using words. Facts and events associated with information of particular time and place are examples of declarative memory. Declarative memory requires conscious effort to recall information. It is easily formed but easily lost. The hippocampus plays an important role in declarative memory (Eichenbaum et al. 1992; Milner et al. 1998; Kandel 2001; Squire and Zola 1996; Squire 2009).

In simplified terms, non-declarative memory is memory that cannot be put into words. Rather, it is procedural and in its most-studied form involves motor skills and movements, such as throwing a ball, riding a bicycle, and swimming. These tasks require coordinated movement of muscles and intensive practice. However, once a person acquires non-declarative memory, such as riding a bicycle, he/she often remembers how to ride a bicycle several decades later without any conscious effort. The cerebellum plays an essential role in non-declarative memory (Ito 2011).

15.3 The Present—Dawn of Memory Research at the Cellular and Molecular Level

Memory has been a major subject of philosophy and psychology for a long time. On the other hand, it is relatively recent that the brain was shown to hold the engram of memory (Penfield 1958; Scoville and Milner 1957; Milner et al. 1998) and that neuronal circuits possess some flexibility to accommodate memory (Bliss and Lømo 1973; Ito et al. 1982).

15.3.1 Discovery of Neuronal Plasticity

In 1949, Donald Hebb proposed in his book "The Organization of Behaviour" that the brain possesses flexibility (plasticity) that is a basis for animals' behaviour and memory (Hebb 1949). In the 1950s, Penfield (1958) presented early experimental evidence on the presence of memory in the human brain by demonstrating that memories could be recalled through the electric stimulation of a patient's medial temporal lobe during surgery. Then, Scoville and Milner (1957) reported the inability for new learning (anterograde amnesia) in patients that received lobectomy of the medial temporal lobe (including the hippocampus and associated areas) for the treatment of epileptic seizures. These observations clearly indicated that memory is processed in the brain and memory traces (engrams) are localized in the brain. This experimental evidence from human subjects greatly accelerated research on neuronal plasticity and learning and memory, and on their underlying cellular and molecular mechanisms in other animals (Eichenbaum et al. 1992; Milner et al. 1998; Kandel 2001).

15.3.1.1 Long-Term Potentiation and Long-Term Depression

In 1973, Bliss and Lømo reported their discovery of electrophysiologically induced synaptic plasticity, a kind of neuronal activity-dependent (or use-dependent) change in neurotransmission efficiency. This so-called long-term potentiation (LTP), first described in rabbit hippocampus, is an increase in neurotransmission efficiency induced by high frequency electrical stimulation of afferent fibers (Bliss and Lømo 1973).

In 1982, Masao Ito and colleagues (1982) reported on another type of neuronal plasticity called long-term depression (LTD). LTD manifests as a use-dependent reduction in neurotransmission. LTD in the cerebellum was induced by simultaneous, electrical stimulation of parallel fibers and climbing fibers at low frequency (Ito 2011). Hippocampal LTP and cerebellar LTD show that, in addition to the normal state, neuronal transmission can be potentiated or depressed. This three-way mode of neurotransmission (LTP-Normal-LTD) results in tremendous complexity in terms of possibilities of information coding using neuronal circuits.

Since the discovery that the hippocampus and associated medial temporal lobe areas are essential for the formation of long-term declarative memory in human subjects (Scoville and Milner 1957; Milner et al. 1998; Squire 2009), a huge amount of research has been carried out on hippocampal LTP. LTP has a variety of characteristics that make it an attractive and suitable cellular mechanism for declarative memory (Eichenbaum et al. 1992; Bliss and Collingridge 1993; Malenka and Bear 2004; Lynch 2004). Hippocampal LTP remains a major topic of research and discussion because of its molecular mechanisms and its role in information processing in the hippocampus (Eichenbaum et al. 1992; Bliss et al. 2003; Lynch 2004; Malenka and Bear 2004; Popov et al. 2004). There are many reviews that focus more on the role of the hippocampus in declarative memory and hippocampal neuronal plasticity (Eichenbaum et al. 1992; Bliss et al. 2003; Lynch 2004; Malenka and Bear 2004; Popov et al. 2004), and on the molecular mechanisms underlying hippocampal LTP and LTD (Mulkey et al. 1994; Silva et al. 1998; Malenka 2003; Klann and Dever 2004; Newpher and Ehlers 2008).

In a complimentary way, the importance of the cerebellum in non-declarative memory has been demonstrated also from human subjects suffering from cerebellar damage (Holmes 1939; Dow and Moruzzi 1958; Ito 2011). Albus and Marr hypothesized that cerebellar neuronal plasticity is the basis of cerebellum-dependent learning and memory (Marr 1969; Albus 1971). Ito et al. (1982) demonstrated electrophysiologically that neuronal plasticity in the form of LTD is indeed present in the cerebellum. Cerebellar LTD is the first type of neuronal plasticity that manifests as a use-dependent "depression" of neuronal transmission. The cerebellum plays roles in behaviours that require quick, accurate and smooth movements (Ito 2011). LTD is hypothesized to actively delete or depress synapses associated with wrong movements. A variety of molecules—including synaptic proteins, neurotransmitters, second messengers, and transcription factors—are required for modulating cerebellar LTD (Ito 2011).

15.3.1.2 Neuronal Plasticity to Behavioural Memory

Neuronal plasticity, such as LTP and LTD, are not memory in themselves but are simply potential cellular mechanisms that underlie behavioural memory (Eichenbaum et al. 1992; Mulkey et al. 1994; Ito 2011; Milner et al. 1998; Malenka and Bear 2004; Lynch 2004). If indeed neuronal plasticity is an underlying mechanism for memory, studies examining the molecular mechanisms responsible for neuronal plasticity may lead to the identification of pathophysiological processes related to memory impairment and dementia. Such research will identify potential molecular targets or genes, leading to the development of treatments for improving impaired memory or drugs to enhance memory in normal, healthy aging.

Figure 15.2 shows the timing of different electrophysiological, biochemical and morphological events associated with memory processes. The memory system is the mechanism by which sensory information, which is coded by brief openings (msec) of ion channels induced by neuronal activity, is converted into a storable form. This stored information, i.e., memory, can remain for minutes or last for the lifetime of an animal. The system also has the ability to retrieve readily the stored information when needed. Since the memory system has an amazing capacity to store large amounts of information (e.g., events of a lifetime) with high fidelity, each molecular step shown in Fig. 15.2 can serve as a potential target for therapeutic treatments aimed at treating diseases affecting memory.

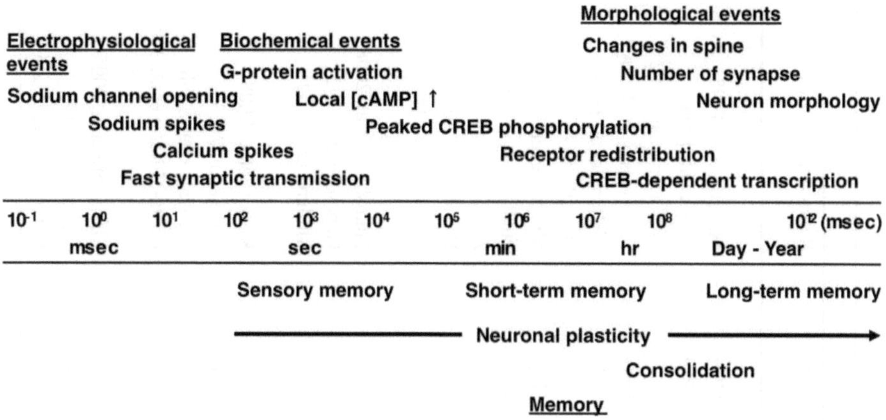

Fig. 15.2 Time course of events during memory formation. Electrophysiological, biochemical, and morphological events associated with memory formation. Neuronal activity starts with the opening of channels that lead to a series of events, ultimately to the formation of memories that can last for the lifetime of an animal. Cyclic AMP-related events are examples of biochemical events that can occur during memory formation. *CREB* cAMP responsive element binding protein

15.3.1.3 Dissection of Molecular Mechanisms Underlying Learning and Memory

In recent years, the advancements of methods to manipulate embryos, novel techniques in reproduction biology have yielded mice that lack a single protein or mice that overexpress a single protein in a particular cell type or tissue. These genetically modified mice are excellent models for studying learning and memory and neuronal plasticity, all contributing tremendously to this research field (Milner et al. 1998; Mayford and Kandel 1999; Ito 2011; Kandel 2001; Morozov et al. 2003).

A variety of genetically manipulated mice are now available: null gene knockout mice that fail to produce a single protein in all of its cells and tissues; conditional gene knockout mice that fail to express a single protein in a particular tissue or cell type during a particular stage of development. With conditional gene-knockout mice, compensatory effects occurring in null gene knockout mice during developmental stages can be avoided, and temporally- and spatially-regulated gene knockout can be achieved (Mayford and Kandel 1999; Morozov et al. 2003).

Although most genetically modified mice generated to study neuronal plasticity-related molecules exhibit impaired or reduced memory functions, some actually display enhanced memory (Table 15.3) (also see Lee and Silva 2009; Monti and Contestabile 2009). Mice with enhanced memory are called “super mice” and were first observed by Manabe et al. (1998) using their Orl1 null knockout mice. After the initial report on Orl1, memory-enhanced mice have been obtained unexpectedly (Table 15.3; also see Lee and Silva 2009). We have recently reported memory enhancement in inducible cAMP early repressor (ICER)-knockout mice (Kojima et al. 2008). The next section is devoted to a detailed review of ICER mutant mice.

Table 15.3 Some genetically modified mice lines with enhanced memory

Gene/protein	Manipulation	Memory tests[a]				
		Water maze	Fear conditioning		Plasticity	References
			Contextual	Cued		
Receptors and channels						
ORL1	KO	(+)			LTP (+)	Manabe et al. 1998
NR2B	OE	(+)	(+)	(+)	LTP (+)	Tang et al. 1999
GABAAα5	KO	(+)				Collinson et al. 2002
GRPR	KO		(+)	(+)	LTP (+)	Shumyatsky et al. 2002
5-HT1B	KO	(+)				Malleret et al. 1999
5-HT3	OE		(+)			Harrell and Allan 2003
Kvβ1.1	KO	(+)			LTP (+)	Murphy et al. 2004
RyR3	KO	(+)			LTP (+)	Futatsugi et al. 1999
Adenosine (A2)	KO	(+)				Zhou et al. 2009
α-2AR	KO			(+)		Davies et al. 2003
BEC1 (KCNH1)	KO	(+)				Miyake et al. 2009
Kinases and phosphatases						
CaMKIV	OE			(+)	LTP (+)	Fukushima et al. 2008
PP1, inducible OE of inhibitor		(+)			LTP (+)	Genoux et al. 2002
Calcineurin (PP2B), inducible OE of autoinhibitory domain		(+)		(+)	LTP (+)	Malleret et al. 2001
Transcription and translation						
ICER	KO	(+)[b]	(+)	(+)		Kojima et al. 2008
ATF4, C/EBP, inducible OE of dominant negative form		(+)			LTP (+)	Chen et al. 2003
C/EBPδ	KO		(+)			Sterneck et al. 1998
eIF2α	OE	(+)	(+)	(+)	LTP (+)	Costa-Mattioli et al. 2007
Miscellaneous						
N-Shc	KO	(+)	(+)	(+)	LTP (+)	Miyamoto et al. 2005
tPA	OE	(+)			LTP (+)	Madani et al. 1999
GAP43	OE	(+)			LTP (+)	Routtenberg et al. 2000

Table 15.3 (continued)

Gene/protein	Manipulation	Memory tests[a]			Plasticity	References
		Water maze	Fear conditioning			
			Contextual	Cued		
SOD	OE	(+)			LTP (+)	Hu et al. 2006
KChIP3	KO		(+)			Alexander et al. 2009
Glial proteins						
S100β	KO	(+)	(+)		LTP (+)	Nishiyama et al. 2002
DAAO	KO	(+)			LTP (+)	Maekawa et al. 2005
Cerebellum-dependent memory						
Delphilin	KO	Optokinetic response adaptation (+)			Cerebellar LTD (+)	Takeuchi et al. 2008
Semaphorin	KO	Motor coordination and swimming (+)				Yukawa et al. 2009
NR2B, inducible OE in granule cells		Motor coordination (+)				Jiao et al. 2008

OE overexpression, *KO* knockout, *LTP* long-term potentiation, *LTD* long-term depression

[a] (+) Indicates enhanced memory or enhanced neuronal plasticity (LTP, LTD)

[b] Borlikova, Kojima, and Endo, unpublished results

15.4 Genetically Modified Mice and Memory Enhancement

Typically, knockout of molecules is expected to yield impaired behaviour, because disruption of essential pathways often causes adverse effects in a highly regulated system. However, this is not always the case for the nervous system. Since memory is an important basis for other higher cognitive functions and for the control of organs and systems in the body, we can expect the presence of alternative, duplicate, or redundant pathways. In addition, animals seem to have a physiological "brake" or a physiological regulatory system that restrains excess neuronal functions (Abel et al. 1998; Borlikova and Endo 2009; Lee and Silva 2009). We will take a look at the latter cases for memory in genetically modified mice.

15.4.1 Inducible cAMP Early Repressor (ICER) Exerts a Powerful Constraint on Long-Term Memory

In general, gene translation and transcription is necessary for the formation of long-term memories (Milner et al. 1998; Kandel 2001). New protein synthesis is hypothesized to induce and support morphological alterations in shape and number of synapse (Milner et al. 1998; Mayford and Kandel 1999; Kandel 2001). The cAMP system is a signal transduction system well conserved throughout evolution and is shown to be important in the neuronal plasticity and memory in invertebrates such as *Aplysia californica*, *Drosophila* and also in mammals (Bourtchuladze et al. 1994; Yin et al. 1994; Frank and Greenberg 1994; Bartsch et al. 1995; Alberini et al. 1999; Schulz et al. 1999; Barco et al. 2002; Lonze and Ginty 2002; Josselyn and Nguyen 2005; Wu et al. 2007). In addition, the cAMP pathway is involved in many disorders affecting cognition, including Alzheimer's disease (Saura and Valero 2011). Although a variety of proteins and signal transduction systems are involved in memory, the cAMP system has been examined heavily in a variety of animal models of memory (Milner et al. 1998; Kandel 2001).

Cyclic AMP activates cAMP-dependent protein kinase (PKA). PKA translocates to the nucleus and phosphorylates cAMP responsive element binding protein (CREB). Phosphorylated CREB facilitates the formation of a transcription complex with CREB binding protein (CBP) and other molecules on the DNA sequence called cAMP responsive element (CRE). This results in the activation of transcription (Fig. 15.3a; Josselyn and Nguyen 2005; Wu et al. 2007). At the same time, phosphorylated CREB induces the transcription of ICER from the internal P2 promoter of the CREM gene (Fig. 15.3b). ICER has CRE-binding ability but lacks transactivation ability. Thus, ICER and phosphorylated CREB compete for CRE. This competition suppresses CREB/CREM-dependent transcription to achieve temporally and spatially regulated gene transcription (Fig. 15.3a; Molina et al. 1993; Mioduszewska et al. 2003; Borlikova and Endo 2009). We have generated ICER-

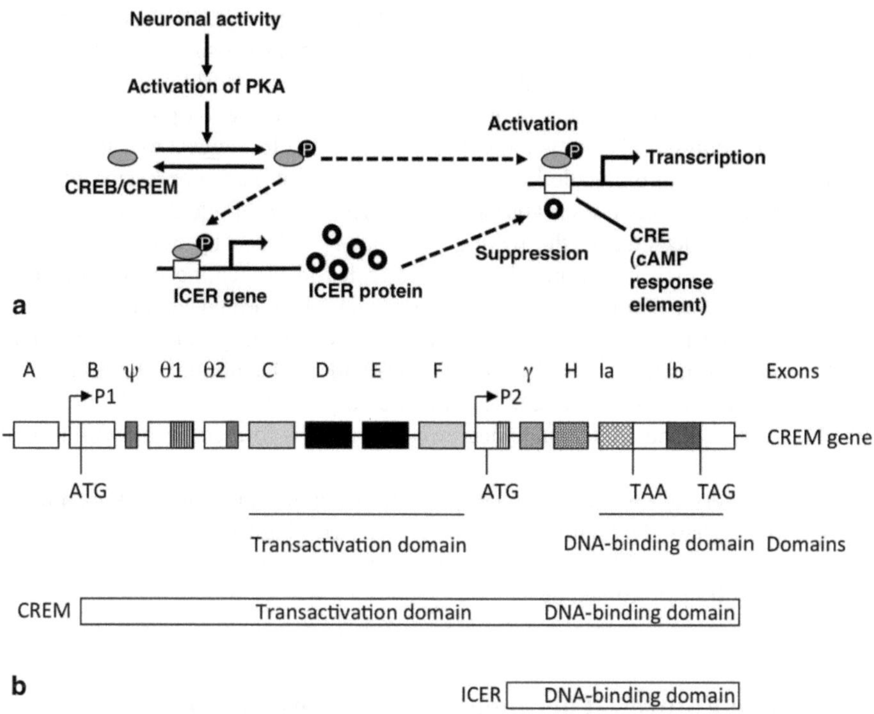

Fig. 15.3 Function and structure of inducible cAMP early repressor (ICER). **a** ICER and CREB compete for CRE. Activation of the cAMP system leads to the phosphorylation of CREB/CREM, and then phosphorylated CREB/CREM activates gene transcription. Phosphorylated CREB/CREM also induces the synthesis of ICER. Although ICER lacks the ability to activate transcription, it does have the ability to bind DNA. ICER and phosphorylated CREB/CREM compete for CRE on the gene, and ICER eventually terminates CREB/CREM-dependent gene transcription. **b** The gene and protein structure of CREMs. CREM mRNA is synthesized when the upstream promoter is used. On the other hand, ICER mRNA is synthesized using the internal P2 promoter of the CREM gene. As a result, ICER lacks a transactivation domain. *CRE* cAMP responsive element, *CREB* cAMP responsive element binding protein, *CREM* cAMP responsive element modulator, *ICER* inducible cAMP early repressor, *PKA* cAMP-dependent protein kinase

knockout mice and ICER-overexpressing mice and have characterized their general behaviours and memory (Kojima et al. 2008; Borlikova and Endo 2009).

ICER-knockout and ICER-overexpressing lines of mice show short-term fear memory similar to control mice (Kojima et al. 2008; Borlikova and Endo 2009). However, ICER-overexpressing mice display significantly reduced long-term fear memory. By contrast, ICER-knockout mice show enhanced long-term memory. Thus, manipulating the amount of ICER expressed—overexpression versus no expression—results in opposing long-term fear memory phenotypes: reduced versus enhanced memory. Since ICER gene manipulation produced (1) no changes in short-term memory, (2) significant changes in long-term memory, and (3) suppression of ICER-induced CREB-dependent transcription, these findings indicate that the manipulation of ICER expression influences the CREB-dependent gene expression necessary for long-term memory. In addition, we also observed opposite phenotypes in mice assessed with the Morris water maze (Borlikova, Kojima and Endo, unpublished results) and in mice subjected to kindling (Kojima et al. 2008), a model for neuronal plasticity and epilepsy. These results suggest that ICER is an extremely important molecule involved in the transcriptional suppression of long-term memory in the central nervous system (Borlikova and Endo 2009).

ICER is not detected in the resting state but is induced by neuronal activity. ICER seems to play important physiological roles in preventing excess memory formation, limiting it only to memories associated with neuronal activation (Kojima et al. 2008; Borlikova and Endo 2009). Excess fear memory, for example, might lead to post-traumatic stress disorder (PTSD) and hinder normal life behaviours (Heim and Nemeroff 2009). Because of the memory "brake" (i.e., ICER), however, PTSD is avoided and an adequate degree of memory is formed, leading to normal behaviours.

The discovery of a memory "brake" provides valuable clues for attacking memory impairment caused by normal aging or certain neurological diseases. We hypothesize that we may be able to enhance memory by releasing the memory brake. This hypothesis will be discussed next.

15.5 The Future—Therapeutic Clues Obtained from Memory-Enhanced Mice

A variety of diseases cause memory impairment (Danion et al. 2007; Pfennig et al. 2007; Kidd 2008; Tröster 2008). Furthermore, the inevitable process of aging often leads to decline of memory and other cognitive functions (Rosenzweig and Barnes 2003; Saura and Valero 2011). Thus, because of rapidly aging demographics, it is urgent to discover ways to improve impaired memory or to delay the onset of age- or disease-related memory decline (Lee and Silva 2009; Monti and Contestabile 2009; Saura and Valero 2011). The aim of current research is to identify the gene responsible for a particular disease, and then generate mice models based on that research. However, diseases sometimes result from multiple rather than single gene mutations; thus, the results of gene mutation experiments may not simply inform therapeutic strategies or development of targeted drugs (Lee and Silva 2009; Monti and Contestabile 2009).

Based on the results obtained from genetically modified mice, a simple working hypothesis has been formulated: loss or reduction of gene X expression improves memory when mice deficient in gene X have enhanced memory (Fig. 15.4a). Table 15.3 provides much evidence to support this hypothesis. A variety of memory-enhancing molecules exist; these reside not only in neurons but also in glial cells. Knowing the details of molecules or genes downstream from memory-enhancing molecules may not be necessary for developing therapeutics that improves memory. For example, even though we do not know the downstream genes regulated by

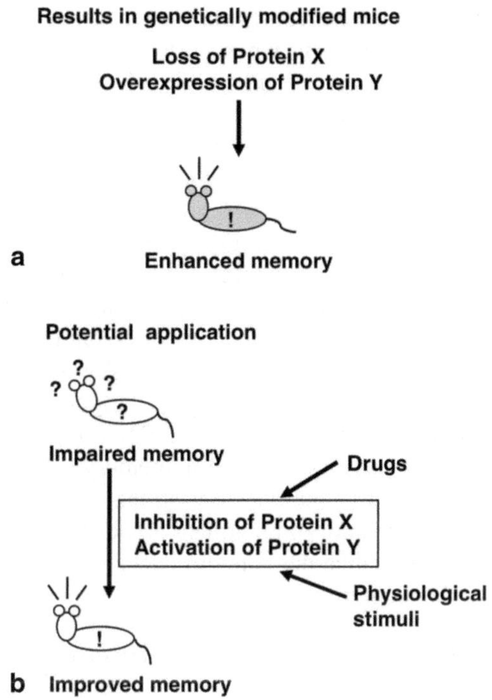

Fig. 15.4 Potential therapeutic strategy obtained from genetically modified mice. **a** Memory-enhanced mice are obtained in mice that have a protein X knockout or that overexpress protein Y. **b** Therapeutic interventions (e.g., drugs or physiological stimuli) that inhibit protein X or activate protein Y can potentially lead to improved memory

ICER, drugs that reduce the physiological function of ICER still have the potential to enhance memory (Fig. 15.4b).

Drugs targeting constitutively expressed proteins would be expected to have harmful effects, as they would alter constantly the functions of constitutive proteins in the entire body. Thus, more reasonable targets for memory improving drugs would be inducible proteins. ICER, on the other hand, is not expressed during resting states but is induced through neuronal activity (Kojima et al. 2008). Thus, any side effects resulting from the inhibition of ICER would be minor. ICER, therefore, is one of the best target candidates for the development of memory-enhancing drugs (Kojima et al. 2008; Borlikova and Endo 2009).

In summary, by critically reviewing memory-enhanced mice lines, we might be able to identify an appropriate combination of genes that can enhance memory (Lee and Silva 2009; Monti and Contestabile 2009). It is this author's desire that the discovery of compounds to modulate gene products and/or physiological stimuli will overcome memory impairments or slow down memory decline.

15.6 Epilogue

Despite the fact that a huge amount of research has been carried out on memory, there is still no example of memory in which its necessary neuronal circuit and engram have been completely established. Recent imaging techniques using PET or fMRI have greatly improved their quality, precision and resolution. These techniques, especially when performed in humans, have contributed significantly to memory research in identifying the location of brain regions activated by memory-inducing neuronal activities (Poeppel and Krause 2008). In addition, a bold project has been undertaken to map all neuronal networks by using billions of serial electron micrographs (Anderson et al. 2009). By combining data obtained from such research, we may be able to answer fundamental questions, such as what memory engram and what memory storage methods are used by the central nervous system.

At the molecular level, the recent emergence of Giga DNA sequencers (or next generation sequencers) sets the stage for obtaining the genetic information of a particular individual in a few days. On the basis of these analyses, we will be able to determine our future disease risks, and maybe even life expectancy on the day we are born (Avent et al. 2009; Toyota et al. 2009). The massive amounts of information obtained with Giga DNA sequencers will also provide us with information about genes involved in memory and genes associated with diseases affecting memory. It is our sincere wish that these modern methods lead to therapeutics for treating memory impairment associated with diseases or aging. On that occasion, we will realize the hope for successful aging by improving memory, the basis for higher cognitive functions.

Acknowledgements I thank Ms. Masako Suzuki for her tremendous technical help throughout the research project and Dr. Shuichi Yanai for the critical reading of an early draft of the manuscript. This work was supported in part by the Naito Foundation, MEXT of Japan, and Japan Foundation for Aging and Health.

References

Abel T, Martin KC, Bartsch D, Kandel ER (1998) Memory suppressor genes: inhibitory constraints on the storage of long-term memory. Science 279:338–341

Alberini CM, Ghirardi M, Huang YY, Nguyen PV, Kandel ER (1999) A molecular switch for the consolidation of long-term memory: cAMP-inducible gene expression. Ann N Y Acad Sci 758:261–286

Albus JS (1971) A theory of cerebellar function. Math Biosci 10:25–61

Alexander JC, McDermott CM, Tunur T, Rands V, Stelly C, Karhson D, Bowlby MR, An WF, Sweatt JD, Schrader LA (2009) The role of calsenilin/DREAM/KChIP3 in contextual fear conditioning. Learn Mem 16:167–177

Anderson JR, Jones BW, Yang J-H, Shaw MV, Watt CB, Koshevoy P, Spaltenstein J, Jurrus E, Kannan UV, Whitaker RT, Mastronarde D, Tasdizen T, Marc RE (2009) A computational framework for ultrastructural mapping of neural circuitry. PLoS Biol 7:e1000074

Aristotle (2012a) On memory and reminiscence (trans: Beare JI), eBooks@Adelaide. http://ebooks.adelaide.edu.au/a/aristotle/memory/. Accessed Nov 2012

Aristotle (2012b) Metaphysics, Book I (trans: Ross WD), eBooks@Adelaide, http://ebooks.adelaide.edu.au/a/aristotle/metaphysics/index.html. Accessed Nov 2012

Avent ND, Madgett TE, Maddocks DG, Soothill PW (2009) Cell-free fetal DNA in the maternal serum and plasma: current and evolving applications. Curr Opin Obstet Gynecol 21:175–179

Bailey CH, Chen M (1988) Long-term memory in Aplysia modulates the total number of varicosities of single identified sensory neurons. Proc Natl Acad Sci U S A 85:2373–2377

Bailey CH, Kandel ER, Si K (2004) The persistence of long-term memory: a molecular approach to self-sustaining changes in learning-induced synaptic growth. Neuron 44:49–57

Barco A, Alarcon JM, Kandel ER (2002) Expression of constitutively active CREB protein facilitates the late phase of long-term potentiation by enhancing synaptic capture. Cell 108:689–703

Bartsch D, Ghirardi M, Skehel PA, Karl KA, Herder SP, Chen M, Bailey CH, Kandel ER (1995) Aplysia CREB2 represses long-term facilitation: relief of repression converts transient facilitation into long-term functional and structural change. Cell 83:979–992

Bliss TV, Collingridge GL (1993) A synaptic model of memory: long-term potentiation in the hippocampus. Nature 361:31–39

Bliss TV, Lømo T(1973) Long-lasting potentiation of synaptic transmission in the dentate area of the anaesthetized rabbit following stimulation of the perforant path. J Physiol 232:331–356

Bliss TV, Collingridge GL, Morris RG (2003) Introduction. Long-term potentiation and structure of the issue. Philos Trans R Soc Lond B Biol Sci 358:607–611

Borlikova G, Endo S (2009) Inducible cAMP early repressor (ICER) and brain functions. Mol Neurobiol 40:73–86

Bourtchuladze R, Frenguelli B, Blendy J, Cioffi D, Schütz G, Silva AJ (1994) Deficient long-term memory in mice with a targeted mutation of the cAMP-responsive element-binding protein. Cell 79:59–68

Chen A, Muzzio IA, Malleret G, Bartsch D, Verbitsky M, Pavlidis P, Yonan AL, Vronskaya S, Grody MB, Cepeda I, Gilliam TC, Kandel ER (2003) Inducible enhancement of memory storage and synaptic plasticity in transgenic mice expressing an inhibitor of ATF4 (CREB-2) and C/EBP proteins. Neuron 39:655–669

Collinson N, Kuenzi FM, Jarolimek W, Maubach KA, Cothliff R, Sur C, Smith A, Otu FM, Howell O, Atack JR, McKernan RM, Seabrook GR, Dawson GR, Whiting PJ, Rosahl TW (2002) Enhanced learning and memory and altered GABAergic synaptic transmission in mice lacking the α 5 subunit of the $GABA_A$ receptor. J Neurosci 22:5572–5580

Costa-Mattioli M, Gobert D, Stern E, Gamache K, Colina R, Cuello C, Sossin W, Kaufman R, Pelletier J, Rosenblum K, Krnjević K, Lacaille JC, Nader K, Sonenberg N (2007) eIF2α phosphorylation bidirectionally regulates the switch from short- to long-term synaptic plasticity and memory. Cell 129:195–206

Danion JM, Huron C, Vidailhet P, Berna F (2007) Functional mechanisms of episodic memory impairment in schizophrenia. Can J Psychiatry 52:693–701

Davies MF, Tsui JY, Flannery JA, Li X, DeLorey TM, Hoffman BB (2003) Augmentation of the noradrenergic system in α-2 adrenergic receptor deficient mice: anatomical changes associated with enhanced fear memory. Brain Res 986:157–165

Dow RS, Moruzzi G (1958) The physiology and pathology of the cerebellum. University of Minnesota Press, Minneapolis

Ebbinghaus H (1885) Memory: a contribution to experimental psychology (trans: Ruger HA, Bussenius CE). Dover, New York

Eichenbaum H, Otto T, Cohen NJ (1992) The hippocampus—what does it do? Behav Neural Biol 57:2–36

Frank DA, Greenberg ME (1994) CREB: a mediator of long-term memory from mollusks to mammals. Cell 79:5–8

Fukushima H, Maeda R, Suzuki R, Suzuki A, Nomoto M, Toyoda H, Wu LJ, Xu H, Zhao MG, Ueda K, Kitamoto A, Mamiya N, Yoshida T, Homma S, Masushige S, Zhuo M, Kida S (2008) Upregulation of calcium/calmodulin-dependent protein kinase IV improves memory formation and rescues memory loss with aging. J Neurosci 28:9910–9919

Futatsugi A, Kato K, Ogura H, Li ST, Nagata E, Kuwajima G, Tanaka K, Itohara S, Mikoshiba K (1999) Facilitation of NMDAR-independent LTP and spatial learning in mutant mice lacking ryanodine receptor type 3. Neuron 124:701–713

Gazzaniga MS (2002) The Cognitive Neuroscience. Norton, New York

Genoux D, Haditsch U, Knobloch M, Michalon A, Storm D, Mansuy IM (2002) Protein phosphatase 1 is a molecular constraint on learning and memory. Nature 418:970–975

Govindarajan A, Kelleher RJ, Tonegawa S. (2006) A clustered plasticity model of long-term memory engrams. Nat Rev Neurosci 7:575–83
Harrell AV, Allan AM (2003) Improvements in hippocampal-dependent learning and decremental attention in 5-HT3 receptor overexpressing mice. Learn Mem 10:410–419
Hebb, DO (1949) The organization of behavior. Wiley, New York
Heim C, Nemeroff CB (2009) Neurobiology of posttraumatic stress disorder. CNS Spectr 14:13–24
Holmes G (1939) The cerebellum of man. Brain 62:1–30
Hu D, Serrano F, Oury TD, Klann E (2006) Aging-dependent alterations in synaptic plasticity and memory in mice that overexpress extracellular superoxide dismutase. J Neurosci 26:3933–3941
Ito M (2011) The cerebellum: brain for an implicit self. FT Press, New Jersey
Ito M, Sakurai M, Tongroach P (1982) Climbing fibre induced depression of both mossy fibre responsiveness and glutamate sensitivity of cerebellar Purkinje cells. J Physiol 324:113–134
Jiao J, Nakajima A, Janssen WG, Bindokas VP, Xiong X, Morrison JH, Brorson JR, Tang YP (2008) Expression of NR2B in cerebellar granule cells specifically facilitates effect of motor training on motor learning. PLoS One 3:e1684
Josselyn SA, Nguyen PV (2005) CREB, synapses and memory disorders: past progress and future challenges. Curr Drug Targets CNS Neurol Disord 4:481–497
Kandel ER (2001) The molecular biology of memory storage: a dialogue between genes and synapses. Biosci Rep 21:565–611
Kidd PM (2008) Alzheimer's disease, amnestic mild cognitive impairment, and age-associated memory impairment: current understanding and progress toward integrative prevention. Altern Med Rev 13:85–115
Klann E, Dever TE (2004) Biochemical mechanisms for translational regulation in synaptic plasticity. Nat Rev Neurosci 5:931–942
Kojima N, Borlikova G, Sakamoto T, Yamada K, Ikeda T, Itohara S, Niki H, Endo S. (2008) Inducible cAMP early repressor acts as a negative regulator for kindling epileptogenesis and long-term fear memory. J Neurosci 28:6459–6472
Lee YS, Silva AJ (2009) The molecular and cellular biology of enhanced cognition. Nat Rev Neurosci 10:126–140
Lonze BE, Ginty DD (2002) Function and regulation of CREB family transcription factors in the nervous system. Neuron 35:605–623
Lynch MA (2004) Long-term potentiation and memory. Physiol Rev 84:87–136
Madani R, Hulo S, Toni N, Madani H, Steimer T, Muller D, Vassalli JD (1999) Enhanced hippocampal long-term potentiation and learning by increased neuronal expression of tissue-type plasminogen activator in transgenic mice. EMBO J 18:3007–3012
Maekawa M, Watanabe M, Yamaguchi S, Konno R, Hori Y (2005) Spatial learning and long-term potentiation of mutant mice lacking D-amino-acid oxidase. Neurosci Res 53:34–38
Malenka RC (2003) Synaptic plasticity and AMPA receptor trafficking. Ann NY Acad Sci 1003:1–11
Malenka RC, Bear MF (2004) LTP and LTD: an embarrassment of riches. Neuron 44:5–21
Malleret G, Hen R, Guillou JL, Segu L, Buhot MC (1999) 5-HT1B receptor knock-out mice exhibit increased exploratory activity and enhanced spatial memory performance in the Morris water maze. J Neurosci 19:6157–6168
Malleret G, Haditsch U, Genoux D, Jones MW, Bliss TV, Vanhoose AM, Weitlauf C, Kandel ER, Winder DG, Mansuy IM (2001) Inducible and reversible enhancement of learning, memory, and long-term potentiation by genetic inhibition of calcineurin. Cell 104:675–686
Manabe T, Noda Y, Mamiya T, Katagiri H, Houtani T, Nishi M, Noda T, Takahashi T, Sugimoto T, Nabeshima T, Takeshima H (1998) Facilitation of long-term potentiation and memory in mice lacking nociceptin receptors. Nature 394:577–581
Marr D (1969) A theory of cerebellar cortex. J Physiol 202:437–470
Mayford M, Kandel ER (1999) Genetic approaches to memory storage. Trends Genet 15:463–470
Milner B, Squire LR, Kandel ER (1998) Cognitive neuroscience and the study of memory. Neuron 20:445–468

Mioduszewska B, Jaworski J, Kaczmarek L (2003) Inducible cAMP early repressor (ICER) in the nervous system—a transcriptional regulator of neuronal plasticity and programmed cell death. J Neurochem 87:1313–1320

Miyake A, Takahashi S, Nakamura Y, Inamura K, Matsumoto S, Mochizuki S, Katou M (2009) Disruption of the ether-a-go-go K^+ channel gene BEC1/KCNH3 enhances cognitive function. J Neurosci 29:14637–14645

Miyamoto Y, Chen L, Sato M, Sokabe M, Nabeshima T, Pawson T, Sakai R, Mori N (2005) Hippocampal synaptic modulation by the phosphotyrosine adapter protein ShcC/N-Shc via interaction with the NMDA receptor. J Neurosci 25:1826–1835

Molina CA, Foulkes NS, Lalli E, Sassone-Corsi P (1993) Inducibility and negative autoregulation of CREM: an alternative promoter directs the expression of ICER, an early response repressor. Cell 75:875–886

Monti B, Contestabile A (2009) Memory-enhancing drugs: a molecular perspective. Mini Rev Med Chem 9:769–781

Morozov A, Kellendonk C, Simpson E, Tronche F (2003) Using conditional mutagenesis to study the brain. Biol Psychiatry 54:1125–1133

Mulkey RM, Endo S, Shenolikar S, Malenka RC (1994) Involvement of a calcineurin/inhibitor-1 phosphatase cascade in hippocampal long-term depression. Nature 369:486–488

Murphy GG, Fedorov NB, Giese KP, Ohno M, Friedman E, Chen R, Silva AJ (2004) Increased neuronal excitability, synaptic plasticity, and learning in aged Kvβ1.1 knockout mice. Curr Biol 14:1907–1915

Newpher TM, Ehlers MD (2008) Glutamate receptor dynamics in dendritic microdomains. Neuron 58:472–497

Nishiyama H, Knöpfel T, Endo S, Itohara S (2002) Glial protein S100β modulates long-term neuronal synaptic plasticity. Proc Natl Acad Sci U S A 99:4037–4042

Penfield W (1958) Some mechanisms of consciousness discovered during electrical stimulation of the brain. Proc Natl Acad Sci U S A 44:51–66

Pfennig A, Littmann E, Bauer M (2007) Neurocognitive impairment and dementia in mood disorders. J Neuropsychiatry Clin Neurosci 19:373–82

Plato (2004) Timaeus (trans: Jowett B), eBooks@Adelaide, http://ebooks.adelaide.edu.au/p/plato/p71ti/index.html. Accessed Nov 2012

Plato (2007) Theaeteus (trans: Jowett B), eBooks@Adelaide, http://ebooks.adelaide.edu.au/p/plato/p71th/index.html. Accessed Nov 2012

Plato (2010a) Crytylus (trans: Jowett B), eBooks@Adelaide, http://ebooks.adelaide.edu.au/p/plato/p71cra/index.html. Accessed Nov 2012

Plato (2010b) Phaedrus (trans: Jowett B), eBooks@Adelaide, http://ebooks.adelaide.edu.au/p/plato/p71phs/index.html. Accessed Nov 2012

Poeppel TD, Krause BJ (2008) Functional imaging of memory processes in humans: positron emission tomography and functional magnetic resonance imaging. Methods 44:315–328

Popov VI, Davies HA, Rogachevsky VV, Patrushev IV, Errington ML, Gabbott PL, Bliss TV, Stewart MG (2004) Remodelling of synaptic morphology but unchanged synaptic density during late phase long-term potentiation (LTP): a serial section electron micrograph study in the dentate gyrus in the anaesthetised rat. Neuroscience 128:251–262

Rosenzweig ES, Barnes CA (2003) Impact of aging on hippocampal function:plasticity, network dynamics, and cognition. Prog Neurobiol 69:143–179

Routtenberg A (2008) The substrate for long-lasting memory: if not protein synthesis, then what? Neurobiol Learn Mem 289:225–233

Routtenberg A, Cantallops I, Zaffuto S, Serrano P, Namgung U (2000) Enhanced learning after genetic overexpression of a brain growth protein. Proc Natl Acad Sci U S A 97:7657–7662

Saura CA, Valero J (2011) The role of CREB signaling in Alzheimer's disease and other cognitive disorders. Rev Neurosci 22:153–169

Schulz S, Siemer H, Krug M, Höllt V (1999) Direct evidence for biphasic cAMP responsive element-binding protein phosphorylation during long-term potentiation in the rat dentate gyrus in vivo. J Neurosci 19:5683–5692

Scoville WB, Milner B (1957) Loss of recent memory after bilateral hippocampal lesions. J Neurol Neurosurg Psychiatry 20:11–21

Shumyatsky GP, Tsvetkov E, Malleret G, Vronskaya S, Hatton M, Hampton L, Battey JF, Dulac C, Kandel ER, Bolshakov VY (2002) Identification of a signaling network in lateral nucleus of amygdala important for inhibiting memory specifically related to learned fear. Cell 111:905–918

Silva AJ, Kogan JH, Frankland PW, Kida S (1998) CREB and memory. Annu Rev Neurosci 21:127–148

Squire LR (2009) Memory and brain systems: 1969–2009. J Neurosci 29:12711–12716

Squire LR, Zola SM (1996) Structure and function of declarative and nondeclarative memory systems. Proc Natl Acad Sci U S A 93:13515–13522

Sterneck E, Paylor R, Jackson-Lewis V, Libbey M, Przedborski S, Tessarollo L, Crawley JN, Johnson PF (1998) Selectively enhanced contextual fear conditioning in mice lacking the transcriptional regulator CCAAT/enhancer binding protein δ. Proc Natl Acad Sci U S A 95:10908–10913

Takeuchi T, Ohtsuki G, Yoshida T, Fukaya M, Wainai T, Yamashita M, Yamazaki Y, Mori H, Sakimura K, Kawamoto S, Watanabe M, Hirano T, Mishina M (2008) Enhancement of both long-term depression induction and optokinetic response adaptation in mice lacking delphilin. PLoS One 3:e2297

Tang YP, Shimizu E, Dube GR, Rampon C, Kerchner GA, Zhuo M, Liu G, Tsien JZ (1999) Genetic enhancement of learning and memory in mice. Nature 401:63–69

Toyota M, Suzuki H, Yamashita T, Hirata K, Imai K, Tokino T, Shinomura Y (2009) Cancer epigenomics: implications of DNA methylation in personalized cancer therapy. Cancer Sci 100:787–791

Tröster AI (2008) Neuropsychological characteristics of dementia with Lewy bodies and Parkinson's disease with dementia: differentiation, early detection, and implications for "mild cognitive impairment" and biomarkers. Neuropsychol Rev 18:103–119

Wu H, Zhou Y, Xiong ZQ (2007) Transducer of regulated CREB and late phase long-term synaptic potentiation. FEBS J 274:3218–3223

Yin JC, Wallach JS, Del Vecchio M, Wilder EL, Zhou H, Quinn WG, Tully T (1994) Induction of a dominant negative CREB transgene specifically blocks long-term memory in Drosophila. Cell 79:49–58

Yukawa K, Tanaka T, Takeuchi N, Iso H, Li L, Kohsaka A, Waki H, Miyajima M, Maeda M, Kikutani H, Kumanogoh A (2009) Sema4D/CD100 deficiency leads to superior performance in mouse motor behavior. Can J Neurol Sci 36:349–355

Zhou SJ, Zhu ME, Shu D, Du XP, Song XH, Wang XT, Zheng RY, Cai XH, Chen JF, He JC (2009) Preferential enhancement of working memory in mice lacking adenosine A(2A) receptors. Brain Res 1303:74–83

Chapter 16
Potential Beneficial Effects of a Diet with Walnuts in Aging and Alzheimer's Disease

Abha Chauhan and Ved Chauhan

Abstract Alzheimer's disease (AD) is a severe neurodegenerative disease that gradually results in loss of memory and impairment of cognitive functions in the elderly people. Amyloid beta (Aβ) is the major protein of amyloid plaques in the brains of patients with AD. Aβ is known to increase the production of free radicals, i.e. reactive oxygen species (ROS) in neuronal cells, leading to oxidative stress and cell death. Oxidative stress and inflammation are prominent features in the aging process and in AD, which may be causally related to neuronal dysfunction and its death. Recently, considerable attention has been focused on dietary antioxidants that are able to scavenge ROS, thereby offering protection against oxidative stress. Walnuts are rich in components that have antioxidant and anti-inflammatory properties. Here, we review the evidence that walnut extract can inhibit the fibrillization of Aβ, solubilise preformed fibrillar Aβ and protects the cells against Aβ-induced oxidative stress and cell death. Walnuts in the diet may offer protection against Aβ-mediated cytotoxicity by (i) reducing the generation of free radicals, (ii) inhibiting membrane damage and (iii) attenuating DNA damage. This effect of walnut extract can be due to the active compounds present in walnuts, which may increase the capacity of endogenous antioxidant defenses and modulate the cellular redox state. A diet rich in walnuts may therefore reduce the risk of developing dementia of Alzheimer's type by inhibiting Aβ fibrillization, Aβ-mediated cytotoxicity and oxidative stress.

Keywords Aging • Alzheimer's disease • Inflammation • Nutrition • Oxidative stress • Walnuts

---

A. Chauhan (✉) · V. Chauhan
NYS Institute for Basic Research in Developmental Disabilities,
1050 Forest Hill Road, Staten Island, NY 10314, USA
e-mail: abha.chauhan@opwdd.ny.gov

M. K. Thakur, S. I. S. Rattan (eds.), *Brain Aging and Therapeutic Interventions,*
DOI 10.1007/978-94-007-5237-5_16,

16.1 Alzheimer's disease (AD)

AD is an age-related neurodegenerative disease that gradually results in memory loss and impairment of cognitive functions over a period of 5–20 years. It is the most common form of dementia in the elderly, and affects an estimated 25 million people worldwide.

The aggregation and fibrillization of amyloid beta-protein (Aβ), leading to the deposition of amyloid plaques in the brain is one of the major pathological hallmarks of AD (Glenner 1983; Masters et al. 1985). In addition, neuronal loss and accumulation of paired helical filaments as neurofibrillary tangles (NFT) in neurons are common features in AD (Iqbal et al. 1998). The mechanisms of neuronal cell loss in AD have not yet been fully elucidated, but increased oxidative stress (Gibson and Huang 2002; Chauhan and Chauhan 2006; Galasko and Montine 2010; Bonda et al. 2010), and inflammation (Rozemuller et al. 2005; Schwab and McGeer 2008; Galasko and Montine 2010) are considered important initiators/mediators of neuronal damage in AD. Extensive evidence indicates that the brains of AD patients are characterized by exaggerated oxidative stress (Gibson and Huang 2002; Chauhan and Chauhan 2006; Bonda et al. 2010), and the overproduction of Aβ leads to Aβ-associated free-radicals production and cell death (Harris et al. 1995; Monji et al. 2001; Sponne et al. 2003). Aβ not only increases oxidative stress, but its generation is also increased as a result of oxidative stress which in turn, causes more oxidative damage.

The neuropathological changes of AD evolve gradually over decades before the clinical symptoms of the disease become evident (Price and Morris 1999; Knopman et al. 2003; Iacono et al. 2008). Increased oxidative damage is also reported in early stages of mild cognitive impairment in the brains of patients with AD, and in cerebrospinal fluid (CSF) from subjects with very early signs of dementia (Keller et al. 2005; Steele et al. 2007).We review in the following sections that early intervention with a diet rich in walnuts may help in reducing the risk of developing AD or delaying its onset because of enhanced oxidative stress and inflammatory response mechanisms involved in aging process and AD, and due to antioxidant and anti-inflammatory components in walnut.

16.2 Age: A Risk Factor for Alzheimer's Disease

Unfortunately, age is the greatest risk factor for AD. AD is ten times more frequent in people over the age of 65. Statistical data show that one in ten over the age of 65, and nearly half of the population over the age of 85 suffers from AD. Increased concentrations of oxidatively- damaged proteins, lipids, and DNA, as well as mitochondrial dysfunction have been reported in aging (Mao and Reddy 2011; Paradies et al. 2011). Aging-related increase in brain oxidative stress has also been reported to correlate with developmental pattern of β-secretase activity (involved in Aβ production) and β-amyloid plaque deposition in the transgenic Tg2576 mice model of AD (Apelt et al. 2004). Constant assault of oxidative stress during aging process may contribute, in part, towards neurogeneration in AD.

16.3 Oxidative Stress in Aging and Alzheimer's Disease

Oxidative stress is a condition in which the generation of free radicals far exceeds its elimination by antioxidant defense mechanism. The free radicals produced in the body are toxic, and if not removed or neutralized, they react with lipids, proteins and nucleic acids and damage cellular functions. Generally, oxidative damage to the cellular components results in alteration of the membrane properties such as fluidity, ion transport, decreased enzyme activities, and protein cross-linking. Excessive oxidant damage eventually results in cell death (Bandopadhyay et al. 1999).

In 1956, Harman had proposed free radical theory of aging (Harman 1956). Since then, it remains a prominent theory. Increased oxidative stress in the aging brain results in increased membrane lipid peroxidation (Montine et al. 2002; Chauhan and Chauhan 2006). Scientists are also focusing on mitochondrial theory of aging, which suggests that oxidative stress within mitochondria can lead to a vicious cycle in which damaged mitochondria produce increased amounts of free radicals, i.e. reactive oxygen species (ROS) leading to progressive augmentation in cell damage (Harman 1972; Miquel et al. 1980; Cadenas and Davies 2000). The free radicals are generated endogenously during oxidative metabolism and energy production by mitochondria, and the electron transport chain (ETC) in mitochondria is a prime source for ROS generation (Cadenas and Davies 2000; Lenaz 2001). The antioxidant defense mechanisms to remove ROS in the cell involve enzymes such as catalase, superoxide dismutase, glutathione peroxidase, glutathione reductase, and nonenzymatic reducing agents such as glutathione, carotinoids, phytochemicals, vitamin E and vitamin C (Bandopadhyay et al. 1999).

Extensive evidence from studies with experimental models and human brain suggests that enhanced oxidative stress plays an important role in neuronal degeneration in AD. In AD, ROS generation is increased due to aging, Aβ production, Aβ fibrillization, neurofibrillary pathology and mitochondrial abnormalities (Chauhan and Chauhan 2006). Imbalance of oxidative homeostasis leading to increased lipid peroxidation is an important factor involved in AD. The brains of patients with AD contain increased levels of lipid-peroxidation products such as 4-hydroxynonenal (HNE) or 2-propenal (acrolein), and enhanced lipid peroxidation can also be detected in CSF and plasma of AD subjects (Lovell et al. 1995; Montine et al. 2002; Arlt et al. 2002). In addition, ROS-mediated oxidative damage of proteins and DNA is also an important event in AD pathology (Smith et al. 1991; Lyras et al. 1997; Gabbita et al. 1998; Lovell et al. 1999; Nunomura et al. 2010).

There is increasing evidence that both soluble and fibrillar Aβ can induce oxidative stress. Several studies suggest that ROS are involved in Aβ fibrillization and NFT formation in AD. Evidence also exists that ROS generation increases with the increase in Aβ and NFT pathology in AD, thereby creating vicious cycle of ROS generation that far exceeds the antioxidant defense system (Chauhan and Chauhan 2006). Some of the age-related changes in neuronal functions are subtle, and may involve calcium dysregulation (Landfield 1987; Khachaturian 1994). The loss of calcium homeostasis induced by oxidative stress can also lead to increased vulnerability to oxidative stress, thus resulting in a vicious cycle of oxidative stress, loss of calcium homeostasis, and further generation of oxidative stress and cell death (Annunziato et al. 2002; Waring 2005). Loss in calcium homeostasis, increased oxidative stress, and mitochondrial dysfunction have been reported in several age-related neurodegenerative diseases, such as AD (Chauhan and Chauhan 2006; Aliev et al. 2009; Wang et al. 2009; Bonda et al. 2010; Galasko and Montine 2010), Parkinson's disease (Dexter et al. 1994; Navarro et al. 2009) and Huntington disease (Chen 2011).

16.4 Inflammation in Aging and Alzheimer's Disease

Several studies have reported neuroinflammation as a prominent feature in aging and AD (Wyss-Coray 2006; Heneka and O'Banion 2007; Parachikova et al. 2007). Glial cells mediate the endogenous immune system in the central nervous system, and their activation is the marker of inflammation in the brain (Kreutzberg 1996). An increase in activated glial cells and immunoreactivity in markers of both microglia and astrocytes has been reported in normal aging brains and AD-affected brains (Rozovsky et al. 1998; Sheng et al. 1998). Activated microglia and astrocytes produce inflammatory molecules such as cytokines (interleukin (IL)-1β, IL-6, and tumor necrosis factor-α (TNF-α), growth factors, and complement proteins in AD (McGeer and McGeer 1995; Chen et al. 1996; Luterman et al. 2000; Tarkowski et al. 2003). The expression of glial fibrillary acid protein is also increased by middle age (Rozovsky et al. 1998) and in elderly (McGeer and McGeer 1995). Several studies have reported increase in TNF-α, IL-6 (Chang et al. 1996; Spaulding et al. 1997), and C-reactive protein (Kushner 2001) in aged mice and humans. Furthermore, IL-1β and TNF-α can also activate microglia and astrocytes, and induce acute phase proteins such as α1-antichymotrypsin, which has been found with amyloid plaques in AD (Kordula et al. 2000).

In vitro studies have shown that Aβ can activate microglia cells, leading to increased production of several cytokines, chemokines, free radicals and proinflammatory enzymes (Lue et al. 2001a; Walker et al. 2006). It activates inflammatory processes in microglia by binding to cell–surface receptors such as the Receptor for Advanced Glycation Endproducts (RAGE) (Lue et al. 2001b) or Toll-like receptor 2 (Jana et al. 2008), or by interacting with complement C1q, the initiating protein of the classical complement pathway (Rogers et al. 1992). In fact, complement activation has been reported in AD brain (McGeer et al. 1989; Chen et al. 1996; Webster et al. 1997). Nitric oxide synthase (NOS) is an enzyme that also plays a pivotal role in inflammation. Several reports have shown that Aβ can stimulate inducible-NOS (iNOS) in microglia and astrocytes, resulting in enhanced NO production (Akama and Van Eldik 2000; Combs et al. 2001).

Cyclooxygenase (COX) is a key enzyme in the prostaglandin (PG) synthesis, which converts arachidonic acid to PGH2. During conversion of PGG2 to PGH2, ROS are generated. In AD, the expression of COX-2 (known to be induced by pro-inflammatory mediators) is upregulated (Pasinetti and Aisen 1998; Ho et al. 1999; Hoozemans et al. 2002), and there is elevated production of inflammatory PGs, especially PGE2 in the brain (Montine et al. 1999). Increase in COX activity and PGE has also been reported in aging brain (Baek et al. 2001). Since pathway of PG synthesis appears to be a major source of ROS in the brain (Baek et al. 2001), inflammation may be partly responsible for increased oxidative stress in aging and AD. Thus factors such as cytokines and PG may act as extracellular signals in generating ROS that are detrimental to neuronal function or glial neuronal interactions, leading to dementia in aging and AD.

The relationship between diet and health benefits has become increasingly obvious with accumulating evidence that those plant foods rich in phenols and flavonoids are important class of defensive antioxidants (Pietta 2000). Recently, potential roles of dietary antioxidants have been emphasized in neurodegenerative diseases including AD. Plant extracts such as green tea, gingko biloba and curcumin were able to prevent oxidative stress-mediated apoptosis in cultured neurons, and reduce the oxidative stress that is associated with AD (Xin et al 2000; Park et al. 2008; He et al. 2011; Mishra et al. 2011). In the following sections, we will present evidence on potential beneficial effects of a diet with walnuts in aging and age-related diseases.

16.5 Antioxidant and Anti-inflammatory Properties of Walnuts

Recent evidence suggests that walnuts (Juglans regia L.) may reduce the risk of age-related diseases because they are rich in nutrients, which have antioxidant and anti-inflammatory properties (Fig. 16.1). Brain needs sufficient amount of water, vitamins (such as folate, thiamine, vitamins B6 and B12), α-lipoic acid, lutein and n-3 fatty acids (Morley 2010). Walnuts contain a number of potential neuroprotective compounds like gamma tocopherol (vitamin E), folate, melatonin, flavonoids, phenolic acid (ellagic acid) and significant amount of n-3 α-linolenic acid (ALA) (a plant based omega-3 fatty acid) (Jurd 1958; Lavedrine et al. 1997; Anderson et al. 2001; Fukuda et al. 2003; Crews et al. 2005; Reiter et al. 2005; Halvorsen et al. 2006). Recommended daily serving of walnuts is one ounce (oz.) i.e. 28 g, which equates to one quarter cup or 12–14 walnut halves. In addition to antioxidants and ALA, walnuts are a good source of protein (4 g/oz.) and fiber (2 g/oz.). Walnuts also contain numerous other vitamins and minerals, and provide magnesium (11 % daily value) and phosphorus (10 % daily value).

Walnut has a high content (3.68 mmol/oz.) of antioxidants such as flavonoids (Pietta 2000; Darvesh et al. 2010; Gutierrez-Merino et al. 2011), ellagic acid (Majid et al. 1991), melatonin (Pappolla et al. 2000; Reiter et al. 2005), gamma tocopherol, and selenium. In terms of antioxidant contents, walnuts ranked second among 1,113 different food items tested (Halvorsen et al. 2006). A recent study investigated the antioxidant efficiency of different dry fruits, and found walnuts to exhibit the best antioxidant properties (Mishra et al. 2010). The highest phenolic content was found in walnuts followed by almonds and cashew nuts, and the least phenolic content was in raisins (Mishra et al. 2010). Another study examined the levels of antioxidants in various foods, and reported at least ten different antioxidants in walnuts. According to this study, 50 g of walnuts have significantly more phenolics [802 mg gallic acid equivalent (GAE) of total phenols] than a 8 oz glass of apple juice (117 mg GAE in 240 ml), a milk chocolate bar (205 mg GAE in 1.5 oz), or a 5 oz glass of red wine (372 mg GAE in 150 ml) (Anderson et al. 2001).

While most nuts contain monounsaturated fats, only walnuts are comprised primarily of polyunsaturated fat (13 g of 18 g total fat in one ounce of walnuts), of which ALA is 2.5 g. ALA is the precursor for eicosapentaenoic acid (EPA, 20:5n-3) and docosahexaenoic acid (DHA, 22:6n-3). DHA is important for neuronal membrane stability, neuroplasticity, synaptic plasticity, gene expression, cell migration and apoptosis. It facilitates signal transduction, neurotransmission, and increases serotonin and dopamine concentrations. EPA regulates the synthesis of arachidonic acid (20:4n-6) and modulates important inflammatory and immune functions (Innis 2007; Heinrichs 2010).

16.6 Health Benefits of Walnuts in the Diet

Green walnuts, shells, kernels and seeds, bark and leaves have been used in the pharmaceutical and cosmetic industries (Stampar et al. 2006). Walnut and its leaves have been used in traditional medicine for treatment of venous insufficiency and haemorrhoidal symptomatology, and for its antidiarrheic, anti-microbial, antihelminthic, depurative and astringent properties (Pereira et al. 2007, 2008; Oliveira et al. 2008). Keratolytic, antifungal, hypoglycemic, hypotensive and sedative activities of walnuts have also been reported (Fukuda et al. 2003; Pereira et al. 2007).

Several studies have suggested that the consumption of walnuts in the diet can reduce the risk of heart disease (Hu et al. 1998; Banel and Hu 2009), and decrease total and low-density lipoprotein (LDL) (Sabate et al. 1993; Abbey et al. 1994; Lavedrine et al. 1999; Zambon et al. 2000; Rajaram et al. 2009; Banel and Hu 2009). In an in vitro study, polyphenol-rich extracts from walnuts was prepared, and LDL was isolated from the plasma of healthy human subjects. Walnut extract (1 μM) inhibited AAPH [2,2′-Azobis (2-amidino propane) hydrochloride, a free radical generator]—induced LDL oxidation by 38 %, and copper-mediated LDL oxidation by 84 % (Anderson et al. 2001). A large cohort study of 83,818 women (age: 34–59 years) showed that consumption of one-ounce of nuts, such as walnuts, or of peanut butter five times or more each week reduced the risk of developing type 2 diabetes (Jiang et al. 2002). An animal study showed that the diet with walnuts could slow the growth of human breast cancers implanted into nude mice (Hardman and Ion 2008).

Recently, Mckay et al. (2010) studied chronic and acute effects of walnuts on antioxidant capacity in a randomized, cross-over pilot study. They reported that walnut consumption did not significantly change the plasma antioxidant capacity of healthy, well-nourished older adults. However, they observed improvement in levels of linoleic acid in red blood cells and total plasma thiols, suggesting that walnuts may have beneficial effects due to increase in linoleic acid in normal subjects. In another study, consumption of walnuts was able to increase total antioxidant capacity and reduce plasma lipid peroxidation (Torabian et al. 2009).

Willis et al. (2009) examined the effect of diet with walnuts on cognitive function in aged rats (19 months old). Aged rats have been reported to show decrements in performance on motor and cognitive tasks that require the use of spatial learning and memory. In this study, the rats were fed a control diet or a diet with 2, 6 or 9 % walnuts for eight weeks, and then examined for motor and cognitive function. It was reported that a diet containing as much as 6 % walnuts (equivalent to one ounce in humans) improved cognitive and motor performance (Willis et al. 2009).

A recent study examined the effects of a short term (8 weeks) dietary supplementation of walnuts on cognitive performance in young adults (Pribis et al. 2011). In this study, 64 college students were randomly assigned to two treatment sequences in a crossover fashion: walnuts–placebo or placebo–walnuts. After 6 weeks, the intervention groups followed the diets in reverse order. Data for non-verbal reasoning, verbal reasoning, memory and mood states were collected at baseline and at the end of the 8-week intervention period. A significant increase (11.2 %) was observed in inferential verbal reasoning with the walnut-supplemented diet. However, no significant difference was observed for mood, non-verbal reasoning or memory, which may be because walnut supplementation in the diet was for only a few weeks.

16.7 Effects of Walnuts on Aβ Fibrillization and Aβ-induced Oxidative Stress and Cell Damage in AD

Fibrillization of Aβ and its deposition as amyloid plaque in the brain is considered the hallmark of AD pathology. Aβ exists in both soluble and fibrillar forms. Aβ fibril formation from soluble Aβ is preceded by oligomerization and aggregation of Aβ, and involves conformational change of the peptide from α-helical to β-pleated sheet structure (Hilbich et al. 1991; Soto et al. 1994). Agents that can inhibit the fibrillization of Aβ may have potential beneficial effects in reducing the risk or delaying the progression of AD. The synthetic peptides homologous to Aβ have been extensively used to study fibril formation in vitro. Aβ 40 or Aβ 42 and some of their shorter derivatives form amyloid-like fibrils in vitro exhibiting a β-pleated sheet conformation that is assayed using Thioflavin T (ThT) fluorescence spectroscopy.

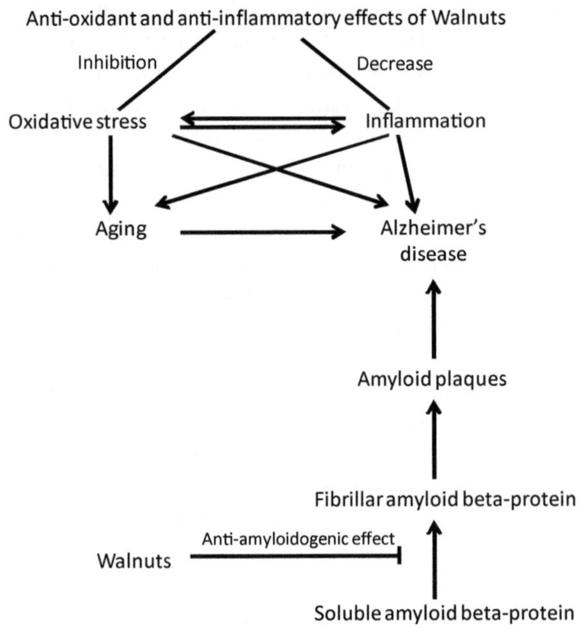

Fig. 16.1 Potential mechanisms of antioxidant, anti-inflammatory and anti-amyloidogenic effects of walnuts in aging and Alzheimer's disease. The role of oxidative stress, inflammation and amyloid beta-protein in Alzheimer's disease is shown in this figure. Oxidative stress and inflammation are commonly observed phenomenon in aging and AD. The fibrillization of amyloid beta-protein is a key event in the amyloid plaque formation in AD brain. Walnuts are rich in antioxidant and anti-inflammatory components, and therefore, inhibit ROS production, reduce inflammation, and also inhibit fibrillization of amyloid beta-protein

Walnut extract has been reported to inhibit the Aβ fibrilization and to solubilize the preformed Aβ fibrils in an in vitro study using ThT fluorescence spectroscopy (to measure degree of Aβ aggregation/fibrillization) and electron microscopy (to assess the morphology of Aβ structure) (Chauhan et al. 2004). ThT fluorescence data showed that the walnut extract inhibited Aβ fibril formation in a concentration- and time- dependent manner. Addition of walnut extract to soluble Aβ after 2 and 3 days of incubation resulted in over 90 % inhibition of Aβ fibrillization. Electron microscopy analysis confirmed that walnut extract has a profound inhibitory effect on the formation of Aβ fibrils. It was also studied whether walnut extract can convert Aβ fibrils back into soluble Aβ (Chauhan et al. 2004). In fact, walnut extract was able to defribrillize the preformed fibrils of Aβ. When preformed Aβ fibrils were incubated with walnut extract for 2 days, up to 91.6 % defibrillization of Aβ fibrils was observed. These results suggest that the compound(s) present in walnuts interact directly with Aβ, resulting in anti-amyloidogenic property of walnut (Fig. 16.1).

Several in vitro studies have shown that Aβ exhibits cytotoxic properties by producing ROS and inducing oxidative stress (Harris et al. 1995; Davis 1996; Sponne et al. 2003; Kadowaki et al. 2005). We recently reported that walnut extract has protective effect against Aβ-induced cell death and oxidative stress (Muthaiyah et al. 2011). In this study, the effect of walnut extract on Aβ-induced cellular damage, ROS generation and apoptosis in PC12 pheochromocytoma cells was studied. The intracellular ROS accumulation resulting from Aβ treatment was significantly reduced when these cells were also treated with walnut extract as compared to control cells treated with only Aβ, which clearly demonstrated that walnut extract has the ability to scavenge oxygen radicals. It is known that flavonoids, ellagic acid, melatonin and gamma tocopherol, which are components of walnuts have antioxidative and free-radical scavenging properties (Majid et al. 1991; Pappolla et al. 2000; Pietta 2000; Darvesh et al. 2010; Gutierrez-Merino et al. 2011). Because constituents of walnuts have strong antioxidant properties, the inhibition of Aβ-induced free radical generation by walnut extract may be attributed to the neutralization of ROS. Walnut extract also reduced Aβ-mediated cell death assessed by MTT (3-(4,5-dimethylthiazol-2-yl)-2,5-diphenyltetrazolium bromide) reduction, release of lactate dehydrogenase (membrane damage), and DNA damage (apoptosis) in a concentration-dependent manner (Muthaiyah et al. 2011). These results suggest that walnut extract can counteract Aβ-induced oxidative stress and associated cell death.

Above studies suggest that consumption of walnuts in the diet may reduce the risk, delay the onset or slow the progression of dementia in AD by maintaining Aβ in the soluble form, preventing it from fibrillization, and protecting against Aβ-induced oxidative stress and cell death.

Acknowledgments This work was supported in part by funds from the New York State Office of People with Developmental Disabilities, and California Walnut Commission.

References

Abbey M, Noakes M, Belling GB, Nestel PJ (1994) Partial replacement of saturated fatty acids with almonds or walnuts lowers total plasma cholesterol and low-density-lipoprotein cholesterol. Am J Clin Nutr 59:995–999

Akama KT, Van Eldik LJ (2000) Beta-amyloid stimulation of inducible nitric-oxide synthase in astrocytes is interleukin-1beta- and tumor necrosis factor-alpha (TNFalpha)-dependent, and involves a TNFalpha receptor-associated factor- and NFkappaB-inducing kinase-dependent signaling mechanism. J Biol Chem 275:7918–7924

Aliev G, Palacios HH, Walrafen B, Lipsitt AE, Obrenovich ME, Morales L (2009) Brain mitochondria as a primary target in the development of treatment strategies for Alzheimer disease. Int J Biochem Cell Biol 41:1989–2004

Anderson KJ, Teuber SS, Gobeille A, Cremin P, Waterhouse AL, Steinberg FM (2001) Walnut polyphenolics inhibit in vitro human plasma and LDL oxidation. J Nutr 131:2837–2842

Annunziato L, Pannaccione A, Cataldi M, Secondo A, Castaldo P, Di Renzo G, Taglialatela M (2002) Modulation of ion channels by reactive oxygen and nitrogen species: a pathophysiological role in brain aging? Neurobiol Aging 23:819–834

Apelt J, Bigl M, Wunderlich P, Schliebs R (2004) Aging-related increase in oxidative stress correlates with developmental pattern of beta-secretase activity and beta-amyloid plaque formation in transgenic Tg2576 mice with Alzheimer-like pathology. Int J Dev Neurosci 22:475–484

Arlt S, Beisiegel U, Kontush A (2002) Lipid peroxidation in neurodegeneration: new insights into Alzheimer's disease. Curr Opin Lipidol 13:289–294

Baek BS, Kim JW, Lee JH, Kwon HJ, Kim ND, Kang HS, Yoo MA, Yu BP, Chung HY (2001) Age-related increase of brain cyclooxygenase activity and dietary modulation of oxidative status. J Gerontol A Biol Sci Med Sci 56:B426–B431

Bandopadhyay U, Dipak D, Banerjee RK (1999) Reactive oxygen species: oxidative damage and pathogenesis. Curr Sci 77:658–666

Banel DK, Hu FB (2009) Effects of walnut consumption on blood lipids and other cardiovascular risk factors: a meta-analysis and systematic review. Am J Clin Nutr 90:56–63

Bonda DJ, Wang X, Perry G, Nunomura A, Tabaton M, Zhu X, Smith MA (2010) Oxidative stress in Alzheimer disease: a possibility for prevention. Neuropharmacology 59:290–294

Cadenas E, Davies KJ (2000) Mitochondrial free radical generation, oxidative stress, and aging. Free Radic Biol Med 29:222–230

Chang HN, Wang SR, Chiang SC, Teng WJ, Chen ML, Tsai JJ, Huang DF, Lin HY, Tsai YY (1996) The relationship of aging to endotoxin shock and to production of TNF-alpha. J Gerontol A Biol Sci Med Sci 51:M220–M222

Chauhan N, Wang KC, Wegiel J, Malik MN (2004) Walnut extract inhibits the fibrillization of amyloid beta-protein, and also defibrillizes its preformed fibrils. Curr Alzheimer Res 1:183–188

Chauhan V, Chauhan A (2006) Oxidative stress in Alzheimer's disease. Pathophysiology 13:195–208

Chen CM (2011) Mitochondrial dysfunction, metabolic deficits, and increased oxidative stress in Huntington's disease. Chang Gung Med J 34:135–152

Chen S, Frederickson RC, Brunden KR (1996) Neuroglial-mediated immunoinflammatory responses in Alzheimer's disease: complement activation and therapeutic approaches. Neurobiol Aging 17:781–787

Combs CK, Karlo JC, Kao SC, Landreth GE (2001) Beta-amyloid stimulation of microglia and monocytes results in TNFalpha-dependent expression of inducible nitric oxide synthase and neuronal apoptosis. J Neurosci 21:1179–1188

Crews C, Hough P, Godward J, Brereton P, Lees M, Guiet S, Winkelmann W (2005) Study of the main constituents of some authentic walnut oils. J Agric Food Chem 53:4853–4860

Darvesh AS, Carroll RT, Bishayee A, Geldenhuys WJ, Van der Schyf CJ (2010) Oxidative stress and Alzheimer's disease: dietary polyphenols as potential therapeutic agents. Expert Rev Neurother 10:729–745

Davis JB (1996) Oxidative mechanisms in beta-amyloid cytotoxicity. Neurodegeneration 5:441–444

Dexter DT, Holley AE, Flitter WD, Slater TF, Wells FR, Daniel SE, Lees AJ, Jenner P, Marsden CD (1994) Increased levels of lipid hydroperoxides in the parkinsonian substantia nigra: an HPLC and ESR study. Mov Disord 9:92–97

Fukuda T, Ito H, Yoshida T (2003) Antioxidative polyphenols from walnuts (Juglans regia L.). Phytochemistry 63:795–801

Gabbita SP, Lovell MA, Markesbery WR (1998) Increased nuclear DNA oxidation in the brain in Alzheimer's disease. J Neurochem 71:2034–2040

Galasko D, Montine TJ (2010) Biomarkers of oxidative damage and inflammation in Alzheimer's disease. Biomark Med 4:27–36

Gibson GE, Huang HM (2002) Oxidative processes in the brain and non-neuronal tissues as biomarkers of Alzheimer's disease. Front Biosci 7:d1007-d1015

Glenner GG (1983) Alzheimer's disease. The commonest form of amyloidosis. Arch Pathol Lab Med 107:281–282

Gutierrez-Merino C, Lopez-Sanchez C, Lagoa R, Samhan-Arias AK, Bueno C, Garcia-Martinez V (2011) Neuroprotective actions of flavonoids. Curr Med Chem 18:1195–1212

Halvorsen BL, Carlsen MH, Phillips KM, Bohn SK, Holte K, Jacobs DR, Jr, Blomhoff R (2006) Content of redox-active compounds (ie, antioxidants) in foods consumed in the United States. Am J Clin Nutr 84:95–135

Hardman WE, Ion G (2008) Suppression of implanted MDA-MB 231 human breast cancer growth in nude mice by dietary walnut. Nutr Cancer 60:666–674

Harman D (1956) Aging: a theory based on free radical and radiation chemistry. J Gerontol 11:298–300

Harman D (1972) The biologic clock: the mitochondria? J Am Geriatr Soc 20:145–147

Harris ME, Hensley K, Butterfield DA, Leedle RA, Carney JM (1995) Direct evidence of oxidative injury produced by the Alzheimer's beta-amyloid peptide (1–40) in cultured hippocampal neurons. Exp Neurol 131:193–202

He Y, Cui J, Lee JC, Ding S, Chalimoniuk M, Simonyi A, Sun AY, Gu Z, Weisman GA, Wood WG, Sun GY (2011) Prolonged exposure of cortical neurons to oligomeric amyloid-beta impairs NMDA receptor function via NADPH oxidase-mediated ROS production: protective effect of green tea (-)-epigallocatechin-3-gallate. ASN Neuro 3:e00050

Heinrichs SC (2010) Dietary omega-3 fatty acid supplementation for optimizing neuronal structure and function. Mol Nutr Food Res 54:447–456

Heneka MT, O'Banion MK (2007) Inflammatory processes in Alzheimer's disease. J Neuroimmunol 184:69–91

Hilbich C, Kisters-Woike B, Reed J, Masters CL, Beyreuther K (1991) Aggregation and secondary structure of synthetic amyloid beta A4 peptides of Alzheimer's disease. J Mol Biol 218:149–163

Ho L, Pieroni C, Winger D, Purohit DP, Aisen PS, Pasinetti GM (1999) Regional distribution of cyclooxygenase-2 in the hippocampal formation in Alzheimer's disease. J Neurosci Res 57:295–303

Hoozemans JJ, Bruckner MK, Rozemuller AJ, Veerhuis R, Eikelenboom P, Arendt T (2002) Cyclin D1 and cyclin E are co-localized with cyclo-oxygenase 2 (COX-2) in pyramidal neurons in Alzheimer disease temporal cortex. J Neuropathol Exp Neurol 61:678–688

Hu FB, Stampfer MJ, Manson JE, Rimm EB, Colditz GA, Rosner BA, Speizer FE, Hennekens CH, Willett WC (1998) Frequent nut consumption and risk of coronary heart disease in women: prospective cohort study. BMJ 317:1341–1345

Iacono D, O'Brien R, Resnick SM, Zonderman AB, Pletnikova O, Rudow G, An Y, West MJ, Crain B, Troncoso JC (2008) Neuronal hypertrophy in asymptomatic Alzheimer disease. J Neuropathol Exp Neurol 67:578–589

Innis SM (2007) Dietary (n-3) fatty acids and brain development. J Nutr 137:855–859

Iqbal K, Alonso AC, Gong CX, Khatoon S, Pei JJ, Wang JZ, Grundke-Iqbal I (1998) Mechanisms of neurofibrillary degeneration and the formation of neurofibrillary tangles. J Neural Transm Suppl 53:169–180

Jana M, Palencia CA, Pahan K (2008) Fibrillar amyloid-beta peptides activate microglia via TLR2: implications for Alzheimer's disease. J Immunol 181:7254–7262

Jiang R, Manson JE, Stampfer MJ, Liu S, Willett WC, Hu FB (2002) Nut and peanut butter consumption and risk of type 2 diabetes in women. JAMA 288:2554–2560

Jurd L (1958) Plant polyphenols: the polyphenolic constituents of the walnut (Juglans regia). J Am Chem Soc 80:2249–2252

Kadowaki H, Nishitoh H, Urano F, Sadamitsu C, Matsuzawa A, Takeda K, Masutani H, Yodoi J, Urano Y, Nagano T, Ichijo H (2005) Amyloid beta induces neuronal cell death through ROS-mediated ASK1 activation. Cell Death Differ 12:19–24

Keller JN, Schmitt FA, Scheff SW, Ding Q, Chen Q, Butterfield DA, Markesbery WR (2005) Evidence of increased oxidative damage in subjects with mild cognitive impairment. Neurology 64:1152–1156

Khachaturian ZS (1994) Calcium hypothesis of Alzheimer's disease and brain aging. Ann N Y Acad Sci 747:1–11

Knopman DS, Parisi JE, Salciati A, Floriach-Robert M, Boeve BF, Ivnik RJ, Smith GE, Dickson DW, Johnson KA, Petersen L E, McDonald WC, Braak H, Petersen RC (2003) Neuropathology of cognitively normal elderly. Exp Neurol 62:1087–1095

Kordula T, Bugno M, Rydel RE, Travis J (2000) Mechanism of interleukin-1- and tumor necrosis factor alpha-dependent regulation of the alpha 1-antichymotrypsin gene in human astrocytes. J Neurosci 20:7510–7516

Kreutzberg GW (1996) Microglia: a sensor for pathological events in the CNS. Trends Neurosci 19:312–318

Kushner I (2001) C-reactive protein elevation can be caused by conditions other than inflammation and may reflect biologic aging. Cleve Clin J Med 68:535–537

Landfield PW (1987) 'Increased calcium-current' hypothesis of brain aging. Neurobiol Aging 8:346–347

Lavedrine F, Ravel A, Poupard A, Alary J (1997) Effect of geographic origin, variety and storage on tocopherol concentrations in walnuts by HPLC. Food Chem 58:135–140

Lavedrine F, Zmirou D, Ravel A, Balducci F, Alary J (1999) Blood cholesterol and walnut consumption: a cross-sectional survey in France. Prev Med 28:333–339

Lenaz G (2001) The mitochondrial production of reactive oxygen species: mechanisms and implications in human pathology. IUBMB Life 52:159–164

Lovell MA, Ehmann WD, Butler SM, Markesbery WR (1995) Elevated thiobarbituric acid-reactive substances and antioxidant enzyme activity in the brain in Alzheimer's disease. Neurology 45:1594–1601

Lovell MA, Gabbita SP, Markesbery WR (1999) Increased DNA oxidation and decreased levels of repair products in Alzheimer's disease ventricular CSF. J Neurochem 72:771–776

Lue LF, Rydel R, Brigham EF, Yang LB, Hampel H, Murphy GM Jr, Brachova L, Yan SD, Walker DG, Shen Y, Rogers J (2001a) Inflammatory repertoire of Alzheimer's disease and nondemented elderly microglia in vitro. Glia 35:72–79

Lue LF, Walker DG, Brachova L, Beach TG, Rogers J, Schmidt AM, Stern DM, Yan SD (2001b) Involvement of microglial receptor for advanced glycation endproducts (RAGE) in Alzheimer's disease: identification of a cellular activation mechanism. Exp Neurol 171:29–45

Luterman JD, Haroutunian V, Yemul S, Ho L, Purohit D, Aisen PS, Mohs R, Pasinetti GM (2000) Cytokine gene expression as a function of the clinical progression of Alzheimer disease dementia. Arch Neurol 57:1153–1160

Lyras L, Cairns NJ, Jenner A, Jenner P, Halliwell B (1997) An assessment of oxidative damage to proteins, lipids, and DNA in brain from patients with Alzheimer's disease. J Neurochem 68:2061–2069

Majid S, Khanduja KL, Gandhi RK, Kapur S, Sharma RR (1991) Influence of ellagic acid on antioxidant defense system and lipid peroxidation in mice. Biochem Pharmacol 42:1441–1445

Mao P, Reddy PH (2011) Aging and amyloid beta-induced oxidative DNA damage and mitochondrial dysfunction in Alzheimer's disease: implications for early intervention and therapeutics. Biochim Biophys Acta 1812:1359–1370

Masters CL, Simms G, Weinman NA, Multhaup G, McDonald BL, Beyreuther K (1985) Amyloid plaque core protein in Alzheimer disease and Down syndrome. Proc Natl Acad Sci U S A 82:4245–4249

McGeer PL, McGeer EG (1995) The inflammatory response system of brain: implications for therapy of Alzheimer and other neurodegenerative diseases. Brain Res Rev 21:195–218

McGeer PL, Akiyama H, Itagaki S, McGeer EG (1989) Activation of the classical complement pathway in brain tissue of Alzheimer patients. Neurosci Lett 107:341–346

McKay DL, Chen CY, Yeum KJ, Matthan NR, Lichtenstein AH, Blumberg JB (2010) Chronic and acute effects of walnuts on antioxidant capacity and nutritional status in humans: a randomized, cross-over pilot study. Nutr J 9:21

Miquel J, Economos AC, Fleming J, Johnson JE Jr (1980) Mitochondrial role in cell aging. Exp Gerontol 15:5755–5791

Mishra N, Dubey A, Mishra R, Barik N (2010) Study on antioxidant activity of common dry fruits. Food Chem Toxicol 48:3316–3320

Mishra S, Mishra M, Seth P, Sharma SK (2011) Tetrahydrocurcumin confers protection against amyloid beta-induced toxicity. Neuroreport 22:23–27

Monji A, Utsumi H, Ueda T, Imoto T, Yoshida I, Hashioka S, Tashiro K, Tashiro N (2001) The relationship between the aggregational state of the amyloid-beta peptides and free radical generation by the peptides. J Neurochem 77:1425–1432

Montine TJ, Sidell KR, Crews BC, Markesbery WR, Marnett LJ, Roberts LJ, Morrow JD (1999) Elevated CSF prostaglandin E2 levels in patients with probable AD. Neurology 53:1495–1498

Montine TJ, Neely MD, Quinn JF, Beal MF, Markesbery WR, Roberts LJ, Morrow JD (2002) Lipid peroxidation in aging brain and Alzheimer's disease. Free Radic Biol Med 33:620–626

Morley JE (2010) Nutrition and the brain. Clin Geriatr Med 26:89–98

Muthaiyah B, Essa MM, Chauhan V, Chauhan A (2011) Protective effects of walnut extract against amyloid beta peptide-induced cell death and oxidative stress in PC12 cells. Neurochem Res 36:2096–2103

Navarro A, Boveris A, Bandez MJ, Sanchez-Pino MJ, Gomez C, Muntane G, Ferrer I (2009) Human brain cortex: mitochondrial oxidative damage and adaptive response in Parkinson disease and in dementia with Lewy bodies. Free Radic Biol Med 46:1574–1580

Nunomura A, Tamaoki T, Tanaka K, Motohashi N, Nakamura M, Hayashi T, Yamaguchi H, Shimohama S, Lee HG, Zhu X, Smith MA, Perry G (2010) Intraneuronal amyloid beta accumulation and oxidative damage to nucleic acids in Alzheimer disease. Neurobiol Dis 37:731–737

Oliveira I, Sousa A, Ferreira IC, Bento A, Estevinho L, Pereira JA (2008) Total phenols, antioxidant potential and antimicrobial activity of walnut (Juglans regia L.) green husks. Food Chem Toxicol 46:2326–2331

Pappolla MA, Chyan YJ, Poeggeler B, Frangione B, Wilson G, Ghiso J, Reiter RJ (2000) An assessment of the antioxidant and the antiamyloidogenic properties of melatonin: implications for Alzheimer's disease. J Neural Transm 107:203–231

Parachikova A, Agadjanyan MG, Cribbs DH, Blurton-Jones M, Perreau V, Rogers J, Beach TG, Cotman CW (2007) Inflammatory changes parallel the early stages of Alzheimer disease. Neurobiol Aging 28:1821–1833

Paradies G, Petrosillo G, Paradies V, Ruggiero FM (2011) Mitochondrial dysfunction in brain aging: role of oxidative stress and cardiolipin. Neurochem Int 58:447–457

Park SY, Kim HS, Cho EK, Kwon BY, Phark S, Hwang KW, Sul D (2008) Curcumin protected PC12 cells against beta-amyloid-induced toxicity through the inhibition of oxidative damage and tau hyperphosphorylation. Food Chem Toxicol 46:2881–2887

Pasinetti GM, Aisen PS (1998) Cyclooxygenase-2 expression is increased in frontal cortex of Alzheimer's disease brain. Neuroscience 87:319–324

Pereira JA, Oliveira I, Sousa A, Ferreira IC, Bento A, Estevinho L (2008) Bioactive properties and chemical composition of six walnut (Juglans regia L.) cultivars. Food Chem Toxicol 46:2103–2111

Pereira JA, Oliveira I, Sousa A, Valentao P, Andrade PB, Ferreira IC, Ferreres F, Bento A, Seabra R, Estevinho L (2007) Walnut (Juglans regia L.) leaves: phenolic compounds, antibacterial activity and antioxidant potential of different cultivars. Food Chem Toxicol 45:2287–2295

Pietta PG (2000) Flavonoids as antioxidants. J Nat Prod 63:1035–1042

Pribis P, Bailey RN, Russell AA, Kilsby MA, Hernandez M, Craig WJ, Grajales T, Shavlik DJ, Sabate J (2011) Effects of walnut consumption on cognitive performance in young adults. Br J Nutr 107:1393–1401

Price JL, Morris JC (1999) Tangles and plaques in nondemented aging and "preclinical" Alzheimer's disease. Ann Neurol 45:358–368

Rajaram S, Haddad EH, Mejia A, Sabate J (2009) Walnuts and fatty fish influence different serum lipid fractions in normal to mildly hyperlipidemic individuals: a randomized controlled study. Am J Clin Nutr 89:1657S–1663S

Reiter RJ, Manchester LC, Tan DX (2005) Melatonin in walnuts: influence on levels of melatonin and total antioxidant capacity of blood. Nutrition 21:920–924

Rogers J, Schultz J, Brachova L, Lue LF, Webster S, Bradt B, Cooper NR, Moss DE (1992) Complement activation and beta-amyloid-mediated neurotoxicity in Alzheimer's disease. Res Immunol 143:624–630

Rozemuller AJ, van Gool WA, Eikelenboom P (2005) The neuroinflammatory response in plaques and amyloid angiopathy in Alzheimer's disease: therapeutic implications. Curr Drug Targets CNS Neurol Disord 4:223–233
Rozovsky I, Finch CE, Morgan TE (1998) Age-related activation of microglia and astrocytes: in vitro studies show persistent phenotypes of aging, increased proliferation, and resistance to down-regulation. Neurobiol Aging 19:97–103
Sabate J, Fraser GE, Burke K, Knutsen SF, Bennett H, Lindsted KD (1993) Effects of walnuts on serum lipid levels and blood pressure in normal men. N Engl J Med 328:603–607
Schwab C, McGeer PL (2008) Inflammatory aspects of Alzheimer disease and other neurodegenerative disorders. J Alzheimers Dis 13:359–369
Sheng JG, Mrak RE, Griffin WS (1998) Enlarged and phagocytic, but not primed, interleukin-1 alpha-immunoreactive microglia increase with age in normal human brain. Acta Neuropathol 95:229–234
Smith CD, Carney JM, Starke-Reed PE, Oliver CN, Stadtman ER, Floyd RA, Markesbery WR (1991) Excess brain protein oxidation and enzyme dysfunction in normal aging and in Alzheimer disease. Proc Natl Acad Sci U S A 88:10540–10543
Soto C, Branes MC, Alvarez J, Inestrosa NC (1994) Structural determinants of the Alzheimer's amyloid beta-peptide. J Neurochem 63:1191–1198
Spaulding CC, Walford RL, Effros RB (1997) Calorie restriction inhibits the age-related dysregulation of the cytokines TNF-alpha and IL-6 in C3B10RF1 mice. Mech Aging Dev 93:87–94
Sponne I, Fifre A, Drouet B, Klein C, Koziel V, Pincon-Raymond M, Olivier JL, Chambaz J, Pillot T (2003) Apoptotic neuronal cell death induced by the non-fibrillar amyloid-beta peptide proceeds through an early reactive oxygen species-dependent cytoskeleton perturbation. J Biol Chem 278:3437–3445
Stampar F, Solar A, Hudina M, Veberic R, Colaric M (2006) Traditional walnut liqueur-cocktail of phenolics. Food Chemistry 95:627–631
Steele M, Stuchbury G, Munch G (2007) The molecular basis of the prevention of Alzheimer's disease through healthy nutrition. Exp Gerontol 42:28–36
Tarkowski E, Liljeroth AM, Minthon L, Tarkowski A, Wallin A, Blennow K (2003) Cerebral pattern of pro- and anti-inflammatory cytokines in dementias. Brain Res Bull 61:255–260
Torabian S, Haddad E, Rajaram S, Banta J, Sabate J (2009) Acute effect of nut consumption on plasma total polyphenols, antioxidant capacity and lipid peroxidation. J Hum Nutr Diet 22:64–71
Walker DG, Link J, Lue LF, Dalsing-Hernandez JE, Boyes BE (2006) Gene expression changes by amyloid beta peptide-stimulated human postmortem brain microglia identify activation of multiple inflammatory processes. J Leukoc Biol 79:596–610
Wang X, Su B, Zheng L, Perry G, Smith MA, Zhu X (2009) The role of abnormal mitochondrial dynamics in the pathogenesis of Alzheimer's disease. J Neurochem 109:153–159
Waring P (2005) Redox active calcium ion channels and cell death. Arch Biochem Biophys 434:33–42
Webster S, Lue LF, Brachova L, Tenner AJ, McGeer PL, Terai K, Walker DG, Bradt B, Cooper NR, Rogers J (1997) Molecular and cellular characterization of the membrane attack complex, C5b-9, in Alzheimer's disease. Neurobiol Aging 18:415–421
Willis LM, Shukitt-Hale B, Cheng V, Joseph JA (2009) Dose-dependent effects of walnuts on motor and cognitive function in aged rats. Br J Nutr 101:1140–1144
Wyss-Coray T (2006) Inflammation in Alzheimer disease: driving force, bystander or beneficial response? Nat Med 12:1005–1015
Xin W, Wei T, Chen C, Ni Y, Zhao B, Hou J (2000) Mechanisms of apoptosis in rat cerebellar granule cells induced by hydroxyl radicals and the effects of EGb761 and its constituents. Toxicology 148:103–110
Zambon D, Sabate J, Munoz S, Campero B, Casals E, Merlos M, Laguna JC, Ros E (2000) Substituting walnuts for monounsaturated fat improves the serum lipid profile of hypercholesterolemic men and women. A randomized crossover trial. Ann Intern Med 132:538–546

Chapter 17
Smart Dietary Interventions and Prevention of Cognitive Decline with Aging

S. Asha Devi

Abstract Brain aging results in the development of cognitive and motor deficits in animals and humans that are manifested by middle-age. These deficits evolve from neuronal damage as a consequence of oxidative stress. Various preclinical and clinical studies have proved the significance of dietary interventions in improving cognitive loss with age. Basic scientists have evaluated the mechanisms involved in improving the cognitive performance in aging animals by using dietary supplements, though human studies lack in understanding the mechanisms. However, observational data support the benefits derived from the nutritional supplementation of specific antioxidants in slowing cognitive loss with age. This article is a record of the recent progress made on oxidative stress and cognitive decline with age on animal models and human subjects showing the importance of non-polyphenolic and polyphenolic-rich plant products in alleviating age-related cognitive loss.

Keywords Age • Brain • Hippocampus • Cognition • Oxidative stress • Proanthocyanidin • Vitamin E

17.1 Introduction

Cognitive decline in past middle-age is a complex process involving many underlying morphological changes that are due to various biochemical and molecular mechanisms. As the older segment of the population continues to grow, it has become absolutely necessary to develop strategies to prevent or lessen age-associated cognitive decline. 'Cognition', in this article is defined as a range of physiological processes that permit one to acquire, evaluate, manipulate and store the acquired information from the surroundings. Basically, cognitive function consists of mainly six domains such as executive function, memory, attention, perception, psychomo-

S. Asha Devi (✉)
Laboratory of Gerontology, Department of Zoology, Bangalore University,
Bangalore 560056, Karnataka, India
e-mail: asuba@blr.vsnl.net.in; sambe.ashadevi@gmail.com

M. K. Thakur, S. I. S. Rattan (eds.), *Brain Aging and Therapeutic Interventions*,
DOI 10.1007/978-94-007-5237-5_17,

tor and language skills and, each of these domains has its own subdivisions. For example, memory is not a single factor but a multi-dimensional unit. Memory involves storage of information for many decades. It is known that memory could be declarative and non-declarative with the former being verbal while the latter type of memory cannot be expressed such as how to drive a car. On a gross scale, the term 'dementia' means the inability to retain all of the above memory functions. Humans experience dementia of two types: semantic and episodic dementia, while the former reflects knowledge that is not something unusual to us and usually not recalled in relation to time, the later encompasses events in relation to time, as examinations based on specific time and even site.

Since, all of the cognitive functions are affected by age, it is essential to alleviate age-related cognitive loss and eventually several behavioral declines such as motor and cognitive functions and ultimately to neuronal degenerative disorders, for example, Alzheimer's (AD) and Parkinson's disease (PD). However, patients receiving diet and nutrient supplements experience less cognitive loss. Recent studies have suggested that cognitive loss during normal aging may be prevented through physical exercise, calorie restriction and dietary supplements—all of which are non-pharmacological interventions.

The focus is on the role of oxidative stress on the cognitive ability of the aging brain in experimental models and humans. Further, attempts have been made to summarize the current status of research on humans and animal models of aging in our lab as well as of others on one particular type of intervention, dietary antioxidant supplements that are beneficial in lessening age-related cognitive loss. In this article, only the most relevant biochemical, morphological and molecular changes during cognitive loss are discussed. Two of the most important antioxidants belonging to non-phenolic and phenolic groups that are of relevance to cognitive function in the aged have been selected. It is expected that the information from preclinical studies from our laboratory as well as from others on humans will assist older adults, to select specific dietary supplements for improving their cognitive ability as well as the middle-aged in preventing cognitive loss.

17.2 Aging of the Brain

The brain is a vital organ since it modulates all the involuntary functions like the heart beat, pulmonary breathing and cognitive functions and hence is more vulnerable to several aging effects. Aging, inflammation and oxidative stress are important factors in brain aging with concomitant cognitive decline particularly decreased memory such as recognition memory (James et al. 2008), short term recall (Gilchrist et al. 2008) and long-term memory (Park et al. 2002) in aged subjects. Wen et al. (2011) from New South Wales have recently reported that the human brain functions as an interconnected world network and not as a collection of discrete regions. In their study, the researchers performed magnetic resonance imaging (MRI) scans on 342 healthy individuals aged 72–92, using a new imaging technique called diffusion tensor imaging (DTI). The information flow within and between regions as well is extremely crucial for cognitive functions. With age, human brain network involving complex neural connectivity deteriorates leading to slowing down of information processing and impacting the cognitive functions. With the advent of new MRI technology and increased computational power, neural maps have been developed. These techniques have resulted in a paradigm shift in the way neuroscientists understand the brain anatomy, in particular the hippocampus and cerebral cortex, the grey outer layer of the brain where most mental functions associated with learning takes place. Wen et al. (2011) have shown that discrete neuroanatomical networks are associated with specific cognitive abilities in old age.

An important change that we see during normal aging is the loss of neurons in the brain. The loss of neurons over time is speculated to be an evolutionary trade-off. Several biological changes characterize normal brain aging in humans. Although some of the age-associated neural alterations are also found in other closest species such as the chimpanzees, the volumetric decline of specific brain structures, such as the hippocampus and frontal lobe, has only been observed in humans ranging from 22 to 88 years of age (Sherwood et al. 2011) although the functional capacity of the brain deteriorates over time in animals as well. In contrast to the previous dogma, the present understanding is that a fully developed brain can replace the lost neurons even into old age. The hippocampus is the "memory hub" but shrinks from middle-age onwards even in healthy people. Basically, the decline in the ability for neurogenesis from adult neural stem cells (NScs) results in reduced brain function, such as spatial learning and memory. The NSCs are located as dormant cells in the subventricular region of the lateral ventricle, and the subgranular zone (SGZ) of the hippocampal dentate gyrus (DG) of the brain (Kempermann et al. 2008). It is known that the hippocampal volume reduces more in patients suffering from depression and other psychiatric conditions compared to healthy subjects. Supporting these observations, are the studies that have demonstrated increased neurogenesis in the hippocampus through administration of antidepressant drugs that in fact results in behavioral changes in stress-induced models and patients (Lee et al. 2007).

Normal brain aging over the years is characterized by the perennial efforts of the brain to battle against accumulation of several insults and oxidative stress is one among them. Experimental studies in our laboratory (Asha Devi 2009) suggest that one of the crucial factors mediating the effects of normal aging on neuronal function and behaviour is oxidative stress. During normal aging, events such as oxidative stress due to elevated reactive oxygen species (ROS), reactive nitrogen species (RNS), followed by increased oxidative modification of lipids, proteins and nucleic acids contribute to lowered cognitive performance of the brain even in the absence of neurodegenerative diseases (Farooqui and Farooqui 2009; Asha Devi and Kiran 2004; Calabrese et al. 2004). The loss in mitochondrial function has important role in aging and neurodegenerative disorders (Lopez-Lluch et al. 2008). In mammalian brain aging, more precisely in rats and mice, the gradual conversion of healthy to dysfunctional mitochondria with decreased rates of electron transfer in complexes

I and IV and hence of ATP generation is associated with the accumulation of oxidation products of phospholipids and proteins, and these characteristics appear as determining factors in brain aging (Boveris and Navarro 2008). In addition, many regions of the brain undergo morphological and functional modifications resulting in a gradual deterioration in memory (Christensen 2001) and motor performance (Sastry and Rao 2000).

Behavioral, cellular and molecular studies in aging rats have shown the possibilities of dramatically reducing the increase in the oxidative stress-related biochemical markers not only in the plasma (Asha Devi et al. 2003) but also in the specific brain regions through physical activity as one of the interventions for improving cognitive performance past middle-age (Jolitha et al. 2006). Interestingly, although cognitive loss is lowered in aged rats by exercise, it is more effective when combined with a non-phenolic antioxidant such as vitamin E (Jolitha et al. 2009; Asha Devi and Prathima 2005). The mechanisms of physical activity alone as an anti-aging factor that can modify brain and behavior, and the benefits derived out of this intervention have been reviewed comprehensively elsewhere (Asha Devi et al. 2011a).

17.3 Nutrition and Cognitive Aging

The identification of neuroprotective antioxidants in food is useful for developing anti-aging natural products and managing cognitive deficits during normal aging. In fact, the synthetic and natural food supplements known as nootropics are known to enhance brain function in terms of enhanced cognition, concentration, short-term and long-term memory capacity and work performance. Interestingly, the tendency of accumulating genetic defects that influence the regenerative capacity of the NSCs such as telomere shortening, DNA oxidations and mitochondrial function, DNA deletions and point mutations are often a result of deficient nutrient supplies such as folate and vitamin B12 that are much needed for genome maintenance(Hamilton et al. 2001). It is known that when free radicals attack delicate brain cells, they disrupt optimal cellular function and often cause age-related cognitive decline.

Among animal models, cognitive ability and motor function are conventionally quantified through various tests such as those that assess the time a rodent can remain on an accelerod. T-maze and Y-maze experiments are used to assess learning in terms of acquisition, working (short-term) and reference (long-term) memory. A good reference memory suggests consistency among trials that is required for learning a task such as swim to a platform. Working memory explains the ability to hold specific information such as places earlier visited. Old rats show reduced reference and working memory in water-maze (Rex et al. 2004), radial arm maze (Shukitt-Hale et al. 2004) and T-maze tests (Jolitha et al. 2009). In an experimental rat model, Bickford et al. (2000) have shown that a diet supplemented with plant-derived antioxidants can reverse age-related decline in memory and cognition.

17.3.1 Antioxidants as Smart Dietary Supplements

While the body produces natural antioxidants such as glutathione (GSH), often it requires an additional supply to prevent the increased damage caused by oxidative stress. An aging brain consumes 30 % of our daily calories and hence a right antioxidant should provide the fuel to the brain to think, concentrate, remember and react even in the aged. For instance, glutathione is the body's most potent antioxidant, and particularly important to the brain. However, GSH levels have been shown to decrease with aging which may contribute as one of the compounds for the increased vulnerability of the neurons to oxidative stress and subsequent damage (Ayden et al. 2007). The antioxidant use in humans has often resulted in mixed results. The notion that dietary antioxidants may have therapeutic role in preventing age-associated neurodegenerative diseases in humans have stemmed from the experiments showing blockage of neuronal death from *in vitro* studies of animal models of Alzheimer's disease (AD), Parkinson's disease (PD) and amyotrophic lateral sclerosis (ALS) (Esposito et al. 2002). In addition, it is known that mental acuity and cognition are two aspects of health that become increasingly important to disease-free older adults. As is the case of many diseases, oxidative stress has been implicated in the etiology of cognitive dysfunction in normal aging. The following sections will focus on the role of dietary antioxidants, in particular vitamin E, a non-phenolic antioxidant and grape seeds, a phenolic antioxidant as smart interventions in maintenance of cognitive function throughout life.

17.3.1.1 Vitamin E and Brain Aging

Vitamin E has received a huge amount of public interest of late, due to its property of destructing free radicals and more so as an antioxidant that is capable of crossing the blood brain barrier (BBB), and its fat-solubility property is exceedingly valuable in protecting cell membranes from oxidative damage. The benefits derived from vitamin E certainly go well beyond that.

Vitamin E is the most studied non-phenolic antioxidant supplement. Actually, vitamin E is not a single compound, but a group of eight closely related compounds: four tocopherols and four tocotrienols. All these eight molecules have biological activity, but the most active one is alpha-tocopherol. Another one, gamma-tocopherol contributes significantly to human health in ways that have not yet been completely evaluated. Several evidences exist for an improvement in the physiology of brain health in rodents, e.g., alpha-tocopherol can improve age-related impairments in long-term potentiation (LTP) and improve cognitive behaviors (Takatsu et al. 2010). Vitamin E has also been shown to have actions such as reducing oxidation of lipids through *in vitro* studies of aging cerebral cortex of mouse brain (Kan et al. 1991), one of the mechanisms for the development of neurodegenerative diseases with aging *in vivo*. Vitamin E is neuroprotective in apoE-deficient mice (Veinbergs et al. 2001) and modifies Aβ toxicity in cultured hippocampal neurons. In their study, they could prevent the onset of behavioral deficits induced by infusions of Aβ into the cerebroventricles. Vitamin E is reported to increase cognitive performance in T-maze in old male rats of 18-months of age and reduced the amount of hydrogen peroxide generation, and free radical mediated reactions such as protein oxidation and lipid peroxidation in the hippocampus and cerebral cortex regions when compared with the unsupplemented rats (Jolitha et al. 2009). Researchers have also noted that vitamin E supplementation in mice at 2 age points, i.e. 13 months and 19.5 months prevents the decrease in activities of mitochondrial markers of aging such as mtNOS, Mn-SOD, NADH-cytochrome c reductase and cytochrome oxidase activity (Navarro et al. 2005).

The following is a selective discussion of vitamin E supplementation in human trials to treat or prevent cognitive decline. Longitudinal studies have shown that vitamin E intake as foods or supplements, is associated with less cognitive decline with age (Morris et al. 2002). Knowing that dietary tocopherols consist of different individual tocopherols, a follow-up report that included six-year data found that the intake of both individual tocopherols and total tocopherols was protective against AD and cognitive decline (Morris et al. 2005). Although there are conflicting results on the effect of antioxidants on cognitive function in the elderly, the search for suitable antioxidant has always been of interest to neurobiologists, neurophysiologists as well as nutrition biochemists for assisting the human population in retaining a healthy brain in their grey years. In a population-based cohort study conducted in Italy, a total of 1033 participants aged at least 65 years underwent clinical and neuropsychological examinations of their blood vitamin E analysis and diets assessed. The study revealed that the higher levels of vitamin E in plasma might provide significant protection against cognitive impairment and dementia in elderly subjects. This conclusion was drawn based on the observation that participants with plasma vitamin E levels in the bottom tertile had a significantly higher probability of being demented (OR 2.6, 95 % CI 1.0–7.1) and also of suffering from cognitive impairment (OR 2.2, 95 % CI 1.2–4.2) compared to those in the highest vitamin E tertile after adjustment for age, gender, education, lipid levels, energy intake, vitamin E intake, and smoking (Cherubini et al. 2005). The Honolulu-Asia Aging Study (Masaki et al. 2000) has shown significant protective effect when vitamin E and vitamin C are given as a combined supplement for non-AD dementias but not for AD. A striking observation has been among those without dementia; use of either vitamin E or vitamin C alone was associated with better cognitive performance. Similar results have been found in the Canadian Study of Health and Aging (Maxwell et al. 2005).

17.3.1.2 Polyphenols and Brain Aging

Grape seeds contain lipids, proteins, carbohydrates, and 6 % polyphenols depending on the variety. Polyphenols in grape seeds are mainly flavonoids, including gallic acid, the monomeric flavan-3-ols catechin and epicatechin, gallocatechin, epigallocatechin and epicatechin 3-o-gallate, and procyanidin dimmers, trimers, and highly polymerized procyanidin. Grape seeds contain mainly phenols such as proanthocyanidin (oligomeric proanthocyanidin). Flavonoids are polyphenolic compounds present in vegetables, fruits, berries and beverages such as tea, red wine and fruit juices, having effects as antioxidants. Flavonoids form a group of many different compounds, of which more than 5,000 have been currently characterised. Flavonols from red wine, mainly catechin monomers and procyanidin dimers and trimers have been shown to have a significant *in vitro* antioxidant activity in many lipid systems and in particular against oxidation of low density lipoprotein (LDL), and higher than the well known α-tocopherol (Santos-Buelga and Scalbert 2000). The beneficial effects of flavonoids are well recognized in the prevention of neurodegenerative alterations with age (Ramassamy 2006; Schmidt-Schilling et al. 2005; Sun et al. 2002; Moosmann and Behl 2002). Considering its neuroprotective function after supplementation in human (Bagchi et al. 2000) subjects, it is imperative to understand metabolites involved that can prevent the loss in cognitive performance in normal aging subjects. Flavonoids such as delphinidin is known to have significant impact on cell signalling mechanisms such as inhibition of endothelial cell proliferation and cell cycle progression via extracellular signal-regulated kinase (ERK)-1/2 activation (Martin et al. 2002). Studies of Joseph et al. (2009) on animals fed with blue berry and spinach dietary supplementation have demonstrated increases in muscarinic receptor sensitivity and reversal in age-related dysregulation and Ca^{2+}–buffering ability, both of which are indices of neuronal dysregulation observed in aging. Studies have demonstrated that dietary supplementation with fruits and vegetable extracts can reduce the susceptibility to oxidative stress as assessed by *in vivo* reductions in neuronal signaling and behavioral deficits and *in vitro* H_2O_2-induced reductions in striatal synaptosomal calcium buffering (Galli et al. 2002). Polyphenolic compounds identified in fruits such as blue berries can improve signal transduction and neuronal communication and thereby improve cognitive and motor functions in the elderly even in the absence of neurodegenerative diseases (Lau et al 2007).

Oligomeric proanthocynidins (OPCs) are a class of flavanoids found in grape seeds. OPCs and procyanicolic oligomers (PCOs) are a class of nutrients belonging to the bioflavanoid family. Oligonol is a technology product emanating from the oligomerization of polyphenols, typically proanthocyanidin from a variety of fruits (grapes, apples, persimmons, etc.) that has optimized bioavailability. It is an optimized phenolic product containing catechin-type monomers and oligomeric proanthocyanidins, the easily absorbed forms. Typically the constituents of Oligonol are 15–20 % monomers, 8–12 % dimers and 5–10 % trimers. Supplementation of mice with Oligonol prior to the administration of ferric-nitrilotriacetic complex, a Fenton chemistry model, significantly reduces the extent of lipid peroxidation in the kidney, brain and liver (Aruoma et al. 2006).

Proanthocyanidins are known to cross the blood-brain barrier and scavenge free radicals in the blood vessels resulting in increased cognitive acuity. Glutamate excitotoxicity is one of the events that is seen during free radical injury. Experiments on GSE from two different varieties containing high amounts of polyphenols were analysed in primary culture of neonatal mouse hippocampal neurons treated with an excitotoxic glutamate. The results have suggested the presence of high affinity molecular targets for polyphenols in hippocampal neurons, which may be different from brain–derived neurotrophic factor (BDNF), and the significance of low molecular weight polyphenols or procyanidin oligomers for neuroprotection from free radicals (Narita et al. 2011). Data obtained from experiments in young and old albino rats have shown that grape seed extract has an inhibiting effect on the accumulation of age-related oxidative DNA damages in spinal cord and in various brain regions such as cerebral cortex, striatum and hippocampus (Balu et al. 2006).

In vivo studies in adult female rats supplemented with GSPE for 8 weeks in our laboratory have suggested neuroprotective effects of GSPE in the cerebral cortex, hippocampus and cerebellum. Experiments from our laboratory on adult female rats have shown increased activity of superoxide dismutase, an important antioxidant enzyme and decreased levels of malondialdehyde (MDA), an oxidation product of lipids by ROS. The study also demonstrated increased choline acetyltransferase (ChAT) activity in the above regions of the brain (Asha Devi et al. 2006). Proteomic analysis by Deshane et al. (2004) using 2D electrophoresis and mass spectrometry of the brain of normal adult female rats supplemented with 5 % GSPE for 6 weeks show 13 altered proteins in amount or charge. Since these proteins are quantitatively less in mouse models of Alzheimer's disease, the data might suggest not only the neuroprotective ability of GSPE but also the association of such proteins with diseases of the brain. An interesting finding from our lab is on the effectiveness of GSPE in reducing the blood glucose in the middle-aged female rats to that of the adults. This reduction was accompanied by improved cognitive ability when these rats were tested in a T-maze. Hence GSPE could impact the hippocampal neurons either in terms of improved regulatory mechanisms for glucose uptake or by altered storage mechanism through chemical or structural components (Asha Devi et al. 2011b). GSPE was effective in reducing lipofuscin granules, a peroxidation product, of mitochondrial degeneration in the hippocampal neurons of middle-aged animals (Fig. 17.1). Blood glucose regulation is also made possible by blue berry extracts which can inhibit α-glucosidase and α–amylase (McDougall et al. 2005). Experiments on young and old rats have demonstrated that blue berries have anti-inflammatory and antioxidant properties (Malin et al. 2011; Galli et al. 2006; Andres-Lacueva et al. 2005). Blue berries can restore memory in aged rats by lowering the nuclear factor-kappa beta (NF-kB) (Goyarzu et al. 2004). A marked finding of Casadesus and his co-scientists (2004) is on the capacity of hippocampus neurons for neurogenesis in the berry supplemented Alzheimer-bred rat and hence its potential for overcoming the genetic predisposition to the disease. Similar to grape seeds, studies have demonstrated that procyanidins extracted from lotus seed (LSPC) can ameliorate memory impairment in cognitively deficient and aged rats (Xu et al. 2009). Their studies were on young female rats, and aged unimpaired and aged impaired rats were chosen from aged female rats. Aged rats also showed a decline in antioxidant defense capacities and a significant increase in lipid peroxidation and protein oxidation levels in hippocampus and cerebral cortex than young rats. LSPC supplementation (50,100 mg/kg BW, p.o.) for 7 weeks significantly improved learning and memory impairments in AI animals in the Morris water maze test, as evaluated by shortened escape latency and swimming distance.

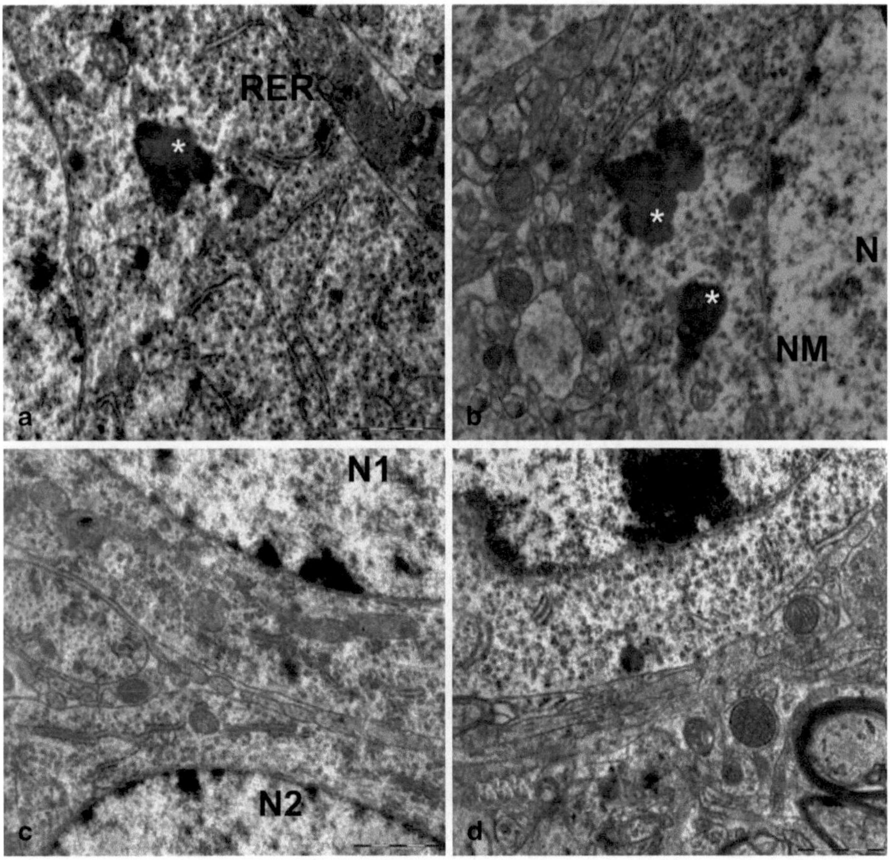

Fig. 17.1 Accumulation of lipofuscin deposit (*asterix*) in adult (**a**) and middle-aged (**b**) female *Wistar* rats. Note the absence of these deposits in GSPE-supplemented adult (**c**) and middle-aged (**d**) rats (× 18,500). *N1* and *N2* are two neuronal cell bodies, *RER* Rough endoplasmic reticulum, *NM* Nuclear membrane, *N* Nucleus

LSPC was effective in restoring acetylcholine (ACh) contents and acetylcholinesterase (AChE) activities in hippocampus and cerebral cortex of AI animals. Overall, polyphenols improve cell survival by directly interacting with receptors or enzymes related to signal transduction.

17.4 Conclusion

Chronological aging and oxidative stress play an important role in brain aging. The increase in oxidative stress parameters in the hippocampus and cortex is accompanied by a decline in cognitive performance in the elderly population. This is true even in the absence of any neurological disorders. Evidences from research have

Table 17.1 Responses of the brain to polyphenols in animals and humans

Species	Age (months)	Effects	References
Fischer rats	3–4	Irradiation decreased performance on a learning and memory maze and decreased the measure of dopamine, a brain chemical, release one month following radiation, these deficits were protected by the antioxidant	Shukitt-Hale et al. 2007
Rodent	3–18	Blueberry and strawberry lowers oxidative stress directly by altering the signaling in neuronal communication and calcium buffering capacity	Shukitt-Hale et al. 2008
Fischer 344 rats	19	Considerable degree of age-related decline in memory loss can be prevented prevented by blue berry extracts	Shukitt-Hale et al. 2009
SHR female rats	1	Grape proanthrocyanidin supplementation significantly reduced arterial pressure and significantly improves cognition	Peng et al. 2005
Transgenic mice APP+ PS1	4, 12	Protective mechanisms are derived from BB-induced enhancement of memory-associated neuronal signaling (e.g. extracellular signal-regulated kinase) and alterations in neutral sphingomyelin-specific phospholipase C activity. Indicate that it may be possible to overcome genetic predispositions to Alzheimer disease through diet	Joseph et al. 2003
129S1/ SvImJ mice	3–3.5	Diet rich in polyphenols and PUFA can modulate neurogenesis in adult mice	Valente et al. 2009
Male *Wistar* rats	22	GSE is effective in preventing AD-type of dementia and acts as an antioxidant	Farbood et al. 2009
Rats	18–22	MAPK is required fore LTP which is important as a cellular signaling and as candidates for memory	Mazzuchelli and Brambilla 2000
Humans	65	A 10-year study period showed that dietary flavonoid intake is associated with better cognitive evolution	Letenneur et al. 2007

suggested that vitamins such as vitamin E in the form of α- and γ-tocopherols and flavanoid-rich compounds from berries provide benefits through improved signal transduction and neuronal communication in the aging animal and human subjects (Table 17.1). This method of smart dietary interventions especially past middle-age and beyond with natural products has proved beneficial in terms of increased alertness and cognition by cleansing the neurons of free radicals. Compared to drugs, therapies based on natural compounds promise to be safer, easier to accomplish their bioavailability, are less toxic, and well tolerated by human subjects, even for longer periods.

Acknowledgements The author wishes to acknowledge, the University Grants Commission (F. No. 3-356/2007 (SR 2008), which provided financial support for the work performed in the author's laboratory. Thanks to Prof. S. Venkateswaran at the Regional Institute of English, Bangalore, for editing the initial draft of this article.

References

Andres-Lacueva C, Shukitt-Hale B, Galli RL, Jauregul O, Lamuela-Raventos RM, Joseph JA (2005) Anthocyanins in aged blue-berry-fed rats are found centrally and may enhance memory. Nutr Neurosci 8:111–120

Aruoma OI, Sun B, Fujii H, Neergheen VS, Bahorun T, Kang K, Sung M (2006) Low molecular proanthocyanidin dietary biofactor oligonol: its modulation of oxidative stress, bioefficacy, neuroprotection, food application and chemoprevention potentials. Biofactors 27:245–265. doi:10.1002/biof.5520270121

Asha Devi S, Prathima S, Subramanyam MVV (2003) Dietary vitamin E and physical exercise: I. Altered endurance capacity and plasma lipid profile in aging rats. Exp Geron 38(3):285–290. doi:10.1016/S0531-5565(02)00206-1

Asha Devi S, Kiran TR (2004) Regional responses in antioxidant system to exercise training and dietary vitamin E in aging rat brain. Neurobiol Aging 25:501–508. doi:10.1016/S0197-4580(03)00112-X

Asha Devi S, Prathima S (2005) Synergistic effects of physical exercise and antioxidants in aging mammalian brain. In: Thakur MK, Prasad S (eds) Molecular and cellular neurobiology. Narosa, New Delhi, p 123–134

Asha Devi S, Jolitha AB, Ishii N (2006) Grape seed proanthocyanidin extract (GSPE) and antioxidant defense in the brain of adult rats. Med Sci Monit 12:BR124–BR129

Asha Devi S (2009) Aging brain: prevention of oxidative stress by vitamin E and exercise. Sci World J 9:366–372

Asha Devi S, Manjula KR, Shankaranarayana Rao BS (2011a) Healthy brain and well-being: sedentary lifestyle can impact cognitive ability adversely. In: Bergin MG (ed) Sedentary behavior: physiology, health risks and Interventions. NOVA, USA, p 1–27

Asha Devi S, Sagar Chandrasekar BK, Manjula KR, Ishii N (2011b) Grape seed proanthocyanidin lowers brain oxidative stress in adult and middle-aged rats Exp Geron. doi:10.1016/j.exger.2011.08.006

Ayden M, Özkök Cengis S, Ağchan B, Yilmaz H, Öztürk O, Yaylim I, Isbir T (2007) Changes in oxidative stress in Wistar albino rats during senescence. Adv Mol Med 3:171–175. doi:10.2399/amm.07.171

Bagchi D, Bagchi M, Stohs SJ, Das DK, Ray SD, Kuszynski CA, Joshi SS, Pruess HG (2000) Free radicals and grape seed proanythocyanidin extract: importance in human health and disease prevention. Toxicol 148:187-192. doi:10.1016/S0300-583x(00)00210-8

Balu M, Sangeetha P, Murali G, Paneerselvam C (2006) Modulatory role of grape seed extract on age-related oxidative DNA damage in central nervous system of rats. Brain Res Bull 68:469–473. doi:10.1016/j.brainresbull.2005.10.007

Bickford PC, Gould T, Briederick L, Chadman K, Pollock A, Young D, B Shukitt-Hale B, Joseph J (2000) Antioxidant-rich diets improve cerebellar physiology and motor learning in aged rats. Brain Res 866:211–217. doi:10.1177/1534582304270783

Boveris A, Navarro A (2008) Brain mitochondrial dysfunction in aging. IUBMB Life 60:308–314. doi:10.1002/iub.46

Calabrese V, Scapagnini G, Ravagna A, Colombrita S, Spadaro F, Buterfield DA (2004) Increased heat shock proteins in rat brain during aging: relationship with mitochondrial function and glutathioine redox state. Mech Aging Dev 125:325–335. doi:10.1016/j mad.2004.01.003

Casadesus G, Shukitt-Hale B, Stellwagon HM, Zhu X, Lee HG, Smith MA, Joseph JA (2004) Modulation of hippocampal plasticity and cognitive behavior by short-term blue berry supplementation in aged rats. Nutr Neurosci 7:309–316

Cherubini A, Martin A, Andres-Lacueva C, Lorio A, Lamponi M, Patrizia Mecocci P, Bartali B, Annamaria Corsi A, Senin U, Ferrucci U (2005) Vitamin E levels, cognitive impairment and dementia in older persons: the InCHIANTI study. Neurobiol aging 26:982–994. doi:10.1016/j.neurobiolaging.2004.09.002

Christensen H (2001) What cognitive changes can be expected with normal aging? Aust N Z J Psychiatry 35:768–775

Deshane J, Chaves L, Sarikonda KV, Isbell S, Wilson L, Kirk M, Grubbs C, Barnes S, Meleth S, Kim H (2004) Proteomics analysis of rat brain protein modulations by grape seed extract. J Agric Food Chem 52:7872–7883

Esposito E, Rotilio D, Di Matteo V, Di Giulio C, Cacchio M, Algeri S (2002) A review of specific dietary antioxidants and the effects on biochemical mechanisms related to neurodegenerative processes. Neurobiol Aging 23:719–735. doi:10.1016/S0197-4580(02)00078-7

Farbood Y, Sarkaki A, Badavi M (2009) Preventive effect of grape seed hydroalcholic extract on dementia type of Alzheimer's disease in aged male rats. Int J Pharmacol 5:257–262. doi:10.3923/ijp.2009.257.262

Farooqui T, Farooqui AA (2009) Aging: an important factor for pathogenesis of neurodegenerative diseases. Mech Age Dev 130:203–215. doi:10.1016/j.mad.2008.11.006

Forman JJ, Torres M, Fukuto J (2002) Redox signaling. Mol Cell Biochem 234:49–62

Galli RL, Bielinski DF, Szprengiel A, Shukitt-Hale B, Joseph JA (2006) Blueberry supplemented diet reverses age-related decline in hippocampal HSP70 neuroprotection. Neurobiol Aging 27:344–350

Galli RL, Shukitt-hale B, Youdim KA, Joseph JA (2002) Fruit polyphenolics and brain aging: nutritional interventions targeting age-related neuronal and behavioral deficits. Ann N Y Acad Sci 959:128–132

Gilchrist AL, Cowan N, Naveh-Benjamin M (2008) Working memory capacity for spoken sentences decreases with adult aging: recall of fewer but not smaller chunks in older adults. Memory 16:773–787. doi:10.1080/09658210802261124

Goyarzu P, Malin DH, Lau FC (2004) Blueberry supplemented diet: effects on object recognition memory and nuclear factor-kappa B levels in aged rats. Nutr Neurosci 7:75–83

Hamilton ML, Van Remmen H, Drake JA, Yang H, Guo ZM, Kewitt K, Walter CA, Richardson A (2001) Does oxidative damage to DNA increase with age? Proc Natl Acad Sci U S A 98:10469–10474

James LE, Fogler KA, Tauber SK (2008) Recognition memory measures yield disproportionate effects of aging on learning face-name association. Psychol Aging 23:657–664. doi:10.1037/a0013008

Jolitha AB, Subramanyam MVV, Asha Devi S (2006) Modification by vitamin E and exercise of oxidative stress in regions of aging rat brain: studies on superoxide dismutase isoenzymes and protein oxidation status. Exp Gerontol 41:753–763. doi:10.1016/j.exger.2006.04.007

Jolitha AB, Subramanyam MVV, Asha Devi S (2009) Age-related responses of the rat cerebral cortex: influence of vitamin E and exercise on the cholinergic system. Biogerontology 10:53–63. doi:.1007/s10522-008-9154-6

Joseph JA, Denisova NA, Arendash G, Gordon M, Diamond D, Shukitt-Hale B, Morgan D (2003) Blueberry supplementation enhances signaling and prevents behavioral deficits in an Alzheimer disease model. Nutr Neurosci 6:153–62

Joseph JA, Cole G, Head et al (2009) Nutrition, brain aging and neurodegeneration. J Neurosci 29:12795–12801

Kan S, Asha Devi S, Kawashima S (1991) Effect of vitamin E on the accumulation of fluorescent material in cultured cerebral cortical cells of mice. Exp Gerontol 26:365–371. doi:10.1016/0531-5565(91)90048-Q

Kempermann G, Krebs J, Fabel K (2008) The contribution of failing adult hippocampal neurogenesis top psychiatric disorders. Curr Opin Psychiatry 21:290–295

Lau F, Shukitt-Hale B, Joseph B (2007) Nutritional intervention in brain aging. Reducing the effects of inflammation and oxidative stress. Inflammation in the pathogenesis of chronic diseases. Subcell Biochem 42:299–318. doi:10.1007/1-4020-5688-5-14

Lee BH, Kim H, Park SH, Kim YK (2007) Decreased plasma BDNF level in depressive patients. J Affect Disord 101:239–44

Letenneur L, Proust-Lima C, Le Gauge A, Dartigues JF, Barberger Gateau P (2007) Flavanoid intake and cognitive decline over a 10-year period. Am J Epidemiol 165:1364–1371

Lopez-Lluch G, Irusta PM, Navas P, de Caba R (2008) Mitochondrial biogenesis and health aging. Exp Geron 43:813–819

Malin DH, Lee DR, Goyarzu P, Chang Y, Ennis LJ, Becket E, Shukitt-Hale B, Joseph JA (2011) Short-term blueberry-enriched antioxidant diet prevents and reverses object recognition memory loss in aged rats. Nutrition 27:338–342

Martin S, Favot L, Matz R, Lugnier C, Andriantsitohaina R (2002) Delphinidin inhibits endothelial cell proliferation and cell cycle progression through a transient activation of ERK-1/2. Biochem Pharmacol 65:669–675

Masaki KH, Losonczy KG, Izmirlian G, Foley DJ, Ross GW, Petrovitch H, Havlik R, White LR (2000) Association of vitamin E and C supplement use with cognitive function and dementia in elderly men. Neurology 54:1265–1272

Maxwell CJ, Hicks MS, Hogan DB, Basran J, Ebly EM (2005) Supplemental use of antioxidant vitamins and subsequent risk of cognitive decline and dementia. Dement Geriatr Cogn Disord 20:45–51

Mazzucchelli C, Brambilla R (2000) MAPK signaling in neuronal plasticity and memory formation. Cell Mol Life Sci 57:604–611

McDougall GJ, Shapiro F, Dobson P, Smith P, Blako A, Stewart D (2005) Different polyphenol components of soft fruits inhibit α-amylase and α–glucosidase. J Agric Food Chem 53:2760–2766

Moosmann B, Behl C (2002) Antioxidants as treatment for neurdegenartive disorders. Expet Opin Investig Drugs 11:1407–1435

Morris MC, Evans DA, Bienias JL, Tangney CC, Wilson RS (2002) Vitamin E and cognitive decline in older persons. Arch Neurol 59:1125–1132

Morris MC, Evans DA, Tangney CC, Julia L, Bienias JL, Wilson RS, Aggarwal NT, Scherr PA (2005) Relation of the tocopherol forms to incident Alzheimer disease and to cognitive change. Am J Clin Nutr 81:508–514

Moskaug JO, Carlsen H, Myhrsted MCW (2005) Polyphenols and glutathione synthesis regulation. Am J Clin Nutr 8:2778–2783 (suppl)

Narita K, Hisamoto M, Okuda T, Takeda S (2011) Differential neuroprotective activity of two different grape seeds. PLoS One 6:e4574

Navarro A, Gomez C, Sanchez-Pino M, Gonzalez H, Bandez MS, Boveris Ad, Boveris A (2005) Vitamin E at high doses improves survival, neurological performance, and brain mitochondrial function in aging male mice. Amer J Physiol Regul Integr Comp Physiol 289:R1392–R1399

Park DC, Lautenschlager G, Hedden T, Davidson NS, Smith AD, Smith PK (2002) Models of visuospatial and verbal memory across adult life span. Psychol Aging 17:299–320

Peng B, Clark JT, Prasain J, Kim H, White CR, Wyss JM (2005) Antihypertensive and cognitive effects of grape polypheols in estrogen-depleted female spontaneously hypertensive rats. Am J Physiol Regul Integr Comp Physiol 289:R771–775

Ramassamy C (2006) Emerging role of polyphenolic compounds in the treatment of neurodegenerative diseases: a review of their intracellular targets. Eur J Pharmacol 545:51–64

Rex A, Spychalla M, Fink H (2004) Treatment with reduced nicotinamide adenine dinucleotaide (NADH) improves water maze performance in old Wistar rats. Behav Brain Res 154:149–153

Santos-Buelga C, Scalbert A (2000) Proanthocyanidins and tannin-like compounds-nature, occurrence, dietary intake and effects on nutrition and health. J Sci Food Agric 80:1094–1117. doi:10.1002/(SICI)1097-0010(20000515)

Sastry PS, Rao KS (2000) Apoptosis and the nervous system. J Neurochem 74:1–20

Schmidt-Schilling S, Schaeffer S, Weber CC (2005) Flavanoids and brain aging. J Phy Pharmacol 1:23–36

Sherwood CC, Gordon AD, Allen JS, Phillips KA, Erwin JM, Hof PR, Hopkins WD (2011) Aging of the cerebral cortex differs between humans and chimpanzees. doi:10.1073/pnas.1016709108 PNAS. 25 July 2011

Shukitt-Hale B, Carey AN, Jenkins D, Rabin BM, Joseph JA (2007) Beneficial effects of fruit extracts on neuronal function and behavior in a rodent model of accelerated aging. Neurobiol Aging 28:1187–1194

Shukitt-Hale B, Lau FC, Joseph JA (2008) Berry fruit supplementation and the aging brain. J Agric Food Chem 56:636–641

Shukitt-Hale B, Cheng V, Joseph JA (2009) Effects of black berries on motor and cognitive function in aged rats. Nutr Neurosci 12:135–40

Shukitt-Hale B, McEwen JJ, Szprengiel A, Joseph JS (2004) Effect of age on the radial arm water maze: a test of spatial learning and memory. Neurobiol Aging 25:223–229. doi:10.1016/S0197-4580(03)00041-1

Sun AY, Simonyi A, Sun GY (2002) The 'French Paradox' and beyond: neuroprotective effects of polyphenols. Free Radic Biol Med 32:314–318. doi:10.1016/S0819105849(01)00803-6

Takatsu H, Owada K, Abe K, Nakano M, Urano S (2010) Effect of vitamin E on learning and memory deficit in aged rat. J Nutr Sci Vitaminol 55:389–393

Valente T, Hidalgo J, Bolea I, Ramirez B, Anglěs N, Jordi R, Morelló JR, Guetiĕrrez C, Boada M, Unzeta M (2009) A diet rich in polyphenols and polyunsaturated fatty acids, LMN diet induces neurogenesis in the subventricular and hippocampus of adult mouse brain. J Alzheimer's Dis 18:849–865. doi:10.3233/JAD-2009-1186

Veinbergs I, Uden EV, Mallory M, Alford M, McGiffert C, DeTeresa R, Orlando R, Masliah E (2001) Role of apolipoprotein E receptors in regulating the differential *in vivo* neurotrophic effects of apolipoprotein E. Exp Neurol 170:15–26. doi:10.1006/exnr.2001.7684

Wen W, Zhu W, He Y, Kochan NA, Reppermund S, Slavin MJ, Brodaty H, Crawford J, Xia A, Sachdev P (2011) Discrete neuroanatomical networks are associated with specific cognitive abilities in old age. J Neurosci 31:1204–1212. doi:10.1523/JNEUROSCI.4085-10.2011

Wiegant FA, Surinova S, Ytsma E, Langelaar-Makkinje M, Wikman G, Post JA (2009) Plant adaptogens in lifespan and stress resistance in C. elegans. Biogerontology 10:27–42

Xu J, Rong S, Xie B, Sun Z, Zhang L, Wu H, Yao P, Zhang X, Zhang Y, Lie L (2009) Rejuvenation of antioxidant and cholinergic systems contributes to the effect of procyanidins extracted from the lotus seedpod ameliorating memory impairment in cognitively impaired aged rats. Eur J Neuropsychopharmacol 19:851–860

Chapter 18
Herbal Cognitive Enhancers: New Developments and Challenges for Therapeutic Applications

Andrea Zangara and Keith A. Wesnes

Abstract Current developments in the search for novel treatments for preserving cognitive function include those for slowing down the progression of the decline in mental ability associated with normal aging as well as treating various dementias. Many natural products possess properties of relevance to the quality of cognitive function, and interest in their use is increasingly driven by a number of factors including the standardization of their production, growing evidence of their mechanisms of action, and improvements in the quality of clinical trials with such products. Of particular interest are products from plants (herbal medicines), due to their potential synergistic complexity and also the ability to interact with multiple mechanisms within the body. However, herbal preparations can vary considerably in their effects and safety, particularly if the 'seed to patient' process is not properly controlled and standardized. The challenge is even greater when targeting human cognitive function, a multi faceted process which is demanding to measure and hard to improve. However, good progress is being made in this field; standardized cognitive tests are available and gold-standard experimental designs and methodologies are being increasingly utilised in clinical trials. Encouraging findings are now emerging in treating cognitive aging and dementia with natural products, and the future holds a great promise for this field.

Keywords Herbal medicines • Natural medicinal products • Standardization • Brain • Cognitive enhancers • Alzheimer's disease • Psychopharmacology • Cognitive functions • Cognitive tests

---

A. Zangara (✉)
SOHO-Flordis International, Level 4, 156 Pacific Highway St Leonards, NSW 2065 Australia
e-mail: andre.zangara@sfihealth.com

Centre for Human Psychopharmacology, Swinburne University, Melbourne, Australia

K. A. Wesnes
Bracket, Goring-on-Thames, RG80EN, UK

Centre for Human Psychopharmacology, Swinburne University, Melbourne, Australia

M. K. Thakur, S. I. S. Rattan (eds.), *Brain Aging and Therapeutic Interventions*,
DOI 10.1007/978-94-007-5237-5_18,

18.1 Introduction

Natural Medicinal Products (NMPs) are a broad category that includes herbal medicines, vitamins, mineral supplements, a variety of nutrients, homeopathic medicines, aromatherapy oils and traditional medicines such as Ayurvedic medicines and Traditional Chinese Medicine (TCM). Natural medicinal products have enjoyed a great increase in popularity over the last two decades, and have recently become a source of intense debate on topics ranging from regulatory, quality, safety, efficacy and marketing. The popularity of NMPs can be attributed to the perception by the general public that pharmaceutically derived medicines interfere with natural processes and have secondary effects, many of which are unwanted. NMPs, and particularly herbals, have been used for medicinal purposes by man for many thousands of years; however, herbal therapies have only entered mainstream healthcare systems in the last few decades, and since then their popularity has increased exponentially. Common health concerns in Europe, as in the USA, reflect those of an aging, increasingly industrialized nation; and age-related cognitive decline together with obesity, cardiovascular disease and decreased physical capability are among the most prominent of these concerns.

Herbal remedies are perceived to be safer because they have been used for hundreds or thousands of years. Furthermore, they are viewed to enhance natural processes and to target diseases from multiple angles, due to the large numbers of active ingredients in plants, as opposed to the 'silver bullet' concept of pharmaceutical drugs based almost exclusively on single chemical entities. Certain herbal medicines, because of the complexity of their chemical content and the variety of bioactivities, can provide the poly-pharmacology which orthodox drugs cannot deliver. However, natural products are rarely evaluated in the well-controlled clinical trials that are required to receive approval by regulatory bodies, and therefore tend to have less 'scientific' evidence to support their efficacy. Further, it is important to recognise that 'natural products' are not necessarily equal 'safe products', and ultimately there cannot be two kinds of medicine—conventional and alternative. Once a treatment has been tested rigorously, it no longer matters whether it was considered alternative at the outset: 'If it is found to be reasonably safe and effective, it will be accepted' (Angell and Kassirier 1998). All medicinal compounds are chemicals, whether synthesised in plants, animals or in manufacturing laboratories; and it is important to remember that at least 25 % of pharmaceutical drugs are derived directly or indirectly from plants. Therefore, all medicinal chemical compounds should be held accountable to similar standards of quality (uniformity, purity and stability), clinical effectiveness and safety; irrespective of their source. The growing realization that some medically approved drugs are believed or identified to be no more effective than placebo (antidepressants), and/or associated with unacceptable side effects (e.g. anxiolytics and addiction), highlights the need to take a broader perspective on the validity of conventional versus alternative medicines.

18.2 Major Issues in the Development of Medicinal Products from Plants

The traditional use of plants or plant preparations to treat health conditions dates back thousands of years, and many remedies from TCM, Ayurvedic and Traditional European Medicine have survived until the present day, and this continuum is often sufficient to convince many people of their safety and efficacy. Importantly, scientific research has already supported the transformation of many traditional remedies into safer and more effective therapeutics; some examples of drugs originating from plants that have central nervous system (CNS) effects are ephedrine (Ephedra sinica Stapf), hyoscine (Hyoscyamus niger L.), morphine (Papaver somniferum L.), physostigmine (Physostigma venenosum Balf.), and galantamine from species of Galanthus and Narcissus.

The scientific evaluation of the cognitive psychopharmacology of herbal products delivered via a complex mix of bioactive components certainly presents many challenges including the quality of raw materials, processing, manufacturing, clinical study designs and the outcome measures employed. Moreover, "bioequivalence" is difficult or impossible to achieve with herbal products due to their chemical complexity. However, many of these challenges can be overcome through standardized processes from the plant to the finished product, and also by employing precise instruments to scientifically verify the extent to which herbs and phytochemicals can support and improve aspects of cognitive function.

The development of NMPs presents further controversial issues due to unclear and rapidly changing regulatory frameworks and quality control systems. It is therefore of paramount importance that the health claims which are communicated to customers, particularly when referring to cognitive functions, are supported by validated and reproducible methods.

18.3 The 'Seed to Patient' Process

The evidence of the efficacy and potential applications of herbal medicines should be subject to rigorous scrutiny. Widely used claims for a number of herbal products are that they improve cognitive abilities and psychological 'wellbeing' or delay brain aging; however such claims often lack evidence-based support. Further, modern mass production of herbal products often results in remedies that differ greatly from the traditions of use which form the basis for their perceived safety and effectiveness (for example, products were not used as tablets in past centuries). Natural medicinal products, particularly from plants, are highly variable and complex products with numerous biologically active components; and their active ingredients are rarely completely identified. Consequently, therapeutic results and safety issues vary greatly from product to product, even within a single class; which means that the evidence of both benefits and risks are specific to the product tested, and cannot

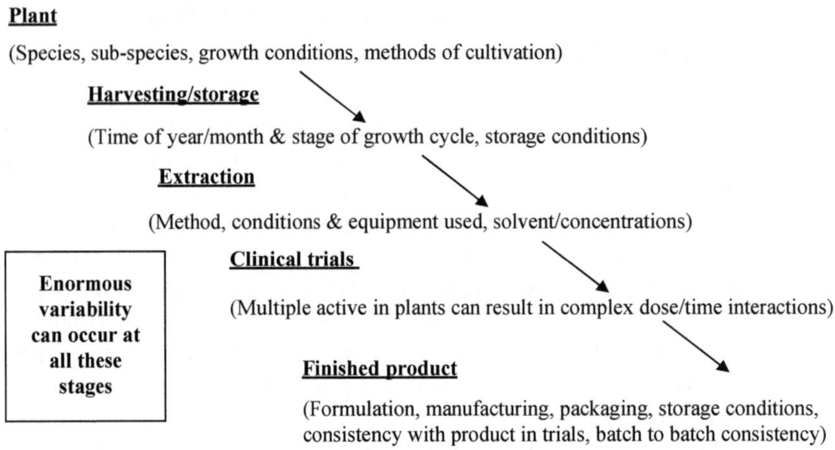

Fig. 18.1 Variabilities in the process 'seed to patient'

necessarily be extrapolated to other products, as is the case for synthetically derived compounds.

Standardization, i.e. the process of delivering a product with specified levels of one or more plant constituents, can ensure that different batches of an herbal product are consistent in terms of their botanical contents. The process of standardization from the original herbal preparation to the finished product (the 'seed to patient' process) includes many variables and challenges (Fig. 18.1), particularly the environmental factors associated with the growth, collection and processing of the raw material. A further issue is related to the need for harmonization and standardization on the use of pesticides and other chemicals on soil and plants, and on the identification of plants from different global sources. The effectiveness of herbal medicine obviously depends on the quantity of the active constituent (or constituents) present, which can be influenced by several factors. The various phytochemicals in plants have often been produced as adaptive mechanisms, for example to enable plants to grow in unfavorable conditions, or to deter insects or to discourage herbivores. Some phytochemicals may also be seasonally dependent, and influenced by where the plant is grown. Another important factor is the method of extraction. This can influence how much of a particular active constituent is present in the herbal product. Some phytochemicals are more soluble in water, while others are soluble in alcohol or oil. The method varies from plant to plant, depending on the types of active constituents.

Identification of all of a plant's constituents often fails because of the complexity of the plant's chemical structure. Plants can be considered to be 'living factories' producing a variety of chemical compounds, including primary metabolites important for the growth of the plants (amino acids, proteins, carbohydrates) and secondary metabolites (alkaloids, terpenoids, phenylpropanoids, polyketides, flavonoids, saccharides); these being promising candidates for herbal cognitive enhancers. Importantly, all these components may work together to deliver a synergistic effect in the finished product. Consequently, ensuring the standardization of not only the finished product, but also the entire journey from the plantation to the consumer, helps to minimize variations in the quality of the product and also to maintain the synergistic potential. It is therefore important that herbal products should be analyzed (generally through chromatographic fingerprint), at various stages of development and particularly at the end stage, to ensure that all of the isolated key biological markers or known active components are at acceptable levels, and are also phyto-equivalent to those of the products that have previously shown safety and efficacy in clinical trials.

18.4 Cognitive Function

Cognitive function relates to the aspects of mental ability which enables us to conduct the activities of daily living. Many aspects of cognitive function are relatively stable and unaffected by, for example, aging, fatigue, drugs, trauma or dementia; while other aspects such as attention and memory are variable by nature and highly susceptible to change. Tests of cognitive function assess how well various cognitive skills are operating in an individual at any particular time. Such evaluations require individuals to perform tasks which involve one or more cognitive domains. It is important to note that the only way to measure cognitive function directly is by assessing the quality of performance on cognitive or behavioural tasks. It is also of interest to assess how the individual feels about his/her levels of cognitive function, but this is simply supportive evidence for the assessment of task performance. Similarly, various measures of brain activity (for example electroencephalography and fMRI scanning) do not measure the quality of cognitive function directly, rather provide us with independent but nonetheless highly valuable information about the activation of certain brain areas and inter-connecting pathways which are crucial for successful completion of various cognitive operations.

It is important that research in this field identifies the appropriate domain of cognitive function to investigate. While ‘cognition enhancement’ is an acceptable generic term, as is ‘health promoting’, both science and regulators require more specific targets; which respect the independence of different domains when considering specific claims. For example, why in medicine would a drug which helped pulmonary function be expected to help the liver? This illustrates the limitation of global scores of cognition for herbal or nutritional claims, and should guide researchers to seek assessments of specifically targeted domains of function. There are a number of core cognitive domains which can be evaluated, including attention, information processing, reasoning, memory, motor control, problem solving and executive function. Taking memory as an example, there are four major types: episodic or declarative memory, working memory, semantic memory and procedural memory (Budson and Price 2005). As Budson and Price illustrate, relatively few conditions are associated with impairments to semantic memory and procedural memory, while working and episodic memory are impaired in a wide variety of neurological, psychiatric, surgical and medical conditions. This creates a rationale for directing testing towards working and episodic memory as a more fruitful potential area to evaluate in novel conditions, and most test systems recognise this approach. Further, tests specific to particular domains are, when available, ideal, as this helps to facilitate the substantiation of any claims made on the basis of the research findings. The most specific tests are attention tests, as well designed tests of attention do not require aspects of memory or reasoning for task performance, and thus changes in performance can be relatively clearly attributable to effects on attention processes. As attention is important for the performance of any task, when seeking to evaluate other domains, it is useful to also assess attention additionally in order that the relative contribution to any effects of changes to attention can be established. Most well established test batteries include assessments of attention, working and episodic memory, motor control, and aspects of executive function.

18.5 Normal and Pathological Cognitive Aging

There has been much historic debate about the decline in the quality of mental functioning which accompanies aging. A traditional approach has been to compare young adults (e.g., 18–25 years) to the elderly (e.g., 65–80 years), and much research has shown that a variety of aspects of cognitive functioning is poorer in the elderly. One consistent criticism of this approach has been that the elderly 'grew up' in a different era, which may have limited their subsequent abilities (for example due to socioeconomic factors such as more limited educational abilities and poorer nutrition), and thus their differences to younger individuals may not simply have been due to aging. A research group based at the University of Virginia, USA, led by Timothy Salthouse, has comprehensively investigated this area over the last few decades. The outcomes of this research programme have been recently summarized (Salthouse 2010). The approach of Salthouse and colleagues has been to assess thousands of healthy individuals across the age range on a variety of traditional neuropsychological tests and to evaluate the pattern of change by decade from early adulthood until the 80s. The consistent finding has been for linear declines to be present in a range of measures of attention, information processing, reasoning and various aspects of memory from the twenties onwards. Using a variety of analytic techniques, the group has established that despite common assumptions to the contrary, age-related declines in measures of cognitive functioning are relatively large, begin in early adulthood, are evident in several different types of cognitive abilities, and are not always accompanied by increases in between-person variability.

This pattern has also been identified over the same age range using computerised tests of cognitive function, linear declines in 5 year cohorts being seen to the speed and accuracy of various aspects of attention, working and episodic memory

(Wesnes 2006). An important aspect of these findings is that the individuals tested had participated in clinical trials as healthy volunteers, and had thus undergone extensive medical screening. These individuals were thus free of major medical or psychiatric conditions and such declines actually represent the best case for normal aging. The same tests have been administered to patients with a wide variety of conditions including hypertension, fibromyalgia, ADHD, epilepsy, narcolepsy, chronic fatigue syndrome, schizophrenia, and multiple sclerosis. When each of these populations is compared to age-matched healthy controls, cognitive deficits of one or more standard deviations are seen, for example, the ability to focus attention (Wesnes 2006). This body of research therefore indicates that major aspects of cognitive function decline with normal aging, and that a variety of mental and physical illnesses will further exacerbate this deterioration. This clearly increases the disease targets in which cognition enhancement would be of relevance, and provides a range of indications in which natural products could be useful in treating such disease induced cognitive deficits.

The fourth edition of the Diagnostic and Statistical Manual of Mental Disorders of the American Psychiatric Association (DSM-IV) identified age-associated cognitive decline (AACD) as a condition which may be a focus of clinical attention (diagnostic code 780.9) (American Psychiatric Association 2000; Maher 2008). The definition was for a 'decline in cognitive functioning consequent to the aging process that is within normal limits given the person's age. Individuals with this condition may report problems remembering names or appointments or may experience difficulty in solving complex problems' (page 684 DSM-IV).

However, to date regulatory bodies in the EU or USA have not accepted AACD or other similar conditions as legitimate conditions for drug registration, and much of the focus of drug development in the last decade has moved to the condition of mild cognitive impairment (MCI; Petersen and Morris 2005). Here the main criterion for an individual to be classified for this condition is to be 1.5 standard deviations poorer than age-matched controls on a recognized test of memory. MCI is believed to be a staging post for Alzheimer's disease. This area has been the subject of numerous trials of novel pharmaceuticals, unfortunately though with very limited success.

The major emphasis of research in cognition enhancers over the last three decades has been to treat the cognitive impairment seen in Alzheimer's disease and other major forms of dementia. Initial success was obtained with anticholinesterases, and there are three compounds now widely used to treat the cognitive symptoms of AD: donepezil, rivastigmine and galantamine. Memantine, a compound which is an NMDA antagonist has also been registered for use in various countries. More recently, treatment has been focused upon disease modification. However, during the last decade all of the Phase III clinical trials on disease modifiers in AD have failed. Partly in response to this, an important stage step in this progress has been two recent publications from workgroups convened by the National Institute on Aging (NIA) and the Alzheimer's Association, one which provides revised guidelines for the diagnosis of MCI due to AD (Albert et al. 2011) and another which proposes a conceptual framework and operational research criteria for the preclinical stage of AD (Sperling et al. 2011). The advantage of the new MCI guidelines is that they extend the definitions beyond simple memory dysfunction to reflect the broader range of cognitive deficits which are known to precede Alzheimer's disease. The guidelines for the assessment of the preclinical stage of AD are particularly exciting as they provide the opportunity to identify declines in cognitive function which precede MCI, and thus occur in otherwise healthy individuals. This will revitalise studies in AACD as the goal is to identify (and subsequently treat) greater rates of decline than would be expected from normal aging in healthy individuals.

18.6 Cognition Enhancement

A recent definition of cognition enhancement is 'the amplification or extension of core capacities of the mind through improvement or augmentation of internal or external information processing systems' (Bostrom and Sandberg 2009). Aspects of cognitive function that are targets for enhancement include attention, information processing, memory, planning, reasoning, decision making and motor control.

The concept of cognitive enhancement can be simply described as an improvement in basic aspects of cognitive function that are essential for the conduct of the activities of daily living. For healthy people, this can represent identifying an improvement on a valid measure of cognitive function recognized to be important for everyday performance, such as attention and memory. The same is true for patients with cognitive impairment, with the provision that for enhancement to have taken place, cognitive function needs to be measurably better than it was before treatment or would have been without treatment.

Our understanding of cognition enhancement is at an early stage, and there are few, if any, established criteria. For a compound to be established as an enhancer of one or more aspects of cognitive function, the following criteria have been recently proposed (Wesnes 2010):

1. Improvements must be identified by well recognised and extensively validated tests of cognitive function.
2. Improvements should be in one or more major domains of cognitive function.
3. Improvements must be seen on core measures of task performance, and any suggestions of speed-accuracy trade-offs should be interpreted with caution.
4. Improvements in one cognitive domain should not occur at the cost to another.
5. The improvements should not be followed by rebound declines.
6. The improvements should be of magnitudes which are behaviourally and clinically relevant.
7. The improvements should not be subject to tachyphylaxis over the period for which the treatment is intended to be used.
8. Self-ratings and consideration of outcomes on everyday living are of interest (particularly in regards to dementia), and may be used as supportive evidence, but are not sufficient in the absence of objective test results.

18.7 Herbal Cognitive Enhancers and Brain Aging

The major bases for brain health are: healthy lifestyle; good diet; balanced social and cultural environments; and efficient cardio vascular and metabolic functions. These will support the normal development, maintenance and protection of the whole nervous system. Some clinical evidence confirms the importance of consuming an antioxidant-rich diet to preserve cognitive ability. Oxidative damage appears to occur as one of the earliest pathophysiological events in AD, therefore an increased intake of antioxidants in patients with first signs of cognitive deficits could be helpful in lowering the rate of progression into dementia; certainly there is some emerging evidence that diets rich in fruits and vegetables reduce the risk of cognitive decline. Oxidative damage is however only one of numerous mechanisms which influence cognition. The CNS is so complex that there is almost no limit to the mechanisms by which cognition enhancement can be achieved, including direct effects on major brain neurotransmitters, effects on free radicals, and effects on the capacity of blood to carry oxygen.

18.8 Phytochemicals

The study of phytochemicals to influence brain functions such as memory and mood can be traced to their historical biosynthesis to deter predators or attract pollinators or disseminators by targeting the nervous system (Perry and Howes 2011). Growing research suggests that anthocyanins, sulforaphane, curcumin and other phytochemicals can effectively counteract brain aging via a range of mechanisms; for example by reducing oxidation and inflammation; decreasing the accumulation of toxic proteins; promoting cell membrane function and the formation of new synapses and brain cells; prolonging the life of existing brain cells; improving the function of the inner lining (endothelial lining) of blood vessels, and thus improving blood and oxygen supply to the brain cells (Kamphuis and Scheltens 2010). However, there is a paucity of randomised controlled trials (RCTs) in this field (van der Beek and Kamphuis 2008), although evidence is emerging; for example of neuroprotective effects of phenolic compounds (Sun et al. 2008), such as resveratrol from grapes and red wine; curcumin from turmeric (Curcuma longa L.); epigallocatechin from green tea (Camellia sinensis Kuntze; relevant to oxidative mechanisms). Further, research data, mainly from in vitro or in vivo models on novel plant extracts and their bioactives with anti-amnesic effects on different neurotransmitter systems are accumulating. Finally, pycnogenol, derived from *Pinus pinaster* or *P. maritime*—the French maritime pine tree—has also shown cognition benefits in an elderly sample (Ryan et al. 2008).

18.9 Herbal Extracts

Plant extracts, due to their multi-component nature can simultaneously interact with various mechanisms to produce cognition enhancement and neuroprotection. A good example is *Ginkgo biloba*, thought to act in several ways including: ability to decrease oxygen radical discharge and proinflammatory functions of macrophages (antioxidant and antiinflammatory), reduce corticosteroid production (anti-anxiety), increase glucose uptake and utilization and adenosine triphosphate production, improve blood flow by increasing red blood cell deformability, decrease red cell aggregation, induce nitric oxide production and inhibit platelet activating factor receptors (Chan et al. 2007). Extracts of *Ginkgo biloba* leaves have been prescribed in Germany, France and Italy for several decades to treat 'cerebral insufficiency', and problems with memory and concentration. *Panax ginseng* is also reported to have multiple actions (for a review see Lee et al. 2009), including effects on vasoconstriction; improved blood flow through modulation of platelet aggregation; roles in both cardio-protection and neuroprotection following a number of insults; shifting of the hormonal balance of the hypothalamic-pituitary-adrenal system; modulation of a number of neurotransmitter systems; and modulation of blood glucose levels in both diabetic and non-diabetic humans. Extracts from the plant *Bacopa monniera* appear to modulate the brain cholinergic system and also possess antioxidant effects, and are supported by a number of well conducted trials (Stough et al. 2011).

18.10 Natural Cognitive Enhancers and AD

AD can be considered as the result of a pathological cascade involving progressively accelerating neurotoxic interactions between cholinergic degeneration, oxidative stress, inflammatory responses, neuroendocrine pathology, compromised cerebral metabolism, neurofibrillary tangle generation, and beta-amyloid (Aβ) deposition, amongst other processes (Kumar and Clark 2002). As mentioned earlier, available treatments for AD are cholinesterase inhibitors and memantine; although these only target specific disease processes in the condition. In addition, Alzheimer's patients may also receive antidepressants or anti-anxiety medicine to control behavioural and psychological symptoms. Preclinical trials with a number of herbal extracts have shown some role in modulating simultaneously a number of these processes, and therefore these herbs are of interest in the clinical development of medicines that could prevent, mitigate or treat AD. Adams et al. (2007) identified over 150 plant species in various preparations and mixtures for age-related cognitive disorders (mainly from European herbals from the sixteenth and seventeenth centuries, alongside traditional Chinese and Indian medicinal practice). Recent reviews have highlighted the broad range of plant extracts and compounds with acetylcholinesterase (AChE) inhibitory activity, as well as evidence for promising species such as sage (Salvia species), lemon balm (Melissa officinalis L.), Huperzia serrata (Thunb.) Trevis., and combinations of other traditional Chinese medicinal herbs, in addition to ginkgo (*Ginkgo biloba* L.). Since 2000, according to the current Anatomical-Therapeutic-Chemical

(ATC) classification, specific *Ginkgo biloba* extracts are listed in the group of anti-dementia drugs together with cholinesterase inhibitors and memantine. A recent systematic review and meta-analysis of nine trials (Weinmann et al. 2010) that met the authors' inclusion criteria using the standardized extract EGb761 in AD as well as vascular and mixed dementia, concluded that *Ginkgo biloba* appears more effective than placebo with moderate effect sizes. Conflicting findings have emerged from the GuidAge study, a 5 year trial run in France in 2,854 elderly people with memory complaints: long-term use of standardised ginkgo biloba extract in this trial did not reduce the risk of progression to Alzheimer's disease; however methodological issues affected the result, because the total number of Alzheimer's cases was unexpectedly low in the study population. A planned evaluation of study participants who had been treated for a minimum of 4 years found a reduction of the Alzheimer's risk of 47 % (Vellas et al. 2012). Man et al. (2008) concluded from a review of controlled clinical studies that herbal medicines "can be a safe, effective treatment for AD", and according to a meta-analyses by May et al. (2009) "There is overall positive evidence for the effectiveness and safety of certain herbal medicines for dementia management."

A detailed review of plants, plant extracts or chemicals with some promising clinical evidence in people with dementia is not in the scope of this chapter, however, some information is provided in Table 18.1, adapted from a recent review on the topic by Perry and Howes (2011).

18.11 The Clinical Assessment of Cognitive Effects of Herbal Extracts

18.11.1 The Cognitive Psychopharmacology of Herbal Extracts

Many trials with natural products that may enhance human cognitive function are not conducted with the rigor required for publication in leading peer reviewed human cognitive psychopharmacology journals. Frequently, claims are based on anecdotal evidence, uncontrolled trials or work with animals. While such evidence is helpful in selecting a substance to study, this evidence cannot alone support a particular claim for its cognition enhancing potential. Precise instruments to scientifically verify the extent to which herbs and other natural products can support and improve the functions of the brain are now available. Overall, it has become clear that some natural products, particularly herbal extracts, can enhance cognitive function. While these products sometimes take longer than pharmaceuticals to work (i.e. weeks or months), they may produce more long-lasting benefits, for example by reducing brain inflammation or improving the brain's antioxidant defense system, or increasing blood flow and oxygen use in the CNS.

The components of the NMPs may act individually and either positively or negatively; and their combination may affect multiple neuronal, metabolic and hormonal systems which themselves modulate behavioural processes. These complex interac-

Table 18.1 Plants with relevance for cognition/dementia. (Adapted from Perry and Howes 2011)

Plant name[a]	Plant part	Phytochemicals associated with biological activities	Clinical effects/observations in humans
Snowdrop *Galanthus* species, daffodil/narcissus, *Narcissus* species, *Leucojum aestivum* L. (Amaryllidaceae)	Bulbs	Alkaloids: particularly galantamine	Numerous multi-center, RCTs show galantamine is well-tolerated and significantly improves cognitive function in AD patients (Howes and Houghton 2009a; Howes et al. 2003). Galantamine may also be of some therapeutic value in Lewy **b**ody disease and Vascular dementia (Howes and Houghton 2009a)
Lemon balm/melissa Melissa officinalis L. (Lamiaceae)	Aerial parts	Essential oil; rosmarinic acid and derivatives	Improved cognitive performance in healthy participants in RCTs following treatment with cholinergically active *M. Officinalis* dried leaf or a standardized extract; cognitive improvements observed in AD patients treated with *M. officinalis* extract for 4 months in a double-blind RCT (Kenndey and Scholey 2006; Howes and Houghton 2009b)
Sage *Salvia* species, in particular: *S. officinalis* L. and *S. lavandulifolia* Vahl. (Lamiaceae)	Aerial parts	Monoterpenoids including1,8-cineole and α-pinene	A standardised oil extract of *S. lavandulifolia* produced significant effects on cognitive ability (immediate word recall scores improved) in healthy young adults (RCT) (Tildesley et al. 2003). A similar study showed positive modulation of mood and cognition in healthy young adults given standardized essential oil of *S. lavandulifolia* (Tildesley et al. 2005). *S. officinalis* extract enhanced secondary memory performance in adults (>65 year age, RCT) (Scholey et al. 2008). In a pilot trial (11 patients with mild to moderate AD) *S. lavandulifolia* oil significantly improved cognitive function, reduced neuropsychiatric symptoms, and improved attention (Perry et al. 2003). In a multi-center RCT, AD patients treated with *S. officinalis* extract had significantly better outcomes in cognitive function (Akhondzadeh et al. 2003)
Lesser periwinkle *Vinca minor* L. (Apocynaceae)	Aerial parts	Alkaloids: vincamine	Double-blind studies have assessed efficacy of vinpocetine in dementia but quality of methods is limited; a 16-week double-blind RCT (203 patients: mild to moderate dementia) showed significant benefit in the vinpocetine treated group (Akhondzadeh and Abbasi 2006). Although a lack of evidence to support clinical use of vinpocetine in cognitive disorders (Szatmari and Whitehouse 2003), it improved cognitive status and cerebrovascular reserve capacity in patients with ischemic stroke and MCI in a pilot study (Valikovics 2007)

Table 18.1 (continued)

Plant name[a]	Plant part	Phytochemicals associated with biological activities	Clinical effects/observations in humans
Ginkgo/maidenhair tree *Ginkgo biloba* L. (Ginkgoaceae)	Leaves	Many studies have focused on a standardized extract of *G. biloba*: EGb 761 (contains flavonoid glycosides and terpenoid lactones amongst other constituents)	Clinical efficacy of extracts (including EGb 761) has been extensively evaluated in numerous RCTs with both AD and healthy subjects (Howes and Houghton 2009b; Hsieh et al. 2010; Howes and Houghton 2003; Napryeyenko and Borzenko 2007). A meta-analysis of RCTs demonstrates clinically relevant positive results with *G. biloba* in AD patients (Ernst 2002). Many trials indicate *G. biloba* can modestly improve cognitive ability, but trial outcomes are not consistently based on objective methods of analysis. One RCT in multiple sclerosis patients (120 mg extract twice daily) showed *G. biloba* to produce no significant improvement in cognition, but it was suggested to influence some cognitive processes (e.g., mental flexibility) (Howes and Houghton 2009b). Generally, oral administration is well-tolerated with no serious adverse effects (Howes and Houghton 2009b). The use of *G. biloba* with antiplatelet or anticoagulant medicines may increase the risk of hemorrhage (Barnes et al. 2007)
Huperzia serrata (Thunb.) Trevis. (Lycopodiaceae)	Moss	Alkaloids: huperzines A and B	In phase IV clinical trials, huperzine A improved memory in elderly, AD, and VaD patients, with few adverse effects (Howes and Houghton 2009a). Clinical efficacy of huperzine A also demonstrated in other RCTs in AD patients with improvements in cognition, behavior, and mood (Zangara 2003; Hsieh et al. 2010). A pro-drug of huperzine, Debio 9902 (ZT-1), was safe and effective in a human scopolamine model of AD (Zangara et al. 2006) and when administered once daily to AD patients in a phase IIa clinical trial; further trials are in progress (Butler 2008). One small trial (14 VaD participants) showed no significant beneficial effect of huperzine A on improvement of cognitive function (Hao et al. 2009)

Table 18.1 (continued)

Plant name[a]	Plant part	Phytochemicals associated with biological activities	Clinical effects/observations in humans
Ginseng *Panax ginseng* C.A.Mey. (Araliaceae). Other species of *Panax* are used for similar indications	Root	Triterpenoid saponins: ginsenosides	Studies in healthy volunteers show improved abstract thinking, attention, information processing, cognitive performance, auditory reaction time, social functioning, and mental health with a standardized ginseng extract (>4 % ginsenosides per oral dose); other studies in healthy volunteers show no quantifiable effects on memory; conflicting trial data are considered to be due to compositional differences in ginsenosides (Leung et al. 2007). A review of RCTs using any type of *P.ginseng* to treat patients with AD focused on two trials assessing the effectiveness of ginseng as an adjunct to drug therapy on cognitive function compared with conventional drug therapy; results (MMSE and Alzheimer's Disease Assessment Scale) were significantly in favor of ginseng; due to methodological limitations, evidence for efficacy of ginseng in AD is inconclusive (Lee et al. 2009)
Polygala tenuifolia Willd. (Polygalaceae)	Root	Only some cinnamic acid derivatives and onjisaponins have shown some relevant activities in vitro (Howes and Houghton 2009b)	An extract (BT-11) enhanced some cognitive functions including memory in elderly humans in a RCT (Shin et al. 2009). In a 12-month RCT (seven AD patients treated with KUT, a Japanese traditional medicine including Polygala) the rate of cognitive decline was significantly slower than patients receiving no medication for AD, with efficacy most obvious at 3 months (Arai et al. 2000). In a 12-week trial, KUT combined with donepezil produced benefits on cognition and brain perfusion in AD patients, compared to donepezil monotherapy (Maruyama et al. 2006)
Saffron *Crocus sativus* L. (Iridaceae)	Stigmas	Carotenoids: crocin	In a 22-week double-blind trial, AD patients treated with saffron showed comparable improvements in cognition compared to donepezil (Akhondzadeh et al. 2010)

[a] Common and Latin names (plant family)

tions may be further modulated by dispositional and situational factors. An additional complication is represented by the possible synergy between these interacting activities, resulting in complex dose and time dependent effects. The difficulty of interpreting some fragile positive effects and negative findings is a clear challenge for the researchers in this field, and a number of authors have called for a set of criteria for assessing any behavioural effects of herbal extracts (Kennedy and Scholey 2003; Wesnes et al. 2004b).

18.11.2 Testing Efficacy of Natural Cognitive Enhancers

To properly evaluate natural cognitive enhancers, including herbal extracts, it has been found to be important to measure cognitive function repeatedly over a study day; and such testing has identified effects which would have been missed by testing only once. This approach can for example capture diurnal effects or effects which emerge due to repeated testing. The use of computerised cognitive assessments such as the CDR System is widespread in this field and has a long history (Wesnes et al. 1987). An advantage of systems designed for use both with healthy and impaired populations is that effects in healthy volunteers often predict to clinical populations.

Natural products can enhance cognitive function even in healthy young volunteers. Attention and memory have been improved with a variety of substances having a wide range of potential mechanisms. Detecting enhancements to cognitive function is much harder than detecting impairments; in normal populations, there is a much smaller window of opportunity to enhance function than there is to impair it. Improvements in normals are rarely greater than 15 %, whereas impairments can be as large as 100 %. Therefore, if enhancements are to be detected, it is necessary to use sensitive instruments.

18.11.3 Methodological Issues: Maximizing the Power of Studies

The first issue is to reduce the variability due to inter-individual differences. Two types of trials can be conducted in this field: single-dose acute studies or studies which involve multiple dosing. Cross-over designs using the volunteer as his/her own control are an ideal way to enhance the sensitivity of the study and to minimize the noise from inter-volunteer differences. In single dose cross-over trials, the sessions can be separated by a week or more, to circumvent any problem with carry-over effects. Crossover designs are the current gold standard for single dose trials in this field. In multiple dosing trials, crossover trials are also applicable; however the issue of the length of the dosing period has practical implications. If the dosing periods are relatively short, say 2–4 weeks, then at least one crossover arm is practical. A washout period needs to be added between the two dosing periods, and for example with two successive 4 week dosing periods separated by a 2 week washout, the study will last 10 weeks. However, with dosing periods longer than a month, it is generally impractical to use crossover design, and the majority of such trials employ parallel group designs.

18.11.4 Repeated Assessments

Repeated assessments of cognitive function, whether in a cross-over or parallel group design, is a key method to further reduce the variability due to individual differences. Each volunteer or patient should be assessed before treatment as well as after, and ideally such testing should be repeated to fully characterize the time profile of any enhancements. In acute trials, repeated testing over the hours immediately following administration can identify clear time-based profiles of effects. In longer trials, testing can be repeated at various stages, e.g., monthly. A further enhancement to this design was seen in a trial in which testing was not only repeated monthly throughout a 12 week period, but was tested at four separate time points on each study day (Wesnes et al. 2000), and testing was repeated two weeks after dosing was stopped. Improvements were only detected at two of the testing times but these effects were seen consistently throughout the study, and were still present two weeks after dosing was stopped.

18.11.5 Training Effects

It has long been known that performance improves with repeated assessments on cognitive tests, independently of the length of the trial or the type of subjects (Wesnes and Pincock 2002). In one trial in an elderly population in which various pencil and paper cognitive tests were administered annually, it was identified that practice effects persisted until at least the third year (Wilson et al. 2002). Training effects may be confounded with treatment effects, and such effects can make the interpretation of any changes identified extremely difficult. Training effects can also 'swamp' enhancements due to treatment. Therefore, to maximize the power of a study, it is important to properly train the volunteers or patients on the cognitive testing procedures prior to the start of the trial. To further prevent training effects, tests should only be repeatedly administered which have alternate or parallel forms (e.g., differing lists of words in recall testing, etc).

18.11.6 Standardized Procedures

Reviews of treatments in cognitive psychopharmacology often cite the absence of standardization of the cognitive tests used in different laboratories as a major limi-

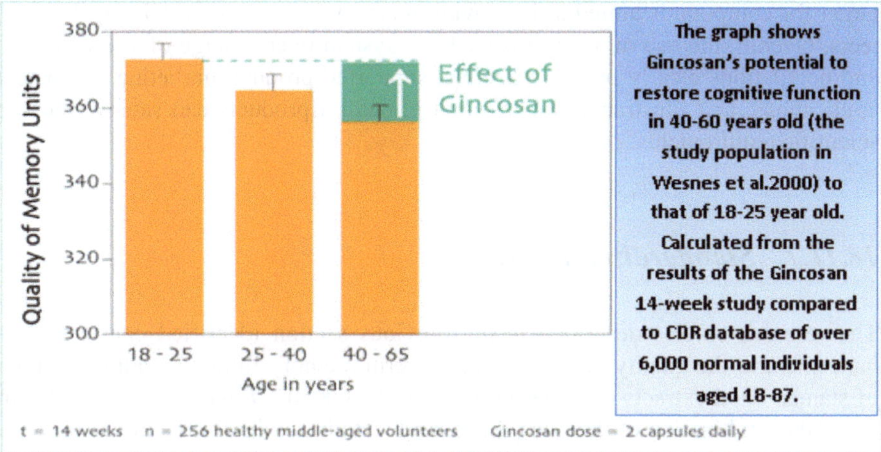

Fig. 18.2 Gincosan® potential to reverse normal cognitive aging

tation, making precise comparisons between trials difficult and often resulting in the reviews been more qualitative in nature than quantitative. Therefore, the use of standardized tests is highly important for the future of research in this field. Test batteries can also be further enhanced by conducting factor analysis to identify the interrelationships between the various measures. There is clearly more power in combining scores from a number of assessments, and avoiding the statistical problems involved in assessing multiple endpoints. Some 'factor scores' which have been derived using such methodology have shown great sensitivity to the effects of natural substances. For example, the Quality of Memory factor from the CDR system combines the scores of the ability to retain and retrieve information from two working memory and four episodic secondary memory tasks into a single measure. This measure has consistently been found to respond positively to standardized extracts of ginkgo and ginseng, whether dosed individually or together. Such effects have been identified in four acute dosing volunteer trials (Kennedy et al. 2000, 2001a, b, 2002) and also multiple dosing trials in young volunteers (Labadorf et al. 2004), middle aged volunteers (Wesnes et al. 2000), elderly volunteers (Wesnes et al. 2004a) and volunteers with neurasthenia (Wesnes et al. 1997). All eight trials tested the same standardized extracts, employed the same cognitive test system, involved pre-study training on the tests as well as repeated testing—both over the study day and for the multiple dosing trials over repeated study days. All trials were randomised, double-blind and placebo controlled. Further, the system used has an extensive normative database, allowing the effects of the compounds to be put into a broader context. For example, the improvements to the Quality of Memory in 256 middle aged volunteers over 14 weeks with the combination of the two extracts (Wesnes et al. 2000) effectively reversed the decline the volunteers would have shown from their early 20s to middle-age (Fig. 18.2). Further the peak overall improvement in the Quality of Memory measure was 7.5 %, which sets a minimum target for compounds aimed at improving memory in healthy middle aged volunteers. Overall, the use of a standardized test system over a range of study designs and populations clearly proved effective, supported product marketing and patent applications, and illustrated that research in natural products can satisfy rigorous scientific requirements.

18.11.7 Standardized Products

The research studies described in the previous section identified consistent enhancement to the quality of short and long term memory following administration of standardized extracts of either *Ginkgo biloba* GK501, *Panax ginseng* G115, or a 60:100 combination of the two (Gincosan®). Both standardized extracts (and the combination) have been developed following a 'seed to patient' process, adhering to international standards starting from the Good Agricultural Process (GAP), Good Laboratory Practice (GLP) through to Good Clinical Practice (GCP). G115 is standardized to an invariable 4 % of ginsenosides, and GK501 is derived by a complex drying process, with concentration in a ratio of approximately 1 part extract to 50 part dried leaves, and standardized to a content of 24–25 % of flavonoids and 6 % of terpenoids.

18.11.8 Promising Recent Work with Natural Products in AACD, MCI and AD Using the Recommendations Made Above

Yurko-Mauroa et al. (2010) evaluated the effects of Docosahexaenoic acid (DHA) on cognitive function in 485 elderly people who fulfilled the DSM-IV criteria described earlier for AACD. Six months of supplementation was found to produce statistically reliable improvements to memory. Though the effect size of the improvement was small (0.19), as with the Wesnes et al. (2000) trial, the computerised cognitive assessment system used in the study had a normative database; and using this database the authors were able to identify that the effect reflected a 7 year reduction in normal aging (3.4 years when compared to placebo), which may well be attractive to the population studied (mean age 70 years). An important aspect of this study was the careful monitoring of safety; the adverse events not being different between the placebo and active treated groups. Besides being conducted to the rigorous standards required in this field and carefully monitoring safety, an important aspect of the study for future research was the presentation of effect sizes as well as an assessment of the potential 'cognitive age-reducing' effect of treatment.

de Jager et al. (2011) conducted a study on MCI patients over a 2 year period, administering a compound containing folic acid, vitamins B6 and B12. The mean plasma total homocysteine was 30 % lower in those treated with B vitamins relative to placebo. B vitamins stabilized a test of executive function relative to placebo. There was significant benefit of B-vitamin treatment among participants with baseline homocysteine above the median (11.3 μmol/L) in global cognition (the Mini Mental State Examination), episodic memory and semantic memory.

Newhouse et al. (2012) conducted a 6 month, randomized, placebo controlled, double blind study of nicotine administered via a patch in MCI patients. One of the outcome measures was the CDR system, and improved delayed word recall was seen over the 6 months period, the nicotine-treated group regaining 46 % of normal performance for age on this aspect of memory, whereas the placebo group worsened by 26 % over the same time period.

Scheltens et al. (2010) studied the effects of a drink named Souvenaid, containing 'Fortasyn Connect' on cognitive function in mild AD. Fortasyn Connect contains EPA, DHA, Phospholipids, Choline, UMP (uridine monophosphate), Vitamin E (alpha-TE), Vitamin C, Selenium, Vitamin B12, B6 and Folic acid. Over 12 weeks compared to placebo, significant improvement in a delayed verbal recall task was identified, though effects were not seen in the AD assessment scale (ADAS-Cog) or other measures. These findings illustrate the progress which can be made in this field when robust trial methodology, standardized extracts and appropriate outcome measures are employed.

18.12 Conclusions

There is a large and growing interest in cognition enhancement. Healthy individuals may want to increase their mental powers, or cognitive endurance, or restore age-related declines. Patients with a wide variety of CNS and general medical disorders may wish to minimize the cognitive dysfunction which accompanies the conditions. Finally of course, there is a huge and growing need to prevent or minimize the cognitive deficits associated with a range of dementias and stroke. Natural products have great potential in all of these areas, and new scientific evidence strongly suggests that particularly products from plants can promote brain health, reduce cognitive aging and slow the course of AD and other dementias. However, the concept that natural products are safe is clearly irrational, given the large number of poisonous substances in nature. Further, the belief that the therapeutic effects of any medicinal product made from a particular herb is the same as any other fails to recognise the complexity of these products. Therefore, assessing both safety and efficacy is vital when evaluating modern natural products. A tightening of the regulations on herbal and other food supplements would help protect the consumer and health professional from products that present risks to health or from misleading claims. "Generic" (untested) products and 'borrowed' science represent a threat to consumers and can put the reputation of the whole market at risk. The level of evidence required in this field should not differ from any other field of clinical science. Therefore, randomised, double-blind placebo controlled trials should be employed where possible, safety should be carefully monitored, and cognitive test systems utilised which are fit-for-purpose for the requirement of detecting enhancements to various aspects of cognitive function. Only properly characterized substances should be tested, and standardized extracts are clearly essential to allow replication in different laboratories.

Acknowledgements We thank Professor Elaine Perry for her thoughtful review of the chapter.

References

Adams M, Gmüdner F, Hamburger M (2007) Plants traditionally used in age related brain disorders—a survey of ethnobotanical literature. J Ethnopharmacol 113:363–381
Akhondzadeh S, Abbasi SH (2006) Herbal medicine in the treatment of Alzheimer's disease. Am J Alzheimers Dis Other Demen 21:113–118
Akhondzadeh S, Noroozian M, Mohammadi M, Ohadinia S, Jamshidi AH, Khani M (2003) Salvia officinalis extract in the treatment of patients with mild to moderate Alzheimer's disease: a double blind, randomized and placebo-controlled trial. J Clin Pharm Ther 28:53–59
Akhondzadeh S, Shafiee Sabet M, Harirchian MH et al (2010) A 22-week, multicenter, randomized, double-blind controlled trial of Crocus sativus in the treatment of mild-to-moderate Alzheimer's disease. Psychopharmacology 207:637–643
Albert MS, Dekosky ST, Dickson D et al (2011) The diagnosis of mild cognitive impairment due to Alzheimer's disease: Recommendations from the National Institute on Aging-Alzheimer's Association workgroups on diagnostic guidelines for Alzheimer's disease. Alzheimers Dement 7:270–279
American Psychiatric Association (2000) Diagnostic and Statistical Manual of Mental Disorders (Revised 4th ed.). Washington DC
Angell M, Kassirier JP (1998) Alternative medicine-the risks of untested and unregulated remedies. N Engl J Med 339(12):839–841. (Editorial)
Arai H, Suzuki T, Sasaki H, Hanawa T, Toriizuka K, Yamada H (2000) A new interventional strategy for Alzheimer's disease by Japanese herbal medicine. Japan J Geriatr 37:212–215
Barnes J, Anderson LA, Phillipson JD (2007) Herbal Medicines, 3rd edn. Pharmaceutical Press, London
Bostrom N, Sandberg A (2009) Cognitive enhancement: methods, ethics, regulatory challenges. Sci Eng Ethics 15:311–341
Budson AE, Price BH (2005) Memory dysfunction. New Engl J Med 352:692–699
Butler MS (2008) Natural products to drugs: natural product-derived compounds in clinical trials. Nat Prod Rep 25:475–516
Chan PC, Xia Q, Fu PP (2007) Ginkgo biloba leave extract: biological, medicinal and toxicological effects. J Environ Sci Health Part C 25:211–44
de Jager CA, Oulhaj A, Jacoby R, Refsum H, Smith AD (2011) Cognitive and clinical outcomes of homocysteine-lowering B-vitamin treatment in mild cognitive impairment: a random-ized controlled trial. Int J Geriatr Psychiatry. doi:10.1002/gps.2758. (Epub ahead of print)
Ernst E (2002) The risk-benefit of commonly used herbal therapies: Ginkgo, St John's wort, ginseng, echinacea, saw palmetto and kava. Ann Internal Med 136:42–53
Hao Z, Liu M, Liu Z, Lv D (2009) Huperzine A for vascular dementia. Cochrane Database Syst Rev 2:CD007365
Howes M-JR, Houghton PJ (2003) Plants used in Chinese and Indian traditional medicine for improvement of memory and cognitive function. Pharmacol Biochem Behav 75:513–527
Howes M-JR, Houghton PJ (2009a) Acetylcholinesterase inhibitors of natural origin. Int J Biomed Pharm Sci 3:67–86

Howes M-JR, Houghton PJ (2009b) Traditional medicine for memory enhancement. In: Ramawat KG (ed) Herbal drugs: ethnomedicine to modern medicine. Springer, New York, p 239–291
Howes M-JR, Perry NSL, Houghton PJ (2003) Plants with traditional uses and activities, relevant to the management of Alzheimer's disease and other cognitive disorders. Phytother Res 17:1–18
Hsieh MT, Peng WH, Wu CR, Ng KY, Cheng CL, Xu HX (2010) Review on experimental research of herbal medicines with anti-amnesic activity. Planta Med 76:203–217
Kamphuis PJ, Scheltens P (2010) Can nutrients prevent or delay onset of Alzheimer's disease? J Alzheimers Dis 20:765–777
Kennedy DO, Scholey AB (2003) Ginseng: potential in the enhancement of cognitive performance and mood. Pharmacol Biochem Behav 75:687–700. (Review)
Kennedy DO, Scholey AB (2006) The psychopharmacology of European herbs with cognition-enhancing properties. Curr Pharm Des 12:4613–4623
Kennedy DO, Scholey AB, Wesnes KA (2000) The dose dependent cognitive effects of acute administration of Ginkgo biloba to healthy young volunteers. Psychopharmacology 151:416–423
Kennedy DO, Scholey AB, Wesnes KA (2001a) Differential, dose-dependent changes in cognitive performance and mood following acute administration of Ginseng to healthy young volunteers. Nutr Neurosci 4(4):295–310
Kennedy DO, Scholey AB, Wesnes KA (2001b) Differential, dose dependent changes in cognitive performance following acute administration of a Ginkgo biloba/Panax ginseng combination to healthy young volunteers. Nutr Neurosci 4(5):399–412
Kennedy DO, Scholey AB, Wesnes KA (2002) Modulation of cognition and mood following administration of single doses of Ginkgo biloba, Ginseng and a Ginkgo/Ginseng combination to healthy young adults. Physiol Behav 75:1–13
Kumar P, Clark M (eds) (2002) Clinical Medicine, 5th edn. WB Saunders, Edinburgh
Labadorf C, Manktelow TC, Labadorf S, Edgar CJ, Wesnes K, Petrini O (2004) The global cognitive effects of ginseng taken by healthy volunteers over a 21 day period. J Psychopharmacol 18(Suppl):A44
Lee MS, Yang EJ, Kim JI, Ernst E (2009) Ginseng for cognitive function in Alzheimer's disease: a systematic review. J Alzheimers Dis 18:339–344
Leung KW, Yung KKL, Mak NK et al (2007) Angiomodulatory and neurological effects of ginsenosides. Curr Med Chem 14:1371–1380
Maher B (2008) Poll results: look who's doping. Nature 452:674–675
Man SC, Durairajan SS, Kum WF et al (2008) Systematic review on the efficacy and safety of herbal medicines for Alzheimer's disease. J Alzheimers Dis 14:209–223
Maruyama M, Tomita N, Iwasaki K et al (2006) Benefits of combining donepezil plus traditional Japanese herbal medicine on cognition and brain perfusion in Alzheimer's disease: a 12-week observer blind, donepezil monotherapy controlled trial. J Am Geriatr Soc 54:869–871
May BH, Lit M, Xue CC et al (2009) Herbal medicine for dementia: a systematic review. Phytother Res 23:447–459
Napryeyenko O, Borzenko I (2007) Ginkgo biloba special extract in dementia with neuropsychiatric features: a randomised, placebo-controlled, double-blind clinical trial. Arzneimittelforschung 57:4–11
Newhouse P, Kellar K, Aisen P et al (2012) Nicotine treatment of mild cognitive impairment: a 6-month double-blind pilot clinical trial. Neurology 78(2):91–101
Perry E, Howes MJ (2011) Medicinal plants and dementia therapy: herbal hopes for brain aging? CNS Neurosci Ther 17(6):683–98
Perry NS, Bollen C, Perry EK, Ballard C (2003) Salvia for dementia therapy: review of pharmacological activity and pilot tolerability clinical trial. Pharmacol Biochem Behav 75:651–659
Petersen RC, Morris JC (2005) Mild cognitive impairment as a clinical entity and treatment target. Arch Neurol 62:1160–1163
Ryan J, Croft K, Mori T, Wesnes KA et al (2008) An examination of the effects of the antioxidant Pycnogenol on cognitive performance, serum lipid profile, endocrinological and oxidative stress biomarkers in an elderly population. J Psychopharmacol 22:553–562

Salthouse T (2010) Major issues in cognitive aging. Oxford University Press. (ISBN13: 9780195372151)
Scheltens P, Kamphuis PJGH, Verheyc FRG et al (2010) Efficacy of a medical food in mild Alzheimer's disease: a randomized, controlled trial. Alzheimer's Dementia 6:1–10
Scholey AB, Tildesley NT, Ballard CG, Wesnes KA, Tasker A, Perry EK, Kennedy DO (2008) An extract of Salvia (sage) with anticholinesterase properties improves memory and attention in healthy older volunteers. Psychopharmacology 198:127–139
Shin KY, Lee J-Y, Won BY, Jung HY, Chang K-A, Koppula S, Suh Y-H (2009) BT-11 is effective for enhancing cognitive functions in the elderly humans. Neurosci Lett 465:157–159
Sperling RA, Aisen PS, Beckett LA et al (2011) Toward defining the preclinical stages of Alzheimer's disease: recommendations from the National Institute on Aging-Alzheimer's Association workgroups on diagnostic guidelines for Alzheimer's disease. Alzheimers Dement 7:280–292
Stough C, Lloyd J, Clarke J, et al (2011) The chronic effects of an extract of Bacopa monniera (Brahmi) on cognitive function in healthy human subjects. Psychopharmacology 156:481–484
Sun AY, Wang Q, Simonyi A, Sun GY (2008) Botanical phenolics and brain health. Neuromolecular Med 10:259–274
Szatmari SZ, Whitehouse PJ (2003) Vinpocetine for cognitive impairment and dementia. Cochrane Database Syst Rev 1:CD003119
Tildesley NT, Kennedy DO, Perry EK, Ballard CG, Savelev S, Wesnes KA, Scholey AB (2003) Salvia lavandulaefolia (Spanish sage) enhances memory in healthy young volunteers. Pharmacol Biochem Behav 75:669–674
Tildesley NTJ, Kennedy DO, Perry EK, Ballard CG, Wesnes KA, Scholey AB (2005) Positive modulation of mood and cognitive performance following administration of acute doses of Salvia lavandulaefolia essential oil to healthy young volunteers. Physiol Behav 83:699–709
Valikovics A (2007) Investigation of the effect of vinpocetine on cerebral blood flow and cognitive functions. Ideggyogy Sz 60:301–310
Van der Beek EM, Kamphuis PJ (2008) The potential role of nutritional components in the management of Alzheimer's disease. Eur J Pharmacol 585:197–207
Vellas B, Coley N, Ousset PJ et al (For the GuidAge Study Group) (2012) Long-term use of standardised ginkgo biloba extract for the prevention of Alzheimer's disease (GuidAge): a randomised placebo-controlled trial. Lancet Neurol 11:851–859
Weinmann S, Roll S, Schwarzbach C, Vauth C, Willich SN (2010) Effects of Ginkgo biloba in dementia: systematic review and meta-analysis. BMC Geriatrics 10:14
Wesnes KA (2006) Cognitive function testing: the case for standardisation and automation. J Br Menopause Soc 12:158–163
Wesnes KA (2010) Cognition enhancement—expanding opportunities in drug development: wake up to the MATRICS. Int Clin Trials 66–72
Wesnes K, Pincock C (2002) Practice effects on cognitive tasks: a major problem? Lancet Neurol 1:473
Wesnes K, Simpson PM, Christmas L (1987) The assessment of human information processing abilities in psychopharmacology. In: I Hindmarch, PD Stonier (eds) Human psychopharmacology: measures and methods, vol I, Wiley, Chichester, pp 79–92
Wesnes KA, Faleni RA, Hefting NR, Hoogsteen G et al (1997) The cognitive, subjective, and physical effects of a Ginkgo biloba/ Panax ginseng combination in healthy volunteers with neurasthenic complaints. Psychopharmacol Bull 33:677–683
Wesnes KA, Ward T, McGinty A, Petrini O (2000) The memory enhancing effects of a Ginkgobiloba/Panax ginseng combination in healthy middle aged volunteers. Psychopharmacology 152:353–361
Wesnes KA, Ferguson J, Petrini O (2004a) The memory enhancing effects of ginkgo biloba in healthy middle-aged volunteers. J Psychopharmacol 18(Suppl):A50 37
Wesnes KA, Zangara A, Scholey A, Kennedy D (2004b) Natural products as cognition enhancing agents. In: Buccafusco JJ (ed) Cognitive Enhancing Drugs. Birkhäuser, p 151–178
Wilson RS, Beckett LA, Barnes LL et al (2002) Individual differences in rates of change in cognitive abilities of older persons. Psychol Aging 17:179–193

Yurko-Mauroa K, McCarthya D, Romb D et al (2010) Beneficial effects of docosahexaenoic acid on cognition in age-related cognitive decline. Alzheimer's Dementia 6:456–464

Zangara A (2003) The Psychopharmacology of Huperzine A: an alkaloid with cognitive enhancing and neuroprotective properties of interest in the treatment of Alzheimer's disease. Pharmacol Biochem Behav 75:675–686

Zangara A, Edgar C, Wesnes K, Scalfaro P, Porchet E (2006) Reversal of scopolamine-related deficits in cognitive functions by ZT-1, a Huperzine A precursor. In: 9th international Geneva/Springfield symposium on advances in Alzheimer therapy, Geneva, Switzerland, 19–22 April 2006 [illegible] Kaur P [illegible] (2010) Beneficial effect of [illegible] of [illegible] related cognitive decline. Alzheimer's Dement [illegible]

Zangara A (2003) The psychopharmacology of huperzine A: an alkaloid with cognitive enhancing and neuroprotective properties of interest in the treatment of Alzheimer's disease. Pharmacol Biochem Behav [illegible]

[illegible] Schaffer [illegible] (2012) [illegible] cognitive function [illegible]

[illegible]

Index

M. K. Thakur, S. I. S. Rattan (eds.), *Brain Aging and Therapeutic Interventions*,
DOI 10.1007/978-94-007-5237-5,

MIX
Papier aus verantwortungsvollen Quellen
Paper from responsible sources
FSC® C105338

If you have any concerns about our products,
you can contact us on
ProductSafety@springernature.com

In case Publisher is established outside the EU,
the EU authorized representative is:
Springer Nature Customer Service Center GmbH
Europaplatz 3, 69115 Heidelberg, Germany

Printed by Libri Plureos GmbH
in Hamburg, Germany